Medicine and Society in Ptolemaic Egypt

Studies in Ancient Medicine

Edited by

John Scarborough

Philip J. van der Eijk
Ann Ellis Hanson
Joseph Ziegler

VOLUME 41

The titles published in this series are listed at brill.com/sam

Medicine and Society in Ptolemaic Egypt

By

Philippa Lang

BRILL

LEIDEN · BOSTON
2013

Cover illustration: Cippus of Horus, 322–280 BCE. Image © The Metropolitan Museum of Art / Art Resource NY.

Library of Congress Cataloging-in-Publication Data

Lang, Philippa, 1974-
Medicine and society in Ptolemaic Egypt / by Philippa Lang.
p. cm. – (Studies in ancient medicine, ISSN 0925-1421 ; v. 41)
Includes bibliographical references and index.
ISBN 978-90-04-21858-1 (hardback : alk. paper) – ISBN 978-90-04-23551-9 (e-book)
1. Medicine, Egyptian. 2. Medicine, Ancient. 3. Medicine, Greek and Roman. 4. Human body–Egypt. 5. Medical logic–History. 6. Physicians–Egypt–History. 7. Medicine–Egypt–Alexandria–History. I. Title.

R137.L36 2012
610.938–dc23

2012026425

This publication has been typeset in the multilingual "Brill" typeface. With over 5,100 characters covering Latin, IPA, Greek, and Cyrillic, this typeface is especially suitable for use in the humanities. For more information, please see www.brill.com/brill-typeface.

ISSN 0925-1421
ISBN 978-90-04-21858-1 (hardback)
ISBN 978-90-04-23551-9 (e-book)

This book is printed on acid-free paper.

CONTENTS

LIST OF ILLUSTRATIONS

PREFACE

The study of medicine in ancient Egypt can be largely divided into two kinds. One group, carried out principally by Egyptologists, has been concerned with the medicine of Egypt from the Old Kingdom to the Late period or Greco-Roman era. The other comes from classicists interested in Greek medicine, chiefly the fragments of the influential elite physicians of Ptolemaic Alexandria, or those using the unusually large amount of papyrological evidence from Greco-Roman Egypt for the study of Greek social history.

Many such works have sought to utilize relevant material from the 'other' tradition as well. This is usually, however, a matter of providing context, comparison or completeness. Thus Egyptian medicine is discussed as a single homogenous entity in works that foreground Greek medicine, or Greeks make an entrance at the end of Egyptian medical history. The chief exception to this division is a sub-genre of argument concerned with the origins of particular views, practices, or drug recipes, and the ways in which Greek and Egyptian medical cultures may have influenced each other.

Medically relevant material also appears in analysis of more general themes, in works on the demography, agriculture, botany and religious-magical practices of this and other periods. These involve medicine only peripherally, as do many works that study cultural identity in Greco-Roman Egypt. This is also a crucial question for medicine, and part of what the current work sets out to examine.

In writing this book, I have tried to utilize all forms of evidence for medicine in Ptolemaic Egypt, whether from Egyptian or from Greek texts and artifacts, as well as those which seem to hybridize elements otherwise labelled as belonging to one culture alone. (For simplicity's sake, however, I have ignored other possible medical cultures, such as Jewish medicine, entirely). I have also attempted, as far as possible, to analyze the structures, beliefs and performances of healing in different social and cultural arenas, from the political elite to the much more obscure world of those of lower social strata, and those silenced by the absence of any evidence at all; to consider all kinds of practice, and to investigate both the patient's and the practitioner's point of view. From this I have tried to develop a multiplying and often tentative exploration of how all kinds of inhabitants of Egypt during the rather arbitrary period of Ptolemaic rule might have experienced, understood and dealt with medicine and illness. Since this history is potentially of interest to readers of diverse expertise and disciplines, I have assumed little prior knowledge of Ptolemaic history, Greek medical practice, or Egyptian medicine, and I apologize to those to whom some of this material is already well-known. Other aspects, I hope, will be less familiar.

The majority of the evidence for the Greco-Roman period of Egypt is in fact Roman in date, and this is also the case in medical history. I have tried to use Roman material cautiously. Roman-era medicine in Egypt supplies evidence for the outcome of Ptolemaic trends, and as such is suggestive for the earlier period, but it may also have evolved considerably since the beginning of Greek rule. In a similar manner, I have often been forced to rely on pharaonic period materials in discussing Egyptian medicine of the Ptolemaic period, sometimes from very early, where a qualified continuity is plausible or directly supported, such as when late or Ptolemaic Egyptian medical texts presume the ideological framework more directly attested in earlier works.

The overall reconstruction, however, is tentative, and represents a set of more or less likely possiblities for Ptolemaic medicine and its functions within wider Greco-Egyptian society. One advantage of this approach to history is that it goes some way toward reflecting the experiential multiplicity of that world: even in the modern world among individuals within a shared linguistic framework, socio-economic group, and scientific culture, medicine and illness is often experienced very differently. This was also the case in Greek-ruled Egypt, but complicated further by socio-economic inequality and a notable degree of linguistic and cultural diversity.

Finally, I offer the usual disclaimer about a lack of consistency in Greek and Egyptian transliteration. As a rule I have tried to keep as close as possible to the original forms, but kept more Latinized names in very familiar cases or where the distinction is useful. For instance, I have used Ptolemy for the kings of Egypt, but Ptolemaios when this name is borne by more ordinary mortals. All dates are BCE if not otherwise stated.

I would like to thank all those who have read earlier drafts of sections of this work, and also my colleagues in Classics and Art History at Emory, for putting up with me while I wrote it. Friends, family and my editors at Brill were also remarkably patient. I am very grateful indeed to Ann Ellis Hanson, who read the whole draft: remaining errors and adverbs are entirely my responsibility.

NOTE ON ABBREVIATIONS

Standard abbreviations have been used for Egyptology journals, and for Classics periodicals according to *L'Année Philologique*. The titles of journals from other fields have been cited in full.

Other abbreviations used:

LÄ	*Lexikon der Ägyptologie*, edited by W. Helck, E. Otto, W. Westendorf. 7 volumes. Wiesbaden: O. Harrassowitz, 1972/5–.
BNP	*Brill's New Pauly, Encyclopaedia of the Ancient World*, edited by H. Cancik, H. Schneider, M. Landfester, C. Salazar. Leiden: Brill, 2006.

For published papyri, the most recent publication has usually been cited, or on occasion the edition most commonly used. For papyri from Greco-Roman Egypt I have given the TM number, referring to its listing in the Trismegistos portal for late Egypt papyrological resources (http://www.trismegistos.org), which lists all other editions.

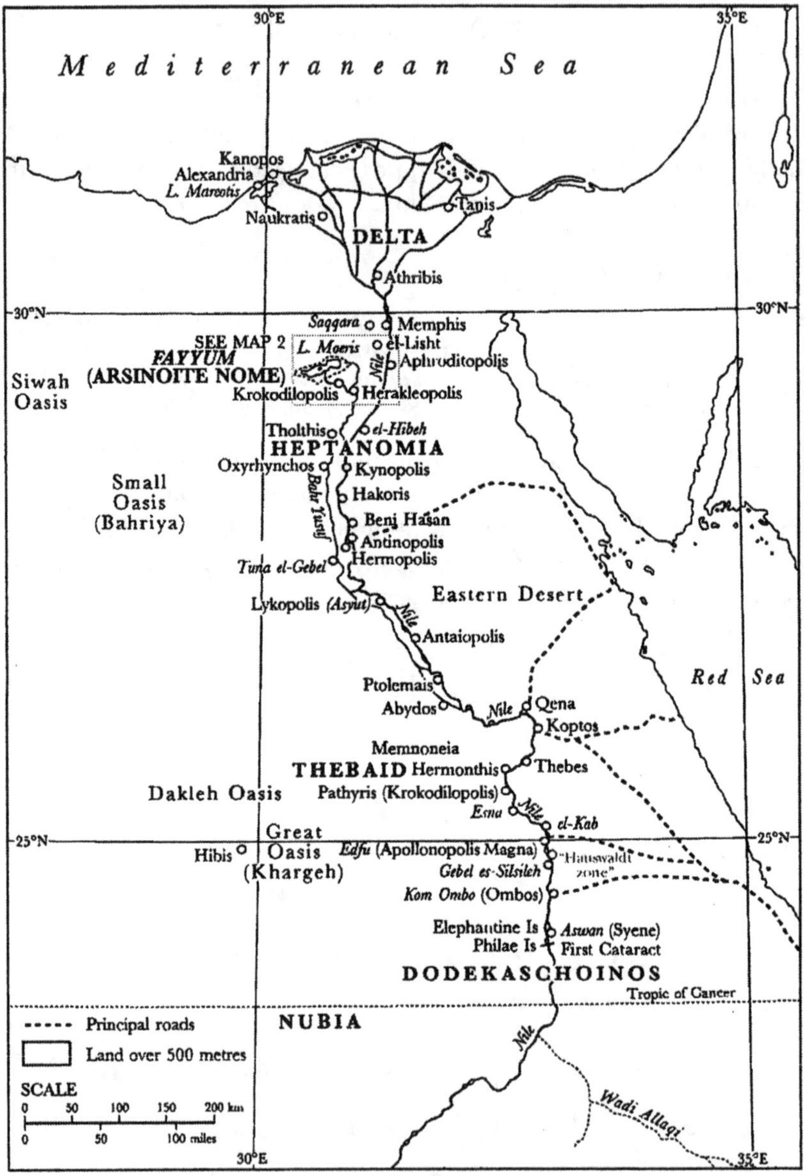

Figure 1. Ptolemaic Egypt.

CHAPTER ONE

GREEKS AND EGYPTIANS

Illness is a sociocultural concept. The meanings imputed to sickness and healing have always varied within and between different societal groups, including different ethnicities. To explore the means and meanings of medicine in Egypt during the rule of the Ptolemies is to investigate both the negotiation of sociocultural identity through health-related choices and beliefs, and, conversely, the effects of history, environment and social structures upon explanatory models of sickness and their behavioral components—medical theories and practices.

In this chapter, I wish to set out, as preliminaries, certain factors that were contingent upon the geographical and historical situation. Part 1.1 summarizes what we can deduce, not about illness in Greek-ruled Egypt, but about diseases. According to this by now standard distinction within anthropology and health care, illness is a state of the patient, understood as some divergence—bodily, behavioral, functional, psychological—from local norms of health. Disease, on the other hand, is the patient's nosologic state according to the orthodoxy of practitioners in medicine, usually those of modern biomedicine (which is how I use it in this chapter. The orthodoxies of antiquity are discussed in chapter 3).[1] The two are related but not co-extensive, and can be sharply divergent.[2]

Paleopathology and comparative epidemiology, for the known geographic, climactic and biological conditions of ancient Egypt, give us some guidance in our own terms for the kinds of illness experienced. Since first generation immigrants would have brought with them both diseases and expectations derived from the epidemiology and biosystems of their previous location, I have included evidence from classical period Greece here.

---

[1] This terminology is now standard. For an early exposition see Kellert, S. (1976). 'A sociocultural concept of health and disease', *The Journal of Medicine and Philosophy* 1 (3), 222–228. Cf. Chrisman, N.J. and T.M. Johnson. 'Clinically applied anthropology', in Johnson, T.M. and C.F. Sargent. (1990, rev. ed. 1996). *Medical Anthropology*, 111.

[2] In the most extreme cases doctors and patients may disagree over whether or not the patient actually has a (non-psychological) condition at all: e.g. chronic fatigue syndrome, fibromyalgia, Gulf War syndrome.

The next section, 1.2, concerns demographics, in terms of both total population and local settlement patterns, which were relevant both to disease epidemiology but also to sociocultural constructions of medicine, through factors including locality, the density and distribution of ethnic groups, diet, and the availability of practitioners.

Ethnicity is a crucial but much disputed concept within the literature on Ptolemaic era Egypt, and its relationship to that society's medical systems is a continuing theme of this book. In 1.3.1, I discuss briefly the leading models for understanding the importance and nature of 'ethnic' identity and interaction that have been proposed, rejected and argued about over the last century, and focus on the relations between the Ptolemaic administration and key Egyptian societal groups. Next, 1.3.2 examines how immigration, foreign rule, and social change were incorporated into and expressed by Egyptian ideological systems and symbols, in particular the construction of political and religious legitimacy through the concepts of *mꜣꜥt* and *jzft*. Greek perceptions of Egypt are considered in 1.4, with particular reference (1.4.2) to Greek views on Egyptian medicine.

1.1. *Physical and Epidemiological Environments*

> Even without this, the Egyptians are the healthiest of all men, next to the Libyans.[3]

The soldiers of Alexander's and Soter's armies who settled in Egypt after 332 came from many of the Greek-inhabited lands and cities of the Mediterranean basin. The family ethnics of one group of settlers reveal significant proportions of people from Macedonia, Kyrenaika, inhabitants of the Balkans, and Greeks from the islands, the north Aegean coast, the Greek mainland from Thessaly and Epiros to the Peloponnese, and the cities of the west coast of Asia Minor and the Propontis.[4] Settlers arriving in Egypt found themselves in a relatively alien landscape on the edge of Africa, to which they brought their own preferences, pathogens and agricultural techniques. They changed the Egyptian environment, and were changed by it.

---

[3] Herodotos 2.77. A.B. Lloyd's efforts to find reasons why this claim might be correct are not convincing. (1976). *Herodotus Book II, Commentary 1–98*, ad loc.

[4] Bagnall, R.S. (1984). 'The origins of Ptolemaic cleruchs', *BASP* 21, 7–20, based on 453 cleruchs over 140 years (until 142). See also Clarysse, W. 'Ethnic diversity and dialect among the Greeks of Hellenistic Egypt', in Verhoogt, A.M.F.W. and S.P. Vleeming. (1998). *The Two Faces of Graeco-Roman Egypt*, 1–13.

The country they entered was essentially a river oasis in the desert of north-eastern Africa, comprising the Nile valley itself and the delta at its head, a total area of about 34,000 km^2, from the first cataracts that marked its most consistent border with Nubia, to the broader east-west axis of the delta and the northern coast. Egypt sits on the edge of the Mediterranean climactic zone, which can be broadly characterized as hot and dry to the point of lengthy drought in summer, but cool, wet and windy in winter, with brief periods of spring and autumn. Syria and Egypt, just west of the Sahara, offer much the hottest and driest variation. As a consequence of the erosion of the river bed and the deposits of silt along its banks, the agricultural land of Egypt dropped away from the relatively high ground beside the Nile. In antiquity, before the modern Aswan dam was completed, floodwater ran through overflow channels into this lower plain, forming a set of agriculturally terraced basins down the very slight incline of the valley and away from the river. Agriculture depended entirely on this annual flooding of the Nile between July and October, which rendered Egypt considerably more fertile than the majority of the Greek mainland and islands, in spite of its much lower annual rainfall.[5] From mid-August to late September the valley floor was almost entirely covered by waters that washed away the salts and deposited a new layer of highly fertile black silt; the inhabitants sometimes called their country *Kmt*, the Black Land. Canals extended this agriculturally productive area. The main crops were grown in the irrigated fields, while villages and smaller settlements were surrounded by gardens of vegetables and other plants.

Beyond the cultivated strip, where the ground level was lowest, the waters never entirely receded, forming marshy areas where fish and other wildlife congregated in large numbers. A similar environment was formed in the delta region as Nile branches and other water channels spread out towards the Mediterranean sea. Accumulated deposits of mud and sand separated the channels, which could be used for crops or for grazing by pastoralists' herds of cattle, sheep and goats. Papyrus reed beds produced a widely used material. Art of the pharaonic period shows the king and other members of the elite hunting wildfowl flocks or even hippopotami, depictions that probably represented the victory of order over chaos as much as they did any actual activity. Marsh areas, in their teeming life and resemblance to the creation environment of Egyptian religion (in which a hill or mound emerges from the waters) were a chaotic, creative space in Egyptian

[5] The average rainfall for most of the Mediterranean basin is 650 mm, in contrast to Egypt's insignificant 100–200 mm.

imagery and myth. The ubiquitousness of this geographic feature—an area of higher ground surrounded, like an island, by flood waters bringing agricultural fertility—is also demonstrated by the fact that many Greek names for Fayum towns and villages end in -νῆσος.

One westward branch of the Nile ended in a lake, called Lake Moeris by the Greeks, that formed an oasis of its own, west of the Nile valley proper and south of the delta region. This was the Arsinoite nome, now known as the Fayum, which in the Ptolemaic era at its maximum agricultural extent formed about 1200 km^2 of cultivated land: the lake itself was reduced in size by its water being siphoned off into irrigation at different levels.

All land not reached by the inundation and additional manmade irrigation was desert, or at best desert savannah. The eastern desert was an important source of minerals. A king of Egypt, at least in times of sufficiently centralized power, was able to embark on large-scale mining expeditions and could also control the trade routes to the Red Sea, dominating the nomadic populations beyond the valley edges proper. The western desert that formed the border with ancient Libya was also important for trade. It contained several oases intermittently controlled by Egypt, including the remote western oasis of Siwa. Buildings, both Greek and Egyptian in style, asserted Ptolemaic control over this land, as far away as Tolmeita in Kyrenaika—about 1000 km from Alexandria.[6] Such control was metaphysical as well as military: the desert borderlands separated off the living space of Egypt and in myth delimited the edges of the ordered universe. Egyptian writings frequently oppose the 'Red Land' (*dšrt*) to the Black Land.[7] The lions and other big cats associated with Sakhmet, Mehit and similar divinities prowled the sands; a danger but also a symbol of the protection of Egypt against the foreigners, demons and diseases that came from outside.

This was the climate, ecology, pathogenic environment, and related set of explanatory models of the cosmos, that first generation immigrants into Egypt encountered. The immigrants, in turn, affected their environment as consumers, agricultural producers, and carriers of disease strains from elsewhere in the world. Epidemic diseases, named in Egyptian texts as the demonic 'arrows of Sakhmet' and other gods, were associated with specific times of year, notably just before the New Year and the inundation. 'Spell for barring the air of a disease year .... It is the year's protection; it is a bitterness repeller in a year of disease', announces the first incantation on the verso

[6] Baines, J. and J. Malek. (2000). *Cultural Atlas of Ancient Egypt*, 19.
[7] See Kemp, B. (1989, 2nd ed. 2006). *Ancient Egypt*, 21–22.

of the Edwin Smith medical papyrus.[8] An 'Asiatic' disease is mentioned in two medical papyri.[9] It is possible that contagious disease in epidemic form was associated with immigrants or minorities, on either an ideological or epidemiological basis.[10]

Scorpions were creatures of the desert, and a notable hazard of living on its fringe. Snakebite and scorpion sting were prevalent in Egyptian imagery, myth and literature; while poisonous animals became a literary *topos* and a virtual sub-genre of their own in Greek didactic, ethnographic and encyclopedic texts of the Hellenistic and early Roman era. The Egyptian landscape provided several of the more exotic examples. Scorpions from Koptos, according to Aelian, are of large size and possess unusually sharp stings causing instant death; however they never harm the women performing rituals in time of mourning at the sanctuary of Isis.[11] This ostensibly biological observation in fact suggests a link with Egyptian myth: the scorpion goddess Serqet aids Isis in protecting her infant son Horus from poisonous animals associated with the usurper god Seth. In turn, Horus' endangerment is also an expression of biology: children are more at risk of serious consequences from scorpion sting.

How lethal these were would have depended on which species were involved. Scorpion stings are painful, but there is normally a good chance of survival. It was certainly a regular and clearly identifiable threat that constituted, together with snakebite, a major subset of perceived health risks. There was an entire category of Egyptian healers linked to the scorpion-headed goddess Serqet, although this did not mean that their practice was limited to the prevention and treatment of stings.[12] Although Greeks would have been familiar with the genus, many varieties of scorpions in Egypt are more toxic than might have been expected by immigrants from southern Europe, where non-venomous species are widespread.[13]

---

[8] V. 1, 1–10. Translated Allen, J. (2005). *The Art of Medicine in Ancient Egypt*, 107. For disease theories see chapter 3.1.2. pp. 108–112.

[9] P. BM 10059 (London Medical Papyrus), spell 32, and the Hearst Medical Papyrus, no. 170. Ritner, R.K. (2000). 'Innovations and adaptations in ancient Egyptian medicine', *JNES* 59, 110–111.

[10] Hearst 11.12–16; London 11.4–6. See Grapow, H., H. von Deines and W. Westendorf. (1954–1973). *Grundriss der Medizin der Alten Ägypter* (henceforth *GdM*) 2.16; Pinch, G. (1994). *Magic in Ancient Egypt*, 141.

[11] Aelian *Nature of Animals* 10.23.

[12] For protection from scorpions see also 4.3.1, pp. 186–187; 4.3.3, 190–192; 5.1.2, pp. 212–213.

[13] Classical evidence and, more usefully, modern distribution patterns, suggest that Egyptian scorpions probably included the severely venomous *Leiurus quinquestriatus*, *Androc-*

Also highly venomous are several of Egypt's numerous snakes, including the horned viper and the hooded cobra. A bite would have been painful and occasionally fatal.[14] The animals were attracted to cultivated areas and villages by the rodents that infested houses, rubbish dumps, granaries and, at certain times of the year, crop-fields. The cobra goddess Renenutet was associated with the harvest and fertility, while the rising cobra, hood extended, provided protective imagery for the king and state as the uraeus on the brow of the king, and as Wadjet, goddess of Lower Egypt. These goddesses symbolized maternal protection and guaranteed the continuation of life and fertility within Egypt. The snake was also construed as significant of chaos, emblematically as the evil underworld constrictor Apophis.

A hieratic papyrus of the early Ptolemaic period lists kinds of snake and classifies their bite into 'can be saved', 'non-fatal,' and 'dies quickly.' Its content, as it claimed, may date from much earlier. Only the bite of the *sdbw* is described as 'harmless', though that of the chameleon (which must be the animal lurking behind the phrase, 'green, changes color according to background'), was wrongly classed as 'non-lethal': it is in fact completely harmless.[15] Actual bites from several species of Egyptian snake would indeed have often been fatal, but the overall incidence of snakebites may well have been less frequent than fear made it.

Less visible hazards for new immigrants involved changes in diet and foodstuffs, often accompanied by local bacteria, viruses and parasites. Descriptions of illnesses in Egyptian and Greco-Roman medical texts are usually difficult to identify with any precision. Most of the evidence for the disease environment of Egypt consists of osteoarcheological samples from two millennia of pharaonic history and prehistory. These provide frequently uncertain indications that a certain condition existed in the area at some time, but estimating the prevalence and possible effects of even attested diseases depends on comparative evidence from similar environments and/or

---

tonus australis, and subspecies of *Buthus occitanicus*; as well as *Androctonus aeneas*, *A. amoreuxi*, and *Buthacus arenicola*. Widespread southern European species are *Euscorpius flavicaudis* and *E. italicus*. See Beavis, Ian C. (1988). *Insects and other Invertebrates in Classical Antiquity*, 21–34; Tod, M. (1939). 'The scorpion in Graeco-Roman Egypt', *JEA* 25, 55–61.

14 Hansen, N.B. 'Snakes', in Redford, D.B. (2001). *The Oxford Encyclopaedia of Ancient Egypt*, 3.296–299.

15 Brooklyn Museum Papyrus 47, 218.48 + 47, 218.85, TM 58496: published by Sauneron, S. (1989). *Une traité égyptien d'ophiologie*. Cf. Nunn, J. (1996). *Ancient Egyptian Medicine*, 183–189.

societies, modern or historical. Temporal, regional, occupational and individual variations in disease are inevitably almost entirely invisible.[16]

In what follows I assume the pathogenic ecology of Ptolemaic Egypt to be similar to that suggested by the pharaonic evidence for Egypt, qualified by what we know of population, agriculture and behavior in the later period. Similar kinds of evidence for archaic and classical Greece allow us to speculate on the differences and similarities encountered by first generation settlers from such areas, or on what disease strains they may have introduced. Some of these differences would have been short-term in their noticeable effects. People usually adapt with relative speed to different diets and, if they initially survive them, to new diseases. Second and subsequent generations, meanwhile, would experience Egyptian conditions as normal and familiar, though for some time the dietary or medicinal preferences of initial settlers might have been preserved within families and communities.

The foodstuffs available were in general terms not very different to elsewhere in the Mediterranean basin. The wealthy presumably ate more animal flesh than the rest of the indigenous population. Beef and wildfowl were the most prestigious meats in pharaonic times and this probably held true later as well: cattle grazing was not easy to find in Egypt. Domestic accounts from residents in a Memphite temple in the mid-second century—a group quite distinct from the majority of the population—show only one instance of the purchase of beef, at a price equivalent to a daily purchase of bread for a year and a half.[17] Mutton, pork, goat, and antelope were also eaten; pigeons, probably raised in dovecots, supplemented ducks and geese. Chickens arrived on a large scale only with the other immigrants from Greek and Roman lands. Fish from the Nile and marshes was, as elsewhere, more widely and readily available than grain-expensive meat.

The basics of the diet were based on cereals and pulses: lentils, chickpeas, and beer made from barley. A kind of porridge and the commonest kind of bread (*kyllestis*) were made from olyra, a form of emmer.[18] Greek

---

[16] Sallares, R.P. (1991). *The Ecology of the Ancient Greek World*, e.g. 123–124 emphasizes nonetheless that there are huge variations in mortality, fertility and morbidity between populations. Some diseases may have been very local: ibid. 227, citing Lucretius' identification of a localized foot condition, points out that Greece's disease ecology differs from that in other parts of Europe.

[17] *UPZ* I 67.4–5, TM 3458 (153/2 BCE). Thompson, D.J. 'Food for Ptolemaic temple workers' in Wilkins, J. et al. (1995). *Food in Antiquity*, 318.

[18] Wild, H. 'Backen', *LÄ* 1.595: up to 40 different kinds of bread. Darby et al. (1977). *Food: the gift of Osiris*, 2.543: up to 17 types of beer. See also Battaglia, E. (1989). *'Artos': il lessico della*

immigrants probably preferred bread made from wheat, and of the many crops that were introduced or experimented with in the early Ptolemaic era, it was wheat and vines that made the major impact. By the advent of the Roman period, olyra had almost disappeared from cultivation and wine consumption and production, which in the pharaonic period had been a marker of the wealthy elite, had expanded significantly among the Egyptian population in addition to its immigrant market (see p. 42). Surpluses in wheat and wine were both exported. The village plots ensured a supply of vegetables like lettuces, turnips, and onions. Egypt has no woodland and had to import most of its timber, but small orchards of fruit and nut trees were not uncommon. The new arrival would have found no shortage of dates, but might have had to buy his olives from further away, and switch to sesame oil for cooking. Castor oil was used for lighting. Beehives provided the main sweetener, though preferred varieties were imported, such as honey from the Greek island of Khios. (Fodder crops, flax, and papyrus constituted the other major agricultural crops of the pharaonic period; flax and papyrus were also exported in large quantities).

Such foods, consumed regularly in sufficient quantities, constitute a usefully varied and nutritious diet, but it is, of course, not at all clear how 'average' the summary of available food given above actually was, or how it varied with occupational group or social status. Records of rations for workers or temple allowances concern distinctive and sometimes temporary populations.[19] Nor did records always corresponded to reality. Two temporary workers at the Memphis Sarapieon, in the mid-second century, were rarely paid their generous bread allowance.[20]

Older male individuals of higher social status are often depicted as carrying excess fat in Egyptian art. This was probably often artistic shorthand for membership of the elite rather than a realistic portrayal, with body fat serving as a marker and result of high socioeconomic status.[21] The later Ptolemies, especially Ptolemy VIII 'Physkon', exploited a similar form of representation.[22] Overall, Ptolemaic landowners and much of the rest of the

---

panificazione nei papiri greci; Thompson, 'Temple workers', for the kinds of foods bought by low-status cult attendants.

19 Miller, R.L. (1991). 'Counting calories in Egyptian ration texts', *JESHO* 34, 257–269.

20 Thompson, 'Temple workers', 323.

21 E.g. Weeks, K.R. 'Art, word and the Egyptian world view', in (1979). *Egyptology and the Social Sciences*, 71–72.

22 Ashton, S.-A. 'The Ptolemaic royal image and the Egyptian tradition', in Tait, J. (2003). *'Never Had the Like Occurred': Egypt's view of its past*, 213–223 esp. 217, 223.

Greek population, like the Egyptian socioeconomic elite, were unlikely to suffer from malnutrition (although this situation was sometimes complicated by parasites).

For farmers and some manual workers the situation was somewhat different. Famines were rare if not unknown in a country famous for its agricultural productivity, but the amount and kind of food available to the population was affected by two principal factors: the size of the harvest and the demands of taxation and rents.[23] The former was crucially dependent on the level of the inundation. Nilometers and temple quays recorded the maximum height of the flood for each year. It is also likely that diseases affected crops on a fairly frequent basis. The Greeks introduced several different wheat strains, reducing the monocultural risk of widespread shortages due to plant disease. On the other hand, replacing barley and emmer crops with wheat might itself have resulted in lower productivity. Husked emmer is resistant to disease both in growth and storage, while statistics for early 20th century Greek Attica show that wheat failed more than one year in four, and barley one year in twenty.[24] Estimates both of population and of Egypt's carrying capacity vary, but shortages in some years combined with taxation were a major contributory factor to the frequent attestations of social unrest in the later Ptolemaic era.[25] Grain prices varied noticeably with region, season and year.[26]

Dietary deficiencies and mild malnutrition stress the body and increase vulnerability to illness. A lack of fat reserves means the body has little to fall

[23] The causeway to the pyramid of Unas at Saqqara carried a 5th dynasty depiction of wasted, weakened figures. The Ptolemaic 'famine stele' carved into the rock on the island of Sehel described a supposed period of starvation in the time of the Old Kingdom king Djoser. A series of poor inundations in the 40s CE, followed by excessive floods in CE 45 and 46, were linked to famine and epidemic disease in succeeding years: Pliny *Natural History* 5.58, Seneca *Natural Questions* 4.2.16; Appian *Civil Wars* 4.61, 108; Bonneau, D. (1971). *Le fisc et le Nil*, 161–163, 235; but see Browne, G.M. (1970). *Michigan Papyri* 10 for evidence of contemporary harvests in the area of Philadelphia. Famines as opposed to shortages were uncommon in antiquity: Garnsey, P. (1988). *Famine and Food Supply in the Graeco-Roman World.*

[24] Plant disease: Sallares *Ecology*, 291–293, with n. 409. Marr, J.L. and P.J. Rhodes. (2008). *The 'Old Oligarch'* 2.6; Theophrastos *Causes of Plants* 3.22.1–2, 4.14.1, *History of Plants* 8.10.2 are among the sources to mention risks of plant or animal disease. Emmer resistant: Braun, T. 'Barley cakes and emmer bread', in Wilkins, *Food in Antiquity*, 35. For 20th century Attic harvests, see Garnsey, *Famine and Food Supply*, 10.

[25] A low inundation was followed by scarcity in 245, prompting imports of grain from Ptolemaic controlled Kyrene, Kypros and Syria. Such relief became unavailable as the empire shrank during the 2nd century. Bonneau, *Le fisc et le Nil*, 125, 223; Hölbl, G. (2001). *A History of the Ptolemaic Empire*, 48.

[26] Bagnall, R.S. and B.W. Frier. (1994). *The Demography of Roman Egypt*, 173.

back on in any lengthy or debilitating illness. About 30% of skeletal remains from the ancient Nile Valley show 'Harris lines' or other skeletal characteristics associated with malnutrition and other physiological stressors such as illness. (A large proportion of this evidence is Nubian and may not be typical of all Egypt).[27] Malnutrition and disease reinforce each other: even in a famine the majority of people die from disease rather than simple starvation.[28]

Enteric diseases such as typhoid and dysentery are thus particularly dangerous during periods of malnutrition. Diarrheal conditions, causing severe dehydration and in extreme cases kidney failure, are a leading cause of mortality among infants and young children in developing countries, although invisible in any osteoarcheological record.[29] A fever described in the Greek medical text *Epidemics* is characteristic of those caused by the salmonella genus of bacteria, possibly *Salmonella typhi* in particular.[30] The typhoid bacillus is transmitted through contaminated water, food or milk. It would have been well suited to the hot dry conditions of Egypt, particularly in the Fayum where the inhabitants relied on lake water and long-distance supplies from the Nile.

The medical texts of both Greece and Egypt contained large numbers of remedies aimed at the gastrointestinal system, but as Scheidel points out (*Death on the Nile*, 65) the majority of these refer not to diarrhea but to purging the belly to remove pathogenic substances in cases of constipation and other diagnoses.[31] P. Ebers, paragraph 207 does suggest that the practitioner examine 'what has gone down from his anus', which may be 'like black lumps' or 'like porridge of beans.' However, the diagnosis and remedy for this condition identified the problem as roast meat that caused a swelling

---

27 See Scheidel, W. (2001). *Death on the Nile*, 104 n. 315 for a survey of studies on evidence for (mal)nutrition in ancient Egypt. 30%: Sandison, A.T. and E. Tapp. 'Disease in ancient Egypt', in Cockburn, A. et al. (2nd ed. 1998). *Mummies, Disease and Ancient Cultures*, 39. Ikram, S. 'Diet', in Redford, *Oxford Encyclopedia*, 1.394 (evidence for malnutrition in childhood is primarily Nubian).

28 Jutikkala, E. and M. Kauppinen. (1971). 'The structure of mortality during catastrophic years in a pre-industrial society', *Population Studies* 25.2, 283–286.

29 Scheidel, *Death on the Nile*, 62–66 esp. 65; Sallares, *Ecology*, 91, 231.

30 [Hipp.] *Epidemics* 7.2 (5.382–386 Littré), see Grmek, M.D. (1989). *Diseases in the Ancient Greek World*, 346–347. Typhoid was often conflated with other fevers until the 19th century. Typhus in antiquity is not confirmed, although lice probably carried the similar 'relapsing fever' (*Borrelia recurrentis*), often accompanied by jaundice. Scheidel, *Death on the Nile*, 66–75.

31 See 3.2.1, pp. 115–116; 4.2.2, pp. 158–159; 4.2.1.1, pp. 159–163; cf, Nunn, *Egyptian Medicine*, 88–91.

in his heart and needed to be purged. This suggests that although diarrhea or abnormal stools may be seen as a symptom of disease, the effluent is not viewed as a problem in itself and may indeed be interpreted as a natural purging and useful response; one that the practitioner tries to strengthen. It is difficult to tell whether the remedies for 'cooling' or 'refreshing' the anus are in response to discomfort caused by diarrhea or constipation, or are meant to treat a gastrointestinal cause of disease.

Acute conditions that resolve early, through death or recovery, rarely leave traces behind. Inflammation from pneumonia can cause fibrous changes in the lungs, as in the body of Nekht-ankh (now in the Manchester museum).[32] Viral and bacterial infections produced the immune response of the 'fevers' that formed the dominant category in Greco-Roman diagnostics, and heat seems to have been an indication of disease in Egyptian medicine as well,[33] but Benson, 'Health in pharaonic Egypt', 21 notes for Greece that there is 'no convincing evidence of any specific viral disease'.[34] A funerary stele showing a doorkeeper with a withered, shortened leg has been interpreted as evidence for poliomyelitis, but a single artistic artifact is a dubious basis on which to declare polio's presence in Egypt, let alone extrapolate its scale.[35] Evidence for smallpox is also weak, though several authors speculate that unrecorded epidemics could have occurred in both pharaonic Egypt and Greece: smallpox is a highly infectious disease, but one that requires a high population density to become endemic.[36] There is no clear evidence for syphilis, though absence of evidence is in this case, as in others, not evidence of absence.[37] The second century CE physician Aretaios

---

32 Tapp, E. 'Disease in the Manchester mummies', in David, A.R. (1979). *The Manchester Museum Mummy Project*, 95–102. Rowling, J.T. 'Respiratory disease in Egypt', in Brothwell, D. and A.T. Sandison. (1967). *Diseases in Antiquity*, 489–493, reviews other possible cases.

33 E.g. Ebers 855d with Bardinet, T. (1995). *Papyrus médicaux de l'Égypte pharaonique*, ad loc. See further chapter 3.

34 Benson, W.H. 'Health in pharaonic Egypt', in Davies, W.V. and R. Walker. (1993). *Biological Anthropology and the Study of Ancient Egypt*, 19–23. For malaria in Greece, see pp. 14–15 below.

35 Nunn, *Egyptian Medicine*, 77; Filer, J. (1995). *Disease*, 74–75.

36 Benson, 'Health', and Nunn, *Egyptian Medicine*, view the evidence for pharaonic Egypt as very doubtful. Scheidel, *Death on the Nile*, allows the possibility for dynastic Egypt and suggests it may have been endemic during high population density in the Roman era. Sandison, A.T. (1972). 'Evidence of infective disease', *Journal of Human Evolution* 1, 213–224, reviews the evidence and argues (Sandison & Tapp, 'Disease in ancient Egypt', 44) that unrecorded epidemics may have occurred. Sallares, *Ecology*, views smallpox as an epidemic disease in Greece.

37 Buikstra, J. et al. 'What diseases plagued ancient Egyptians? A century of controversy considered', in Davies & Walker, *Biological Anthropology*, 24–53.

of Kappodokia described what is clearly diphtheric sore throat as common, probably endemic, in early Roman Egypt and Syria.[38] In more modern times endemic diphtheria has killed at a rate of around 1 in 10.

Characteristic skeletal deformities indicate long-term infection by the tuberculosis bacterium.[39] The remains of Nesparehan, a priest of Amun in the late first millennium, showing angular curvature of the spine (hump-back) in association with a psoas abscess, were recognized in 1910 as typical of Pott's disease, a common pathology of tuberculosis cases. Some 30 other reliable instances of tuberculosis-style pathology are known for ancient Egypt,[40] but although several individuals are depicted as hump-backed in visual representations in tomb chapels these cases might involve other medical conditions. It is also possible that the hump-backed pose depicts not the reality of an individual but their status through an artistic convention: all examples are of servants.[41] The detailed 1993 review by Buikstra et al concluded that, 'the presence of tuberculosis-like pathology' (p. 46) remains convincing. However, as they also point out, the impact and prevalence of such pathologies in the Egyptian population, as opposed to the depicted population, remains unresolved.

There is limited paleo-osteoarcheological evidence for tuberculosis in Greece, but the skeletal deformity was described in classical period medical texts, while references to the characteristic symptoms of pulmonary tuberculosis are common among Greco-Roman writers on medicine. Any layman, said Aretaios, can recognize the disease when he sees a coughing, pale, worn-out invalid.[42] Tuberculosis is not density-dependent and survives quite happily in small populations in endemic form; it can also appear as an

---

[38] Aretaios *Causes and signs of acute diseases* 1.9 (*CMG* 2.10–12 Hude). Grmek, *Diseases*, 337–338 also views diphtheria as the condition in [Hipp.] *Dentition* 24 and 31 (both 8.548 Littré), and as a factor in the cough of Perinthos, [Hipp.] *Epidemics* 6.

[39] Evidence for the other major mycobacterial disease, leprosy, in Egypt before the Roman period (there are two probable examples from 4th century CE Nubia) is scarce, but Dzierzykay-Rogalski, T. (1980). 'Paleopathology of the Ptolemaic inhabitants of the Dakleh Oasis (Egypt)', *Journal of Human Evolution* 9, 71–74, viewed the changes in four skeletons found in a Ptolemaic period cemetery in the Dakhleh oasis as characteristic of the disease.

[40] Nesparehan: Smith, G.E. and M.A. Ruffer. (1910). *Potts'che Krankheit an einer ägyptische Mumie aus der Zeit der 21. Dynastie (um 1000 v. Chr.)*. Buikstra, 'What diseases?' 3, 25 lists 13 confirmatory studies and discusses relatively recent findings at Saqqara and Abydos.

[41] Nunn, *Egyptian Medicine*, 73–74.

[42] E.g. [Hipp.] *Internal Affections* 10, 12 (7.188–190, 192–198 Littré); *Diseases* 2.48 (7.72 Littré). Grmek, *Diseases*, 187 notes possible alternative diagnosis for the first of three consumptives described in *Internal Affections*. Cf. [Hipp.] *Epidemics* 1.3 (2.604–610 Littré), 7 (5.378 Littré); Celsus 3.22; Aretaios *Causes and signs of chronic diseases* 1.8.

epidemic under conditions of rapid population growth and urbanization. The evidence is far from conclusive, but points to endemic rather than epidemic TB for Ptolemaic and early Roman Alexandria.[43]

Water-borne parasites (*Schistosoma haematobium, S. mansoni*) that cause schistosomiasis (bilharzia) have been found in mummies and are very likely to have affected many people who dwelt near, and either drank or bathed, in the water of the Nile and its canals.[44] Parasitic burdens rarely cause death outright, but they cause chronic anemia and alarming symptoms such as hematuria (in the case of schistosomiasis). Conditions in Greece were unfavorable to the *Schistosoma* parasite, but Greek physicians could have known the disease from elsewhere. Schistosomiasis contributes significantly to immune and physical weakness, and so to morbidity and mortality.

The naturally mummified body of an adolescent male weaver from the reign of Setnakht (1187–1185) contained not only schistosomal and tapeworm eggs, but also a parasitic cyst, probably *Trichinella spiralis*. Both tapeworms and Trichinella are obtained through eating meat, in Trichinella's case pork. The individual in question, Nakht, was attached to the staff of a funerary temple, and meat may have been a larger part of his diet than it was for agricultural workers. Malnutrition and complications were likely results of this multiple infestation.[45]

Tapeworms (*Taenia solium, T. saginata*) have been found elsewhere, as have roundworm (*Ascaris lumbricoides*), the parasitic nematode worm *Strongyloides*, and the guinea worm (*Dracunculus sp.*), the last of which, like schistosomiasis, is acquired from water.[46] The relatively high incidence of

---

[43] Scheidel, W. 'Creating a metropolis: a comparative demographic perspective' in Harris, W.V. and G. Ruffini. (2004). *Ancient Alexandria between Egypt and Greece*, 19.

[44] Evidence for schistosomiasis summarized by Sandison & Tapp, 'Disease in ancient Egypt', 40. Ruffer, M.A. (1910). 'Note on the presence of "Bilharzia haematobia" in Egyptian mummies of the Twentieth Dynasty', *BMJ* 1, 16; Millet, 'ROM I' (below n. 45), for a New Kingdom mummy with schistosomal ova and (probably as a result) liver cirrhosis, 100–101; Schistosome antigen: Deelder, A.M. et al. (1990). 'Detection of schistosome antigen in mummies', *Lancet* 335, 724–725.

[45] Nakht: Millet, N.B. et al. 'ROM I: mummification for the common people', in Cockburn, *Mummies*, 91–105. *Taenia* (tapeworm) ovam, 101; *Trichinella*, 102. Harris lines indicating malnutrition: 95, 102. He had also had malaria.

[46] Tapeworms (*Taenia*): above and Tapp, E. 'Disease and the Manchester mummies—the pathologist's role' in David, A.R. and E. Tapp. (1984). *Evidence Embalmed*, 78–95. Roundworm (*Ascaris*): Cockburn et al. 'A classic mummy: PUM II', in Cockburn, *Mummies*, 79 (in mummy of ca. 170). Evidence that this individual had a chronic debilitating illness suggests guinea worm (*Dracunculus*) infestation as well; cf. Tapp, E. 'The unwrapping of a mummy' in David,

these among the minute sample of Egypt's population available as mummies, together with evidence from 19th and 20th century Egypt and similar societies suggests that such parasitic infestation was endemic.[47] The frequent references to worms or snakes in Egyptian medical literature may reflect observation of the more visible of these, such as guinea worms (see 3.1.2, pp. 109–110). Mosquitoes are the vector for various species of filariasis worms, some of which cause blindness and which also tend to cause swelling and thickening of the skin. One example has been found,[48] and Nunn, *Egyptian Medicine*, 71 suggests depictions of individuals with enlarged male genitalia may show the results of filariasis.

Mosquitoes are notoriously also the vector for malaria. The most dangerous kind is caused by infection with *Plasmodium falciparum*, which causes malignant tertian malaria and sometimes blackwater fever (malarial hemoglobinuria).[49] The antigen for malaria has been found in mummies dating from the Predynastic, New Kingdom, and Late periods, as well as from fifth century Nubia.[50] On the other hand, the low modern incidence of sickle-cell anemia in Egypt has been used to argue that malaria has not been long endemic there.[51] It might have been routinely present only in areas in which conditions were particularly well suited to mosquitoes, such as the lakes and canals of the delta and Fayum. Herodotos remarked (2.95) that the dwellers in the marshlands sleep under nets because of the gnats. He might have been referring to mosquitoes; then again he might have meant gnats. Greek biology did not discriminate between the two.

Malaria was certainly widespread in fifth and fourth century Greece, where its characteristic periodic fevers were crucial to diagnosis and prog-

---

Manchester Museum, 83–93. *Strongyloides*: Tapp, E. 'Disease in the Manchester mummies', in David, *Manchester Museum*, 95–102.

47 Though schistosomiasis increased in modern Egypt due to perennial irrigation after the building of the Aswan Dam, which inadvertently created perfect conditions for those parasites that cause it.

48 Tapp, E. and K. Wildsmith. 'The autopsy and endoscopy of the Leeds mummy', in David, A.R. and E. Tapp. (1992). *The Mummy's Tale*, 132–153 (for skin thought to belong to this individual).

49 So called because the internal destruction of red blood cells results in black urine. Grmek, *Diseases*, 295 ff.

50 Miller, R.L. et al. (1994). 'Diagnosis of *Plasmodium falciparum*. Infections in mummies using the rapid manual *Parasight*™-F test', *Transactions of the Royal Society of Tropical Medicine and Hygiene* 88, 31–32.

51 Scheidel, *Death on the Nile*, 76. High rates of sickle-cell anemia tend to correlate with historically endemic malaria. A single copy of the gene that in two copies produces sickle-cell, affords some protection against malaria.

nosis in medical nosology.[52] Three of the four malarial species were probably endemic,[53] but opinions differ on how widespread was *Plasmodium falciparum*. The much less harmful *P.vivax* and *P.malariae* were the commonest forms—probably hyper-endemic, as in the more recent past—in Greece's more seasonal climate, though lesser forms of malaria also have an impact on health, especially that of infants, and on fertility.[54] Scheidel, *Death on the Nile*, 80 observes that the Greeks might have brought new strains of malaria with them, but it remains unclear whether immigrants or indigenes were most at risk of infection by *P.falciparum*. Ancient sources, supported by (a very small sample of) funerary data, suggest that malaria was not a major presence in Alexandria itself. Possibly salinity from seawater made even the local marshes an unhappy environment for mosquito species, as it did in the 19th and early 20th centuries.[55]

Eye conditions constituted a large category of ill health in Egyptian and Greek medical texts. There were also frequent references to blindness in other Egyptian religious and literary materials, although many of these might have been metaphorical. Analysis relies on modern causes of blindness in similar environments. A very likely suspect is endemic infection with *chlamydia trachomatis*. This causes trachoma, a condition that visibly affects the eye; repeated reinfection causes blindness. In early modern Egypt it also led to to fatal neonatal pneumonia. It is transmitted directly as a venereal disease, or through flies. It may be the disease known as *nḥ3t* cited in the Ebers medical papyrus.[56]

---

52 On counting in Greek medicine as a theoretical expectation and an empirical activity, see Lloyd, G.E.R. (1987). *The Revolutions of Wisdom*, 257–270. He notes that cases where fevers are exactly quartan or tertian in periodicity are actually quite rare in the *Epidemics*.

53 There is a long-running debate on whether the skeletal changes of porotic hyperostosis observable in the ancient osteoarcheological record are reliable indicators of thalassemia. Since this is linked to resistance to falciparum malaria, porotic hyperostosis could in that case be used as an index of malaria incidence. Angel, J.L. (1964). 'Osteoporosis: thalassemia?' *American Journal of Physical Anthropology* and in subsequent articles analyzing skeletal populations: for references see Roberts, C. et al. 'Health and disease in Greece', in King, H. (2005). *Health in Antiquity*, 44. The correlation is rejected by Sallares, *Ecology*, 275–277: porotic hyperostosis is the result of iron deficiency.

54 Where it has been hyper-endemic, as in Greece in the more recent past, 50–75% of children and many adults show clinical symptoms including enlarged spleens.

55 Scheidel, 'Creating a metropolis', 18–19. Absence of malaria: Strabo 17.1.7.

56 Benson, 'Health', 21; Nunn, *Egyptian Medicine*, 291. *Nḥ3t* (Ebers 350, 358, 407) is identified with trachoma by Ebbell, B. (1937). *Papyrus Ebers* and Westendorf, W. (1999). *Handbuch der Altägyptischen Medizin*, 151.

The lockjaw effects of tetanus may well be described in case 7 of the Edwin Smith papyrus, which concerns injuries.[57] The alternative prognosis reads:[58]

> One who has a gaping wound in his head, which has penetrated to the bone and violated the sutures of his skull, who has a toothache, whose mouth is clenched, who suffers from stiffness in his neck: an ailment for which nothing is done.

Similarly, in the classical Greek medical text *Epidemics*:[59]

> In the commander of the large ship, whose right forefinger, bone and all, had been crushed by the anchor, an inflammation appeared, a dry gangrene, and some fever .... Prediction: the backward spasm is on its way. The jaw began clenching, then it went to the nape of his neck; on the third day, he was totally convulsed backward with sweating; on the sixth day after prediction he died.

Tetanus usually enters the bloodstream after injury. Major and minor trauma is a daily hazard in most forms of work, and a commonplace in war. The Smith text details many possible injuries to the head and neck before the extant papyrus is broken off, while the tomb of Ipuy at New Kingdom Deir el-Medina illustrated a set of occupational disasters just about to happen. The ostraka found at Mons Claudianus reveal the kinds and frequency of injuries suffered by manual workers in Egypt in the Roman period, which in this regard would not have differed greatly from the Ptolemaic or the pharaonic. Ostrakon 212 (CE 137–145) lists nine workers out of action on a single day: one has an eye infection caused by a stone splinter, four have been injured, one bitten by a scorpion, one is fevered, one is convalescent, and one burnt.[60]

Long-term stress on joints and bones causes the degenerative osteoarthritis and osteophytosis (bony outgrowths on the spine) commonly seen in Egyptian skeletal remains and in early Greek remains. It is less common in Greek skeletons of the archaic and classical eras.[61] In modern times these conditions are predominantly associated with the accumulated wear

---

57 Nunn, *Egyptian Medicine*, 75.

58 Trans. Allen, *Art of Medicine*, 77. The first prognosis has similar features, including the stiffness in the neck but not the clenched mouth: the practitioner will in this case 'fight with' the disease, which may not be fatal.

59 [Hipp.] *Epidemics* 7.36 (5.404 Littré), cf. *Epidemics* 5.74 (5.246–248 Littré). Grmek, *Diseases*, 351–352.

60 Bingen, J. et al. (1997). *Mons Claudianus Ostraca Graeca et Latina II. O. Claud. 191 à 416*, pp. 31–33, nos. 212, 213.

61 Grmek, *Diseases*, 77 ff.

and tear of aging, but in antiquity, when most people lived shorter lives with much more manual work, many such cases were probably due to occupational activities involving heavy objects and repeated movements, such as quarrying, farming, porterage, and so on. Assuming that the sample available to modern investigation reflects a general distribution in the Egyptian population, such disorders were widespread.[62]

Lung damage from smoke inhalation is frequently reported. Certain occupations, like quarrying, may have produced the silica particles and consequent pneumoconiosis observed in several mummies, but in a desert environment the inhalation of sand is another possible culprit.[63]

Sand and stone particles, surviving through the bread-making process, have also been implicated in dental attrition, the most frequent of the numerous dental problems evident in the extant osteoarcheological evidence from Egypt and Greece.[64] Teeth problems are common to both Greek and Egypt. In dental attrition, the enamel is abraded until the pulp is exposed, resulting in the death of living tissue, abscesses and chronic infection.[65] Such abscesses are a feature of every skeletal collection from ancient Egypt and Nubia,[66] and are not restricted by age or socioeconomic group. Rameses II, Amenhotep III and other Egyptian kings all suffered from severe abscessing. Angel saw pronounced attrition in the teeth of 40% of 87 individuals from archeological sites scattered over classical period Greece.[67]

Periodontal (gum) disease was a problem in Egypt second only to attrition. Bacteria in plaque cause painful inflammation (gingivitis) of the gums,

---

62 Buikstra, 'What diseases?' 47, also arguing that the incidence of ankylosing spondylitis has been exaggerated, partly due to terminological confusion in diagnosis; cf. Filer, *Disease*, 78–81.

63 Anthracosis (carbon deposits in lungs): Ruffer, M.A. (1910). 'Remarks on the histology and pathological anatomy of Egyptian mummies', *Cairo Scientific Journal* 3, 1–5; Long, A.R. (1931). 'Cardiovascular renal disease', *Archives of Pathology* 12, 92–96; Millet, 'ROM I', 98. Sand particles and/or pneumoconiosis observed: Tapp, E. et al. (1975). 'Sand pneumoconiosis in an Egyptian mummy', *BMJ* 2, 276; Tapp, 'Disease in the Manchester mummies', 97.

64 A comprehensive review and discussion of the extant literature is Rose, J.C., G.J. Armelagos and L.S. Perry. (1993). 'Dental anthropology of the Nile Valley', in Davies & Walker, *Biological Anthropology*, 61–67; cf. Harris, W.V. et al. 'Dental health in ancient Egypt', in Cockburn, *Mummies*, 59–68. Briefer summaries are Filer, *Disease*, 94–102; Nunn, *Egyptian Medicine*, 202–205.

65 Filce Leek, F. (1972a). 'Bite, attrition and associated oral conditions as seen in ancient Egyptian skulls', *Journal of Human Evolution* 1, 289–295; (1972b). 'Teeth and bread in ancient Egypt', *JEA* 58, 126–132; (1973). 'Further studies concerning ancient Egyptian bread', *JEA* 59, 199–204. However the bread samples analyzed may have been roughly made as funerary offerings rather than for consumption: Filer, *Disease*, 97.

66 Rose & Armelagos, 'Dental anthropology', 62.

67 Angel, J.L. (1971). *The People of Lerna*, 90. Grmek, *Diseases*, 113–115.

as experienced by Amenhotep III, and eventually destroy the bony supports of the teeth. Although the other common modern consequence of plaque, caries (tooth decay) is very unusual in earlier remains, its incidence increased through the pharaonic period and reached its highest level during Roman rule, due perhaps to shifting diets or a decrease in attrition.[68] Caries appears in about 6% of cases from the archaic and classical periods of Greece, but this average proportion varies considerably by location.[69]

Comparative evidence suggests that pregnancy and childbirth were hazards with an outright mortality rate of about 1%.[70] Non-fatal but chronic conditions also resulted from childbirth, including cases in pharaonic Egypt of a vaginal-vesical fistula and uterine prolapse, which would have often increased vulnerability to other conditions.[71]

The unhealthiest places to live throughout the ancient world were large-scale urban environments. Even in Alexandria, which had an ancient reputation as a healthy city, deaths almost certainly exceeded births.[72] Sallares, *Ecology*, detected in the Greek classical medical texts a picture of *poleis* as commonly suffering small scale localized epidemics: a phenomenon repeatable in the major villages of Egypt. Tuberculosis and trachoma were almost certainly endemic, along with some forms of malaria in the Fayum and perhaps parts of the delta. Parasitic infestation was common, causing chronic malnutrition, anemia and weakened immunity. Influenza, typhoid, pneumonia, and tetanus are killers that leave few clues in the archeological record. Local populations, however, were usually too small to allow epidemics of such density dependent diseases as smallpox, measles or mumps to become endemic childhood killers. Smallpox, for instance, needs a pool of around 200,000 to become well established within a local population. Alexandria, and perhaps Memphis and Ptolemais, were the only places in Ptolemaic Egypt with these kinds of numbers.

---

68 From ca. 3% in the Predynastic to about 20% in the early Christian empire: Thornton, F. (1990). 'Oral Pathological Comparison of Discrete Ancient Nile Valley and Concurrent Populations' (M. Phil. thesis, cited by Nunn, *Egyptian Medicine*, 203). For example, 4 Ptolemaic period mummies in the Manchester Museum exhibit caries: Filce Leek, F. 'The dental history of the Manchester mummies', in David, *Manchester Mummies*, 75.

69 Grmek, *Diseases*, 115–118, a relatively high proportion in the ancient world.

70 Benson, 'Health', 20.

71 Derry, D.E. (1935). 'Note on five pelves of women of the eleventh dynasty in Egypt', *Journal of Obstetrics and Gynaecology of the British Empire* 42.3, 490–498; Smith, G.E. and F.W. Jones. (1910). *Archaeological Survey of Nubia-Report 1907–1908* 2: *Human Remains*, 267.

72 Alexandria: Diodoros 17.52.2; Strabo 17.1.7; Ammianus 22.16.8.

The very young, in particular, were extremely vulnerable to dietary lacks, parasite burdens and diarrheal infections. In societies today without easy access to modern sanitation and medicine neonatal loss can be on the order of 20% in the first month of life.[73] Malnutrition and iron deficiency anemia interact with digestive diseases to produce high rates of child mortality, and there are several indicators that malnutrition was commonplace among young children in the Greek mainland. For example, bladder stone in infants occurs in the medical texts, but this is now seen only in cases of severe malnutrition, due to insufficient calorific intake during long-term lactation or weaning.[74]

For many Greeks a move to Egypt may have resulted in improvements in nutrition. Although an adequate diet cannot be assumed for all its inhabitants regardless of harvest, social status and location, lack of food is on average less likely there than almost anywhere else in the area of the Mediterranean basin during classical antiquity. Moreover, Greek settlers were as a group of higher socioeconomic status compared to the rest of the population: more likely to be well nourished on a varied diet, less likely to be working in the fields, or near the waters of the Nile.

Immigration inevitably exposed people to new diseases or viral strains, although millennia of movements between the peoples of the Mediterranean region must have mitigated this effect. The risk of exposure was presumably at its worst in the early years of heavy immigration by settlers in the countryside, especially as internal Egyptian migration seems also to have taken place on a significant scale. It remained a persistent notable feature of urban settings, particularly a maritime trading center such as Alexandria.[75] But contact and individual transmission is not enough for a disease to become either endemic or epidemic in a new population, if for instance the disease kills too quickly or the population is too small to maintain transmission to the non-immune.[76] At all events there is no extant evidence for the catastrophic morbidity of a highly infectious disease encountering a population group with no immunity to it. An argument from silence would suggest that the large-scale immigration in itself did not result in high profile epidemics among either immigrant Greeks or their host population.

---

73 Benson, 'Health', 19–24.

74 Makler, P.T. (1980). 'New information on nutrition in ancient Greece', *Klio* 62, 317–319.

75 A bubonic plague outbreak in Hellenistic Egypt and Syria is described by Rufus of Ephesos: Sallares, *Ecology*, 266.

76 Cf. Sallares, *Ecology*, e.g. 227.

Thus in spite of Sallares' characterization of (classical) Greece as 'a relatively healthy place in which to live' (*Ecology*, 241), Egypt does not seem to have been much worse, especially if you were, in fact, Greek. Many diseases were endemic or occasional throughout the Mediterranean region; new or varying strains were a periodic hazard. The Greek arrival in Egypt thus generally did not result in a noticeably different experience of disease. Being ill remained frequent, dangerous and highly unpleasant.

Evidence from skeletal samples at different periods over the two thousand years or so of pharaonic history, together with the range of possibilities suggested by comparative analysis indicates that, assuming the high risks of early childhood were survived, men lived—on average—into their late thirties.[77] Women tended to have slightly shorter lifespans. Bagnall and Frier (*Demography*, 90) estimate—with a high degree of uncertainty—that females in Roman period Egypt who survived the first 10 years of their life subsequently lived to an average age of 34.5–37.5.

1.2.1. *Demography: The Numbers Game*

> But none is as fertile as low-lying Egypt when the overflowing Nile saturates and crumbles its soil; nor is any country so rich in towns of skilled inhabitants. Three hundred cities are established there; add to these thirty-three thousand and after that twice three and three times nine—and princely Ptolemy is ruler of them all.
>
> Theokritos.[78]

Two estimates for the population of early Greco-Roman Egypt are offered by Diodoros Sikelos and Josephus respectively, the former writing in the second half of the first century BCE and the latter in the second half of the first century CE. Diodoros gave a total population of 3 million, Josephus, of 7.5 million.[79]

---

[77] See e.g. the studies by Masali, M. and B. Chiarelli. (1972). 'Demographic data on the remains of ancient Egyptians', *Journal of Human Evolution* 1, 161–169; Winkler, E.-M. and H. Wilfing. (1991). *Tell el-Dab'a VI: Anthropologische Untersuchungen an den Skelettresten der Kampagnen 1966–1969, 1975–1980, 1985*.

[78] Theokritos *Idyll* 17.77–83. Translation Verity, A. (2002).

[79] Diodoros 1.31.6–9 (ca. BCE 59): 3 million in about 3000 towns and important villages. Josephus *Jewish War* 2.385 (ca. CE 75): 7.5 million. See Rathbone, D.W. (1990). 'Villages, land and population in Graeco-Roman Egypt', *PCPhS* 36, 103–142 esp. 107: arguing that the

Coincidentally, a similarly wide range appears in recent modern estimates. Rathbone's influential 1990 paper concluded that the total population of Egypt during the Greek and Roman eras can be reasonably supposed to have fluctuated between 3 and 5 million, a figure found plausible by Bagnall and Frier, and representing a sharp revision downwards from earlier estimates of 8–10 million. Walter Scheidel estimated 5–7 million for the population of Roman Egypt at its height, with the proviso that real population figures are probably much lower than the possible maximum of 7 million. He suggested that 6 million is, 'is as good a guess as any.'[80] Clarysse and Thompson have recently argued that Egypt as a whole numbered under 1.5 million in the mid third century BCE.[81] This figure was arrived at on the basis of a very detailed study of records from areas of the Fayum oasis on the west bank south of the delta, the chief—almost the only—region which offers significant documentary evidence for the Ptolemaic period. However, the population may have increased significantly by the time Diodoros was assembling his sources in the first century.[82] Similarly, although Clarysse and Thompson allow that 500,000, the usual estimate for the population of Alexandria in the first century, is possible, they suppose that this must have been much lower in the century or so after the city's foundation.[83]

The total average population of Ptolemaic Egypt can therefore be confidently said to be somewhere between 1.5 and 6 million. The reliability of this estimate is sadly not matched by its usefulness.

It is still nonetheless possible to discuss Egyptian demographics in both general and, in a small number of cases, very specific terms. The kinds of documentary evidence from which population totals are extrapolated often give us detailed information about groups of people in a specific location at

---

common emendation of Diodoros' figure to 7 million is a misreading of the passage, and that both reports might well be rhetorical. See also 6.2, p. 249 n. 26.

80 Scheidel, *Death on the Nile*, 246–247.

81 Clarysse, W. and D.J. Thompson. (2006; corrected pb. ed. 2009). *Counting the People in Hellenistic Egypt*, 102.

82 Rathbone, 'Villages', 123, cf. Manning, J. (2003). *Land and Power in Ptolemaic Egypt*, 49; Bagnall & Frier, *Demography*, 54. Scheidel, *Death on the Nile*, 186, 246–247. Clarysse & Thompson, *Counting*, 101–102. For the population of Egypt in the pharaonic period see Rathbone, 104–105; Kemp, *Egypt*, 49–51. Diodoros 1.31.6 offers 7 million in 18,000 cities for this period, allegedly based on 'sacred writings'; this is rounded up in Herodotos 2.177 to 20,000 cities under Amasis.

83 Diodoros 17.52.6: Alexandria has a population of over 300,000 'free' inhabitants. Rathbone, 'Villages', 120 estimates 500,000, cf. Clarysse & Thompson, *Counting*, 102, with the reservations in the main text above. Fraser, P.M. (1972). *Ptolemaic Alexandria*, 2.171–172 n. 358 argues for 1 million, which would mean a city the size of imperial Rome.

a specific time. In chapter 5, this kind of information provides vital evidence for the individuals and numbers categorized by the state administration as members of the medical profession in parts of the Fayum. Moreover, as Bagnall remarks, many of the questions historians ask of this material are those that such records were originally designed to answer, although this begs the question of how well they answered them.[84] For example, 1387 adult civilians are explicitly recorded for the unusually large village of Arsinoe in 230–229, suggesting a total civilian population for the latter of around 2000, plus an unknown number of military residents and their families.[85] Yet in the next year the adult civilian population of the same village dropped drastically, to 915.[86] Settlement size also varied greatly. Hamlets of fewer than 10 individuals were probably common, but settlements with more than 1800 adults were very rare, especially in the third century.[87] Administrative regional capitals were not much more than unusually large villages: at this time the Arsinoite nome capital Krokodilopolis is estimated to have had a population of around 3500 civilians and another 500 or so military residents.[88] In between such documented extremes there is sufficient information to extrapolate plausible figures for an 'average' third century village at around 500 civilians and perhaps another 100 or so military residents, but insufficient to draw a map by population size of the actual non-standard villages of the Fayum.[89] Averaging over longer time scales, such as the entire Greco-Roman period, is even riskier.[90]

Description offers a broader if fuzzier picture than quantification. It is clear from the examples we do have that urbanization was much lower in

---

[84] (1995). *Reading papyri, Writing Ancient History*, 85. It is for example difficult to estimate to what degree male tax-payers migrated temporarily to cities in order to avoid registration for tax purposes.

[85] This is not the nome capital, but a village in the Themistos *meris* of the Arsinoite nome, part of a further sub-division that Thompson & Clarysse call 'district B'. It may also have been known as Arsinoe ἐπι του χωματος': 22–27; for citations and bibliography see Daris, S. (2010). *Dizionario dei nomi geografici e topografici dell'Egitto greco-romano, Supplemento* 5 (2006–2009), p. 18 s.v. "Ἀρσινόη', no. 3.

[86] Clarysse & Thompson, *Counting*, 104, table 4:4, who multiply (94) adult males by 2.909 to arrive at an estimated total population. Cf. Bagnall & Frier, *Demography*, 103 n. 35. Rathbone, 'Villages', uses adult males x 3.1. Arsinoe's startling annual variation was not unusual: Clarysse & Thompson, *Counting*, 109.

[87] Clarysse & Thompson, *Counting*, 106–108, with note 77.

[88] Ibid. 98–100.

[89] Ibid. 106–107.

[90] E.g. Rathbone, 'Villages', 123–124 suggests a Greco-Roman average settlement size of 1000 with others at 2000–4000 + and some approaching the 15,000 level of the smaller Roman era metropoleis.

the early Ptolemaic period than it later became. About 95% of the civilian population of the nome lived outside its capital, and the huge majority dwelt in small villages or even hamlets. This was an overwhelmingly rural society. Urbanization seems to have increased in subsequent centuries and exploded under Roman rule, when some forty Egyptian *metropoleis* may have averaged 15,000 inhabitants each.[91]

Similarly, Strabo's comment that in the late first century Ptolemais is the biggest city in Upper Egypt, around the same size as northern Memphis, supplies us with a relativized picture of the urban distribution among the major cities, even if we are very uncertain as to how many people either Memphis or Ptolemais actually contained at this time.[92]

1.2.2. *Demography: Patterns of Immigration*

There was nothing new about immigration by various ethnolinguistic groups into the Nile Valley: some earlier such cases had also been on a large scale, and/or comprised a politically powerful group. An immigrant community from the southern Levant eventually produced the rule of the Hyksos kings in the delta during the Second Intermediate Period, which was later represented as unwelcome foreign domination resisted and cast out by the Egyptians;[93] the Third Intermediate Period saw rulers of Libyan descent and culture in northern Egypt as well as intermittent Kushite rule in the south; and the resurgent unification of Egypt under the Saite kings in the seventh century was followed by two periods of rule from Persia: 525–404 and 343–332.[94] A sizable group of emigrant Jews formed a community around Elephantine in the fifth century, and may also have entered the country in the first generations of the Ptolemaic period as war captives or soldiers. Jewish immigration grew sharply during the third to first centuries

---

[91] Clarysse & Thompson 2.99 n. 36; Rathbone, 'Villages', 120, 123–124; Bagnall & Frier, *Demography*, 65: 2nd century CE Karanis has 4000 inhabitants.

[92] Strabo 17.1.32, 42, 46. Thompson, D.J. (1988). *Memphis under the Ptolemies*, 32–35 estimates Ptolemaic Memphis as having ca. 50,000–200,000 inhabitants. Rathbone, 'Villages', 141 n. 41 thinks these numbers should be lower.

[93] The name derives from *hkꜣ ḫꜥswt*: rulers of foreign lands. Two steles of Kamose narrate his campaign: '... for my desire is to rescue Egypt and to drive out the Asiatics'. Translated and discussed by Smith, H.S. and A. Smith. (1976). 'A reconsideration of the Kamose texts', *ZÄS* 103, 48–76. Cf. Manetho's version in Josephus, *Against Apion* 1.14.75.

[94] For an overview Taylor, J. 'The Third Intermediate Period', in Shaw, I. (2000). *Oxford History of Ancient Egypt*, 339–341; Lloyd, A.B. 'The Late Period', in ibid., 369–394.

BCE, forming communities that enjoyed a degree of recognition.[95] In more recent centuries settlers in Egypt often originated in the Greek-speaking world. The victory in 664 over the Nubian rulers of Upper Egypt that ushered in the reunified Egypt of the Saite dynasty was heavily reliant on mercenaries from Ionia and elsewhere, resident in Egypt in large numbers and privileged in the military establishment. Among these were probably the Ionians who settled in Memphis in the sixth century. They had their own quarter and temple, the Hellenion. Another part of the town contained settlers from Karia. These Hellenomemphites and Kariomemphites retained some degree of separate identity but in many ways were apparently well integrated into local linguistic and religious behaviors.[96] The trading colony of Naukratis, founded by the Milesians between 664 and 610 on the Kanopic branch of the Nile near the coast supported a largely Greek population. In the Ptolemaic era, a large temple seems to have been built in Egyptian style, possibly to the cult of Amun as lord of Batet.[97] This joined earlier Greek temples, including a Hellenion and a temple to Aphrodite.

Ptolemy I's acquisition of Egypt, at the end of the fourth century, meant Greco-Macedonian military and political control over Egypt and its economic resources. It also resulted in an unprecedented degree of immigration over the next century. Thousands of individuals from the Greek-speaking world settled in Alexandria and throughout the country, with large concentrations, including entirely new villages and towns, in certain parts of the country.[98] Many of the immigrants located themselves in Alexandria, which rapidly developed into an important trading center of the Hellenistic world. The other urban centers run along Greek organizational lines as *poleis* were the pre-existing colony of Naukratis, and Ptolemais in Upper Egypt, possibly founded by Soter as a deliberate counterweight to the regional power of Thebes. The rest of Egypt was the countryside (*chora*): an agrarian economy based on the unit of the village.

The largest and most powerful group among settlers in the chora was composed of the cleruchs and their descendants. Originally former soldiers of the Greek-Macedonian armies of Alexander and his generals, they were

---

[95] Hölbl, *Ptolemaic Empire*, 189–190. War captives of Soter: Josephus *Jewish Antiquities* 12.3–9 and *Against Apion* 1.208–222, Ps.-Aristeas 12–14, 22–25.

[96] Thompson, *Memphis*, 82 ff. esp. 93–97.

[97] Herodotos 2.718, cf. the dedications to Greek gods found by Petrie and Gardner in the late nineteenth century. See Möller, A. (2000). *Naucratis: trade in archaic Greece*, 8–25, 119–133.

[98] Most notably the Fayum. For settlements in that area see Mueller, K. (2006). *Settlements of the Ptolemies.*

given allotments of land (*kleroi*) throughout the Egyptian countryside, particularly in the Fayum.[99] Cleruchs effectively constituted a reserve military force in rural areas, though many of the wealthier ones probably dwelt in the cities or larger towns while renting out their land to other Greek or to Egyptian farmers. As a group they formed a new social and economic elite in their communities, tending to have larger households that included one or more slaves.[100] Signs of a heavily cleruchic presence are the gymnasia known for six of the larger Fayum villages, including the Arsinoite nome capital Krokodilopolis.[101] The gymnasion was a distinctively Greek civic institution strongly associated with both military training and sociopolitical identity. Serving soldiers of the army, resident in garrisons and forts, were also an often notable presence, though their numbers and locations are rarely specified in the papyrus documents. Egyptians were not included in the army until after 217. Cleruchic and military residents ensured both stability and a new, relatively wealthy market for products and services.

The settlers and their descendants were primarily not peasant farmers, but soldiers, ex-military landowners, traders, middlemen, managers and merchants, entrepreneurs and administrators, including most of the central government and court. Greek tax-farmers, irrigation engineers, and traders are the protagonists of the archive of Zenon, himself a classic example of this type of person as the estate manager and agent of Egypt's then chief financial official, the dioikêtês Apollonios. A number of individuals were identified as 'Hellenes' in documentary texts, including tax records, on the basis of some degree of Hellenization. Some individuals had both Greek and Egyptian names (see 1.3.1, p. 28, n. 114). Intermarriage and mixed descent was also a factor, though the head of household in cleruchic families tended to retain at least a Greek name as a marker of his socially significant ethnic origins.[102]

Absolute numbers, or indeed relative percentages reliably averaged over a wide area are as usual difficult to establish. Clarysse and Thompson estimate the total numbers of 'Hellenes' from all these categories in the Arsinoite nome for the mid third century as approximately 29% of the total

---

99 For cleruchs as the soldiers of Soter's army together with Greek and Macedonian deserters from Perdiccas' forces, see Bagnall, 'Ptolemaic cleruchs', 16ff. In the Fayum: e.g. Clarysse & Thompson, *Counting*, 90.

100 Clarysse & Thompson, *Counting*, 238. Bagnall, 'Ptolemaic cleruchs', 4, 18 describes them as almost a 'closed class.'

101 Krokodilopolis, Philadelphia, Samereia, Tebtunis, Theadelphia, Euhermeria. Clarysse & Thompson, *Counting*, 133.

102 Clarysse & Thompson, *Counting*, 246 and below, n. 122.

population, over half of which was serving or former military.[103] Within the nome, however, the proportion of residents with this tax status varied considerably, both between its three sub-divisions (*merides*) and between individual villages. Just over 42% of civilian adults in Trikomia were registered for tax purposes as Hellenes; in Athenas Kome this category constitutes 9% of a much smaller village. They are also a much smaller proportion of the civilian population, around 16.5% in the Arsinoite nome and probably considerably less for much else of Egypt.[104]

In many ways the Ptolemaic Fayum was an atypical region. Although Greek communities are known throughout Egypt, outside the three designated cities of Alexandria, Ptolemais and Naukratis, immigration, and particularly army settlement, was concentrated in the Fayum and north-western delta. Many of the Greek names of the new villages are dynastic, such as Philadelphia and Theadelphia, or derived from Alexandrian demes (e.g. Lysimakhis). Others, including the settlements of Memphis, Oxyrhynkha and Sebennytos, are named after the administrative regions (nomes) from which much of their population derived through an internal, possibly forced, mass series of resettlements; while places which utilize the Egyptian names of the gods, like Soknopaiou Nesos or Kerkeosiris, also suggest a largely Egyptian population, though Greek and Egyptian names for a settlement often differed.[105]

1.3.1. *Ethnicity, Ideology and Identity*

The population of Egypt, especially in the New Kingdom and Late Period, was in many ways much more diverse than dominant, public modes of expression, which emphasized continuity and successfully maintained a core ideology of religious and civil discourse, made it seem. Ray ('Literacy', 51) estimated that over 40 foreign languages were spoken and written in Egypt between the New Kingdom and the Arab conquest; yet hardly any appear in the record apart from Egyptian and Greek, the languages of power.[106]

---

[103] Clarysse & Thompson, *Counting*, 140. The tax-identifier 'Hellene', especially in civilian contexts, can indicate an occupation or status, rather than a simply ethnic categorization: see La'da, C. (2002). *Foreign Ethnics in Hellenistic Egypt*. I discuss the issue fully in chapter 5, section 5.2.2.

[104] Ibid. 138–140, table 5.2.

[105] Ibid. 90–91, and cf. n. 114. For a gazetteer, see ⟨http://fayum.arts.kuleuven.be⟩.

[106] 1% of extant documentation is in Latin. Aramaic document 'archives' of the Jewish

The Persian empire, based overseas, had utilized local forms of government and key elites backed up by military power, not always with complete success. In contrast, the Ptolemaic period saw Greek settlers form a large part of a significantly different governmental and socioeconomic elite; the distinguishing characteristic of which was the capacity to operate within Greek linguistic and administrative contexts. The majority of Egyptians were agrarian, illiterate, and at the wrong end of a stratified hierarchy of power, but the small elite and sub-elites of Egyptian society were to a large degree incorporated within this new governing class and helped to form its ideological and governmental program. In particular, the dynasty of the high priests of Ptah in Memphis, who remained the city's leading family throughout the Ptolemaic period, had close relations of mutual support with the Macedonian dynasty, even during periods of unrest in northern Egypt.[107] At Edfu, too, in spite of its relatively southern location, officials of the temple of Horus remained loyal.[108] There were Egyptian nomarchs and officers under Soter, including a grandson of Nektanebo II.[109] This small number of high-ranking officials formed the upper part of the scribal class of Egypt, the linguistic and political interface between the Greco-Macedonian core of Ptolemy's court and the administration of a country in which Egyptians remained the overwhelming majority. An early example of this mutual

settlers at 5th century Elephantine survive. Ray, J. 'Literacy and language in Egypt in the late and Persian periods', in Bowman, A.K. and G. Woolf. (1994). *Literacy and Power in the Ancient World*, 51–66; cf. Bagnall, *Reading Papyri*, 20.

[107] This particular alliance was of long standing. In 332 Alexander had sacrificed at Memphis to the Apis bull and other gods: Arrian *Campaigns of Alexander* 3.1.2–3. According to the *Alexander Romance* he was crowned in the temple of Ptah at Memphis. There is no contemporary confirmation of such a ceremony for the Greek kings until Ptolemy V Epiphanes in 197, but it is most likely that all the Ptolemies presented and were acknowledged as Egyptian kings in this fashion. Thompson, *Memphis*, 16, 106; Lloyd, A.B. 'The Ptolemaic period', in Shaw, *Oxford History*, 410. The city was the initial capital and residence of Ptolemy I Soter, until around 320/19: Thompson, *Memphis*, chapter 4.

[108] Johnson, J.H. 'Is the demotic chronicle an anti-Greek tract?' in Thissen, H.-J. and K.-T. Zauzich. (1983). *Grammata Demotika*, 115. On the other hand, it is often supposed to be no coincidence that many of the Ptolemaic period rebellions began in the region of Thebes. In the most extreme case, an independent state with an Egyptian king was established in the Theban region between 205 and 186, echoing several previous declarations from the Middle Kingdom onwards of the preeminence of Thebes and the god's servant of Amun in the south. The city of Ptolemais may have been established partly as a counterweight to Thebes in this region.

[109] Peremans, W. (1977). 'Un groupe d'officiers dans l'armée des Lagides', *AncSoc* 8, 175–185. (1983). 'Les Égyptiens dans l'armée de terre des Lagides', in Bengtson, H. *Althistorische Studien*, 92–101; Hölbl, *Ptolemaic Empire*, 25. The grandson of Nektanebo II: *Urk*. 2.24–26; *PP* I 285 and II 2122; Johnson, 'An anti-Greek tract?', 117–118 with n. 64.

guaranteeing of power is the Egyptian Manetho of Sebennytos, who had close connections with the Ptolemaic court, probably during the end of Soter's reign and the earlier years of Philadelphos.[110]

Manetho's history of dynastic Egypt, *Aigyptiaka*, was written in Greek, and its presentation of Egyptian history, inventions and culture played into favorable Greek perceptions of Egypt. His 'Sacred Book' dealt with that Greek obsession, Egyptian religion, and *On festivals, On ancient ritual and religion* and *On the making of kyphi* were either included in his 'Sacred Book', or were written as separate treatises. However, Manetho's efforts to introduce his world to his new audience were partly a corrective to what he perceived as Greek misreadings: he attacked the 'ignorance' of Herodotos.[111]

Other officials also adapted, not least linguistically, to Greco-Macedonian power, not only at the highest levels but throughout the hierarchy. A crucial player in the Ptolemaic and later Roman administration was the village scribe, the *komogrammateus*. The best-known and studied example in the Hellenistic period is Menkhes, who in 119–111/110 was for at least the second time the village scribe of Kerkeosiris, in the Fayum.[112] In one text the bilingual Menkhes also employed a Greek name, Asklepiades (*P. Tebt.* I 164 = TM 3799), a name which appears to have had no relation to the probable meaning of the Egyptian Mnkh, 'He who is perfect.'[113] Other members of his family also employed dual names. Like many officials in the administration he thus effectively had two linguistic identities, both public and presumably easily equated with each other by his local contemporaries, but much more opaque to historians.[114] Other individuals were perhaps more thoroughly

[110] Fraser, *Alexandria*, 1.505–511.

[111] Josephus *Against Apion* 1.73. Later examples of Egyptians working easily in the Hellenic linguistic-cultural world include the *hierogrammateus* and Stoic Khairemon in the first century CE and Apollonides the 'Archprophet-Orapis' of Memphis later that century, who also wrote in Greek on Egyptian religion. For the latter, Parsons, P.J. (1974). 'Ulpius Serenianus', *CdÉ* 49, 153–156 and cf. 143–145. Both appear to have offered a Hellenistically idealized account of priests as virtuous philosophers, rather than as technical experts in the ritual mechanics of the cosmos: Fowden, G. (1986). *The Egyptian Hermes*, 53–56, with note 35.

[112] The Menkhes 'archive', excavated as the cartonnage of mummified crocodiles at the turn of the century in the large Fayum village of Tebtunis, was first published in B.G. Grenfell, A.S. Hunt and J.G. Smyly. (1902). *Tebtunis Papyri* I.

[113] Verhoogt, A.M.F.W. (1998). *Menches, komogrammateus of Kerkeosiris*, 51, note 1.

[114] Greek-Egyptian double names are a well-known phenomenon. Examples by group are described by Peremans, (1971). 'Egyptiens et étrangers dans l'administration civile et financière de l'Egypte ptolémaïque', *AncSoc* 2, 33–45 and subsequent articles in *AncSoc*, reprinted in *Ptolemaica Prosopographia*. Cf. Clarysse, W. (1985). 'Greeks and Egyptians in the Ptolemaic army and administration', *Aegyptus* 65, 57–66; Clarysse & Thompson, *Counting*, 323 ff. The name might be a translation or transliteration of the Egyptian name, or might sound similar,

subsumed under a Greek identity that gave them access into the higher levels of the civil and latterly the army administration. They may have used their Greek name on a more permanent basis; or adopted characteristically Greek cultural practices, such as visits to the gymnasion or theater.

This all raises the much-debated issue of ethnicity. Greek rule in Egypt was, as many have remarked, not characterized by systematic racism or discrimination directed against people of indigenous descent or appearance. The Ptolemaic dynasty ruled as local kings, not as absentee overlords living abroad; revenues were not extracted from the country, only exacted from the countryside. The kings and their officials governed through and with local elites, both Greek and often Egyptian; the economic and ideological power of the temples was not restricted. The new government introduced transformative, centralizing innovations in economic policy and agricultural practice, but J.G. Manning has argued persuasively that these were not imposed from the center, but instantiated slowly and piecemeal through processes of adaptive negotiations with local bureaucracies and farmers. This process can also be seen occurring between local elites and the peasantry in private texts such as those of the Zenon archive, and in the appearance (and sometimes disappearance) of novel crops in the Fayum.[115]

Some of this material may reflect resistance, expressed through refusal or flight, rather than enthusiasm. The revolts in rural parts of the south that occurred intermittently from the end of the third century onwards probably originated in economic unhappiness with local elites rather than in nationalistic sentiment. (Although that does not preclude such unhappiness being partially construed, justified and fueled in ethnocultural oppositional terms, as I argue below in 1.3.2, pp. 36–37).

Colonial or imperial models for ethnically based relations have recently been regarded as having limitations for our grasp of social or ethnic relations in Ptolemaic Egypt. The definitive examples of these societies from relatively modern eras differ in a number of important respects from Ptolemaic Egypt, to which applies neither the concept of the modern nation state,

---

but in many cases there is no obvious connection: Martin, V. (1956). 'L' onomastique comme indice des rapports entre indigènes et occupants dans l' Égypte gréco-romaine', *Akten des VIII Internationalen Kongresses für Papyrologie*, 85–90. Greek names are mainly but not entirely used in official contexts: Clarysse, 'Greeks and Egyptians'.

115 Manning, *Land and Power*, esp. 129 ff. For resistance through flight see e.g. Bagnall, R.S. 'Decolonizing Ptolemaic Egypt', in P. Cartledge et al. (1997). *Hellenistic Constructs*, 237–238, cf. Manning, *Land and Power*, 115. The failure of some new crops might be seen as a form of resistance. See Thompson, D.J. 'New and old in the Ptolemaic Fayum', in Bowman, A. and E. Rogan. (1999). *Agriculture in Egypt*, 107–122.

nor the relationship between an imperial center and an exploited periphery, nor racism based explicitly on biological characteristics and often codified in law.[116] The chief social and economic impacts of Alexander's conquest resulted not from the behavior of Egypt's kings, but from the new wave of socially and economically powerful migrants.

An alternative conceptualization of the situation is the separatist model, which takes note of the numerous ways in which a kind of duplicate existence could be led:[117] two judicial systems; the existence of dual-identity individuals known from private texts, who utilized Egyptian names and language for their religious behaviors and private lives, but Greek names and script in their official capacity, switching to and fro as context required; to some extent two educational systems; the widespread use of two languages. This model has also been attacked, as downplaying evidence for integration and interaction, and for over-emphasizing the exclusion of Egyptians from government, military and other power structures.[118] Instead, these critics point to the presence of artifacts, including religious objects, that combine both Greek and Egyptian elements;[119] to the evidence for intermarriage; to the presence of Egyptians (albeit often using their Greek names) in official positions and, after 217, in the army; and to the interplay between Egyptian and Greek in literature and religious thought, as well as in more technical subjects such as astrology, 'magic', pharmaceutics, and possibly other areas.[120]

This last kind of evidence should certainly qualify our understanding of how particular groups of Egyptians and Greeks interacted. It demonstrates that ethnic identity in Egypt was not understood as a binary category, persis-

---

[116] But see Malkin, I. (2001). *Ancient Perceptions of Greek Ethnicity*, 12–13, for a persuasive critique of the usefulness of notions of 'center' and 'periphery' in regard to Greek self-definition.

[117] Hence the sub-title of the volume of papers edited by Janet Johnson in 1992: *Life in a Multi-Cultural Society*. Notable exponents of this approach are Préaux, C. (1978). *Le monde hellénistique*; Goudriaan, K. (1988). *Ethnicity in Ptolemaic Egypt*; Samuel, A.E. (1989). *The Shifting Sands of History*.

[118] La'da, C.A. 'Encounters with Egypt: the Hellenistic Greek experience', in Matthews, R. and C. Roemer. (2003). *Ancient Perspectives on Egypt*, 157–169, makes this point clearly, but in my view relies overmuch on (the lack of) overt and consistent ethnic discrimination.

[119] For hybrid archeological forms, including mongoose-headed Egyptian gods wearing Greek garments, see Rottroff, S.I. 'The Greeks and the Other', in Coleman, J.E. and C.A. Walz. (1997). *Greeks and Barbarians*, 221–235. There was also much non-hybridized sculpture in both Egyptian and Greek styles.

[120] Rossi, C. (2004). *Architecture and Mathematics in Ancient Egypt*, 127, cf. 172–173, on the possible use by Egyptian temple builders of the Greek techniques of architectural models and late Hellenistic modular architecture.

tent throughout life and dependent on fixed criteria; in particular, it was not imposed from without by the state. The systems of meaning that we loosely call 'culture' were dynamic and sensitive to evolving social conditions, both within and between ethnolinguistic groups; the term 'syncretic' is inadequate to describe the diversity and multivalency of the symbolic forms thus produced.

They were, however, produced in a context of an asymmetric power relationship that mapped closely, if not exactly, onto ethnocultural categories. The very fact that individuals had alternate social personas for use in official and non-official situations testifies to the overwhelming identification of sociopolitical status with 'Greekness'. This was a category imprecisely defined by linguistic and other sociocultural criteria; it was also in most cases a de facto ethnic group based on descent, in at least the male line, from individuals of Greek origin.[121] The language of socioeconomic advantage is Greek: Soter's pragmatic allowance of demotic as an official language in the first decades of Macedonian government disappeared under Philadelphos as Egyptian literacy in Greek became sufficiently widespread. Known instances of intermarriage were usually cases of Egyptian women marrying Greek men: in the huge majority of societies, women marry 'up' the social scale.[122] There are few clear instances of explicit ethnic-based discrimination or tension in primary texts, but a letter to Zenon complains that its author is being discriminated against by Zenon's agents because he is a 'barbarian' and 'I do not know how to act like a Greek.'[123] Ptolemaios, the son of a Macedonian father and, possibly, an Egyptian mother, resident in the largely Egyptian environs of an Egyptian sanctuary, claimed in an appeal to Greek civic officials that he was beaten up (by Egyptians), 'because I am a Greek'.[124] Csaba La'da sees the relative rarity of such cases as a testimony

---

121 Dubuisson, M. (1982). 'Remarques sur le vocabulaire grec de l'acculturation', *Revue Belge de Philologie et d'Histoire* 60, 5–32: the language used in Greek to describe acculturation reflects the assumption that barbarians can become Greeks through the acquisition of culture, but that Greeks can become barbarians only when their bloodlines are mixed.

122 In Ptolemaic Thebes Greek men married women with Egyptian names in 17 out of 19 cases of intermarriage: Clarysse, W. 'Greeks in Ptolemaic Thebes', in Vleeming, S.P. (1995). *Hundred-Gated Thebes*, 5. Cf. Clarysse, W. 'Some Greeks in Egypt', in Johnson, *Life*, 51; La'da, 'Encounters', 167. For this common social pattern: Buss, D. 1989. 'Sex Differences in Human Mate Preferences: evolutionary hypotheses tested in 37 cultures', *Behavioral and Brain Sciences* 12, 1–49.

123 *P.Col.Zen.* 2.66, TM 1781.

124 Ptolemaios: *UPZ* 1.7, TM 3398; 1.8, TM 3399; 1.15, TM 3406; see further below, 2.3.3, pp. 74–75, cf. 2.3.1, p. 68. For the possibility of other motives see Thompson, *Memphis*, 230.

to the non-racist character of Greek Egypt,[125] but those two examples alone demonstrate a clear familiarity with both ethnic categorization itself, the plausibility of discrimination and violence along ethnic lines, and particular forms of ethnic discourse.[126]

Roger Bagnall points out that societies with hierarchies of power are hardly limited to definite examples of imperialism or colonialism. The usefulness of the imperialist model, I would argue, is as a subset of this category: the relatively well-documented experiences of imperialist societies in the 19th and 20th centuries are illustrative of the huge diversity and complexity of forms in which ethnicities and cultures in a hierarchical power relationship relate to each other; they extend and nuance our awareness of the possibilities for that kind of interplay. Other comparative evidence, for instance in 20th century pluralistic societies, can be used to structure and develop the historical imagination in the same way.

1.3.2. *Government, Foreigners, and the Eternal Struggle between Good and Evil*

At its most powerful Egypt extended beyond the Nile Valley eastwards into Palestine, and especially southwards into Nubia; at other times Meroitic, Libyan, Asiatic or Mediterranean languages and culture became part of Egyptian conceptual space, whether through invasions and political domination, the settlement of war captives, the mercenaries that made up much of the army from the New Kingdom onwards, and economic migrants.[127] In spite of this, political-religious legitimacy and consequent social and environmental stability were defined through a remarkably coherent and consistent ideological system and its related institutions, which even foreign dynasties found they had an interest in upholding.

Mythology and ritual expressed Egypt as an atemporal world perpetually reinscribed. The cosmos of the Nile valley and delta was recreated each day

[125] La'da, 'Encounters', 164, 166, 167 ('free and low-tension interaction'); cf. Goudriaan, *Ethnicity*, 107–108; Ritner, R.K. 'Implicit models of cross-cultural interaction: a question of noses, soap, and prejudice' in Johnson, *Life*, 289.

[126] The writer of the Egyptian's letter to Zenon characterizes the distinction as 'Greek' and 'barbarian', a distinction that is itself Greek and may not be the complainant's own choice of phrase.

[127] For Asiatic immigrants, including large numbers of war captives, in the Middle Kingdom see Bourriau, J. (2000). 'The Second Intermediate Period', in Shaw, *Oxford History*, 186–189. For Libyan mercenaries see Taylor, J. 'The Third Intermediate Period', in ibid., 339–341 and for Greek soldiers see Lloyd, 'Late period', ibid. 372–373, 388.

with the reemergence of the sun, which represented a victory that could never be taken for granted. Egyptian theological time was both circular and continuous. The victory was that of *mꜣʿt*, a word and concept usually translated into English as 'order.' According to this governing ideology, the continued existence of all things depended upon the continual recreation of *mꜣʿt*.[128] Similarly, on one level difficulties and disasters in Egypt's long past and present were not just the contingencies of history, but expressions of the innate tendency towards chaos and dissolution, *jzft*, within the cosmos. The king was a critical component of the universe as cause, part, proof, and defender of *mꜣʿt*, which he maintained through ritual (cult officials acted in lieu of the king); through a just and effective administration, again mediated by officials, of the land and its people; and through his victorious defense of Egypt's borders. The outer walls and great pylon entranceways of Egyptian temples depicted the king towering above his Lilliputian enemies, bound and trampled underfoot. This kind of scene is one of the most long-standing typologies in Egyptian monumental art, with examples known from the Predynastic to the Roman periods.[129] It also occurs in tombs and on luxury items. It is probable that such depictions in word and image are not only historical propaganda, but also the defensive creation of such victories for *mꜣʿt* through the effective power called *ḥkꜣ*.[130]

Successful kings of foreign or new dynasties inserted themselves into this narrative through the production and maintenance of both social order and proper ritual, including such appropriate behaviors as offerings to the gods and the building or restoring of temples.[131] These exercises in royal decorum were also political negotiations; they positioned the king in relation to the gods, leading families, and temple officials. The Libyan families that produced the 21st–24th dynasties, the Kushite kings of the 25th dynasty, and even the Persian emperors all attempted, with varying degrees of success and acculturation, to integrate their rule into the political and ideological

[128] See e.g. Allen, J.P. (1988). *Genesis in Egypt*, or more briefly, 'The Egyptian concept of the world' in O'Connor, D. and S. Quirke. (2003). *Mysterious Lands*, 23–30.

[129] van Dijk, J. 'The Amarna period and the later New Kingdom', in Shaw, *Oxford History*, 315–316.

[130] *Ḥkꜣ* is often translated 'magic': see 4.3.1, pp. 185–186. On the power of this scene to create the reality it depicts see Ritner, R.K. (1993). *The Mechanics of Ancient Egyptian Magical Practice*, 113ff.

[131] In the Hermopolis stele of Nektanebo I the king makes offerings to Thoth and Nehmetawy in return for their assistance in his successful military coup against his equally indigenous uncle.

systems of Egypt according to this template.[132] Kambyses (525–522) presented himself in appropriate ideological terms and seems to have sought the co-operation of the elite; Dareios I (522–486) followed a similar policy, patronizing the temple cults and largely restricting Persian interference to the insertion of a satrap at the top of the national administrative hierarchy.[133] The trilingual decrees of Kanopos and Memphis (the Rosetta stone) in 238 and 196, respectively, are epigraphic, public statements of thanks by Egyptian synods for Ptolemaic *philanthropia* to the country and temples. As in earlier periods, a king's Egyptian legitimacy was presented in terms of his relationships with the temple officials, especially at a time when individuals of Greek language and—usually—descent, dominated the other powerful institutions of Egypt: the court and the military.

The perception of metaphysical propriety was thus not readily separable from political concerns and socioeconomic security. Unsuccessful kings, as embodiments and products of disorder, were delegitimized. Hatshepsut, the female king, and the 'heretic' Akhenaten maintained sufficient political power and religious authority during their lifetimes to retain and enforce their power. After their deaths, however, their successors tried to eradicate them as though they had never been.[134] In particular, the foreigner

[132] Rulers from Libyan families retained their nomenclature, as well as Libyan customs such as wearing an ostrich feather in their hair, but intermarried extensively with the previous royal family, which itself had dynastic connections with the high priesthood of Thebes, and with the family of the high priests of Memphis: Baines, J. 'Contextualising Egyptian Representations of Society and Ethnicity', in Cooper, J.S. and G.M. Schwartz. (1996). *The Study of the Ancient Near East in the Twenty-First Century*, 378–382. The Nubian Kushite overlords of Egypt in the 25th dynasty articulated their rule according to the archaizing, legitimizing Egyptian templates of the Old Kingdom: O'Connor, D. 'Egypt's views of 'others'', in Tait, *'Never Had the Like Occurred'*, 176–178.

[133] According to Herodotos 3.29 and Plutarch (*Isis and Osiris* 44, cf. 31) Kambyses killed the Apis bull, but the Apis stele of Year 6 of his reign shows him personally dedicating the bull's sarcophagus: Thompson, *Memphis*, 106 n. 3. The steles dedicated by two high-ranking Egyptian officials, Udjahorresnet and Somtutefnakht under, respectively, Dareios I and Dareios II, testify both to elite Egyptian collaboration with Persian rule, and to the Persians' support of Egyptian religious elite institutions: Udjahorresnet: Vatican Museum 158 (113) and see chapter 5, appendix. Somtutefnakht: Naples Museum 1035. Translations in Lichtheim, M. (1978). *Ancient Egyptian Literature* 3.36–44.

[134] Tutankhamun's restoration stele promised a return to the old world order (*Urk.* IV, 2027f.; cf. *Urk.* IV, 2155ff.), but he is left out of the New Kingdom king-lists along with Akhenaten and several other figures from this problematic period until Horemheb, whose reign is backdated to include their regnal years: Redford, D.B. (1986). *Pharaonic King-Lists, Annals and Day-Books.* The eradication was not complete: in the 3rd century Manetho knew enough to include Hatshepsut and the Amarna pharaohs in his 18th dynasty king-list: Josephus *Against Apion* 1.15.93ff. Hatshepsut also disappears from the lists, and images and

stereotype provided a readily available language of hostility and resistance, through the assimilation of invading or unwelcome forces to those of *jzft* and its malcontents.[135] Official history and imagery attests to massacres, corpse mutilation, and the enslavement of war captives. At best, the foreigner is assimilated as an inferior part of the ordered cosmos: a loyal subject or payer of tribute. Those who do not speak Egyptian are 'barbarians', in Herodotos' understanding of the concept (2.158), and the motif of invaders from the north became a recurrent feature of Egyptian literature.[136]

The Persians were easily fitted into such accounts of invading foreigners and illegitimate rule. Revolts broke out on Kambyses' death and throughout the Persian period until the successful insurrection of Nektanebo I. The reconquest, in 343, was accompanied by plunder of the temples and the destruction of city defenses, while Xerxes is portrayed in Egyptian sources as dismissive of indigenous temple cults.[137] Ptolemaic propaganda took advantage of their Persian predecessors' categorization as an incarnation of chaotic malevolence to which Alexander had brought a welcome end. There were repeated references to the recovery on various Syrian campaigns of statues of the gods stolen by the Seleucids' predecessors in Asia Minor, the Persians.[138]

The Macedonians' own claims to be the legitimate and necessary kings of Egypt were also susceptible to the disproof of revolt, although most of these were local or regional rather than national uprisings.[139] There is also

---

cartouches were erased or re-identified at some point late in the reign of her immediate successor Tuthmosis III, perhaps either as a dynastic power play or a rejection of female kingship: Roth, A.M. 'Erasing a Reign', in Roehrig, C.H. et al. (2005). *Hatshepsut. From Queen to Pharaoh*, 281. Akhenaten's new palace at Amarna and the temples built to the Aten under his reign were systematically destroyed and removed. At Karnak and Luxor Tutankhamun's name is replaced by Horemheb's on temple monuments: Redford, *King-Lists*, 190.

135 Conceptualizations of the foreigner: O'Connor, 'Egypt's view'. Acculturation by immigrants: Kemp, *Egypt*, 33–46.

136 E.g. *Urk.* IV, 383 ff.: an example of royal anti-invasion propaganda eighty years after the invasion in question.

137 Lloyd, 'Late Period', 384.

138 Hölbl, *Ptolemaic Empire*, 81, nn. 14–18. The recovery of religious artifacts plundered by foreign invaders had a Late period precedent in the demotic 'prophecy of the lamb' concerning the chapels taken by the Assyrians to Nineveh.

139 The first rising was in 245. A long-running series of uprisings in the north from soon after 217 until 185 overlaps with the southern rebellion that produces a native state and two kings in the Thebaid, ca. 205–186; the 160s see the rebellion of Petosarapis in Alexandria, social unrest in the Fayum and another revolt in the Thebaid; in 130–131 Harsiese declares himself king at Thebes; 91–88 sees another Theban rebellion; uprisings also occur in ca. 63 and in 55. Hölbl, *Ptolemaic Empire*, 49, 153–159, 181–182, 198–199, summary 306–307; Préaux,

some evidence for at least localized elite disenchantment in the form of several retroactive prophecies, a genre in which forecasts are composed after the events described. Three are known from the Greco-Roman period: the so-called, 'Prophecy of the Lamb', 'Demotic Chronicle' and 'Oracle of the Potter'.

All described a period of disasters for Egypt until eventually some kind of order and good kingship was restored: they can be read both as 'universalizable' accounts of the relationship between kingship and the state of the country, or as applicable to specific historical situations. The 'Oracle of the Potter' referred to the destruction of 'the city of the foreigners', usually read as Alexandria, and possibly to Greeks in the guise of 'followers of Tryphon (Seth)'; the undoubtedly hostile view of the 'Demotic Chronicle' about Persian 'foreigners' could have applied equally to the Greeks.[140]

These writings, like the history of revolts against the Persians, used to be thought to have expressed the popular resentment of Egyptians against exploitative colonists, visible also in periodic strikes, flights into the desert and marshes, or actual revolts. But it is very difficult to gauge the extent of the role actually played by nationalistic sentiment in these cases. Internal power struggles were a notable feature of Egypt whenever central authority was insufficient, and the 29th and 30th dynasties involved military conflict between rival indigenous claims to the throne; kings of the 29th dynasty generally did not hold the throne for long.[141] Much of the evidence, especially at its most forceful, for the assimilation of the foreigner to the chaotic and non-human, comes from either the profoundly ideological functions of the temples or the related sphere of royal legitimization. As David O'Connor notes for the pharaonic period ('Egypt's view', 160), it is difficult to establish to what degree this anti-foreigner, *mꜣʿt*-preserving ideology was shared by the larger population. Moreover, even within the elite sphere diplomacy, trade, immigration, and the deliberate assimilation of native elites, were also long-standing features of Egyptian relations with the foreign. Hatshepsut's vizier had an Asiatic name. Thus several scholars have argued that these examples of resistance were directed not against Greeks *qua* Greeks,

Cl. (1936). 'Esquisse d'une histoire des révolutions égyptiennes sous les Lagides', *CdÉ* 11, 522–552; Pestman, P.W. 'Haronnophris and Chaonnophris. Two Indigenous Pharaohs in Ptolemaic Egypt (205–186 B.C.)', in Vleeming, S.P. (1995). *Hundred-Gated Thebes*, 101–137.

[140] Summaries and bibliographies of these 3 texts: Depauw, M. (1997). *A Companion to Demotic Studies*, 97–99. At least the latter two were composed in demotic during the Ptolemaic era, although the 'Potter's Oracle' survives only in Greek.

[141] Lloyd, 'Late period', 377.

but against the elite establishment in general, in which indigenous officials worked closely with the court and administration. Revolutionaries on occasion attacked the temples, and there is little specific evidence for inter-ethnic violence.[142] The pseudo-prophecies, meanwhile, provided a framework within governing ideology for understanding disaster and recovery in terms of good and bad kings; categories that were not necessarily co-extensive with indigenous versus foreign.[143]

Social and economic motivations for revolt do not, however, rule out the possibility that it was often couched in ethnic terms.[144] The 'Demotic Chronicle' probably emerged, not from ethnically-neutral rural resentment of the powerful, but out of an aristocratic milieu surrounding the temple of Harsaphes at Herakleopolis in Middle Egypt. The 'Oracle of the Potter' viewed Memphite power favorably. The category of the foreign was not systematically applied on the basis of birthplace or nomenclature; but in Egypt its long-standing association with disorder rendered ethnocultural positioning a readily available mode of resistance within governing ideological frameworks.

1.4.1. *Ethnocultural Perceptions*

> But concerning Egypt I will now speak at length, because nowhere are there so many marvelous things, nor in the whole world beside are there to be seen so many works of unspeakable greatness.
>
> Herodotos 2.35

Through the formulations discussed in 1.3.2, changes in historical fortune were assimilated to a story that was at once an atemporal metaphysical drama and a continuous display of Egypt's inexorable survival, outstripping and persisting through the brief lives of other civilizations. Annals and other records offered an apparently tidy accumulation of kings and their mortuary

---

142 E.g. Goudriaan, *Ethnicity*, 108–115. For the older view e.g. Lloyd, A.B. (1982). 'Nationalist propaganda in Ptolemaic Egypt', *Historia* 31, 33–55.

143 Johnson, 'An anti-Greek tract?': references to Greeks in the 'Chronicle' are neutral, perhaps even favorable. See also Johnson, J.H. and R.K. Ritner. 'Multiple meaning and ambiguity in the "Demotic Chronicle"', in Israelit-Groll, S. (1990). *Studies in Egyptology presented to Miriam Lichtheim*, 1.494–506.

144 Cf. Pestman, 'Haronnophris and Chaonnophris'.

temples, officials and their tombs, piling up history like a drift of sand. Egyptian priests, said Herodotos, read to him from a papyrus roll a list of 331 kings for 331 generations.[145] This chronological accounting took a Hellenized form in Manetho's third century history of Egypt for a Greek audience, in the formulation of the dynastic record still largely in use today. Texts of ritual and technical knowledge, often written in archaic, 'classical' forms of the language, proclaimed their origins in and continuity with the distant past.[146] Actual innovation and variation in many fields, including medicine, was concealed by this rhetoric of continuity, itself one of the most unchanging features of ideological expression, so that absence of change became a standard part of the depiction of Egypt in other societies, including that of classical and Hellenistic era Greeks.

As early as the Homeric poems, written down in the eighth century but derived from earlier oral traditions, Egypt appeared as a semi-magical world on the borders of Greek experience: self-contained, ancient, and full of knowledge and power not readily available elsewhere.[147] In the *Laws*, Plato praised its supposed proscription of change in art and music:[148]

> And if you look there, you will find that the things depicted or graven there 10,000 years ago (I mean what I say, not loosely but literally 10, 000) are no whit better or worse than the productions of today, but wrought with the same art.

Plato's insistence on a specific amount of time transforms a vague impression of a long period of time into a circumstantial (if fictional) actuality, reinforcing his point.[149] Aristotle and Diodoros of Sicily reported Egyptian proscriptions against change in medicine.[150] Egypt was presented as not only unchanging but isolated and insular: Herodotos remarked on their closing themselves off from all foreign customs.[151]

---

[145] Herodotos 2.100: 330 kings between Min and Sethos (probably Shabataka of the 25th dynasty); cf. Manetho, who has 323 kings up to that reign: Jacoby, F. (1923–1958). *FGrH* no. 609, 58 ff.

[146] Archaism, while a recurrent feature of Egyptian literature and artistic representation, is especially prevalent during the Late period. For archaism in art, see e.g. Morkot, R. (2003). 'Archaism and innovation in art from the New Kingdom to the twenty-sixth dynasty', in Tait, *'Never Had the Like Occurred'*, 79–100. Egyptian literature: e.g. Loprieno, A. (1996). 'Defining Egyptian literature: ancient texts and modern theories', in Loprieno, *Ancient Egyptian Literature*, 39–58.

[147] *Odyssey* 4.125–135, 14.285–286.

[148] *Laws* 656e–657a, trans. Bury. Cf. Herodotos 2.79.

[149] Plato *Timaeus* 22b: an Egyptian priest told Solon that the Greeks are always children, never old.

[150] See chapter 3, section 3.4.

[151] 2.91, cf. 2.79. Strabo 17.1.19 disagrees.

Much of this is a product of the mutually reinforcing stereotypes of Greek ethnological discourse (a reflective and distorting lens)—and of Egyptian self-presentation. In classical period Greek writings, Egypt was consistently a place of wonders—in its geography, particularly the unparalleled length of the Nile, the great size of its monuments, its antiquity—and of sometimes bizarre curiosities: animal worship, its inhabitants' purgative habits, the mummification of its dead. Its peculiarities as a civilization are inseparable from its geophysical uniqueness, as Herodotos 2.35–36 makes clear.

> The Egyptians, besides having a climate peculiar to themselves, and a river different in its nature from all other rivers, have adopted customs and usages in almost all respects different from the rest of mankind.

Many famous thinkers, from Homer and Daidalos to Solon and Plato, either visited Egypt or were supplied with this experience, as a necessary fact of intellectual existence, by later biographical tradition.[152] Egypt served as an iconic explanation of wisdom and ideas, both for some well-known individuals and also for arts and knowledge whose origins were totally unknown, such as agriculture, writing, and knowledge about the gods.[153] According to Diodoros, those with the greatest reputation for learning wished to learn of Egypt's 'customs and usages, as being worthy of attention' (1.69.3–4). Approached this way, Egypt functioned as a collective culture hero for younger civilizations, an approach that might be more or less serious. Socrates, having just claimed writing was invented by the god Theuth (Thoth), is promptly accused of making up stories about Egypt and other places as it suits him.[154] It also continued to be a suitable fantasy setting: Euripides took the real Helen from the *Iliad* and put her into this self-enclosed world until Menelaus, returning from Troy, was blown off course into the same text.

The central text for the Greco-Roman discourse of Egypt is that of Herodotos, who stated explicitly that his account of Egypt was derived from his own observations and from talking to Egyptian priests.[155] Similarly,

---

[152] As well as Lykourgos, Orpheos, Musaios, Melampos, Pythagoras, Herodotos, Eudoxos.

[153] Lefkowitz, M.R. 'Some ancient advocates of Greek cultural dependency', in Coleman and Walz, *Greeks & Barbarians*, 237–253, convincingly demolishes both the biographical and etiological claims.

[154] Plato *Philebus* 18b–c; *Phaedrus* 274c–275a.

[155] Herodotos and Egyptian priests: e.g. 2.10, 2.99.1, cf. Egyptians of the cultivated lands, 2.77. Priests of specific temples are sometimes specified, e.g. 2.3. The translator of hieroglyphics at 2.125 was unreliable: Lloyd, *Commentary*, ad loc. On a visit to the country he may

Hekataios of Abdera, author of an idealizing third century ethnography of Egypt whose work partially survives in Diodoros' first century compilation, claimed to have used information gathered from temple records and his own eyewitness experience.[156] Although Herodotos showed some awareness of the great regional religious diversity of Egypt in his remarks on different attitudes toward the crocodile (2.69, cf. 2.92), in general the Egypt of the ethnographers, the main source of information for Egypt beyond its borders, was a place where difference and change was obscured.[157] The main effect is to confirm and develop preconceived Greek ideas of Egypt through the quasi-empirical reification of the ethnographer. As Harrison 2003 puts it in relation to Herodotos: '... he traveled (if he did) to find out what he already knew.' Plutarch viewed Herodotos as a 'barbarophile', idealizing other cultures, especially that of Egypt, for the purpose of denigrating his own.[158]

Even in this kind of account Egypt was a museum stranded by time, to be visited and wondered at, even sometimes admired, but not necessarily imitated.[159] Other accounts, moreover, relativized the difference as inferiority. Egyptians appeared as deceitful, cunning, slavish, laughable, or primitively

well have spoken in Greek to inhabitants including temple officials, though of what rank or sanctuary is unknown. It is however possible that his 'Egyptian' informants were Greeks resident in Egypt, including priests of Greek temples: Tait, J. 'The wisdom of Egypt: classical views', in Ucko, P. and T. Champion. (2003). *The Wisdom of Egypt*, 29. Certainly he employs material that originated at some point with Egyptian sources, and his summaries of mummification, medicine and animal worship tally with other evidence and appear to supply additional information: see Lloyd, *Commentary*.

156 Diodoros 1.46.7–8. Burton, A. (1972). *Diodorus Siculus Book I: A Commentary*, argued that Hekataios and Agatharkhides of Knidos were not the only principal sources for Diodoros book 1. Against this view see O. Murray's 1975 review of Burton in *JHS* 95, 214–215; Hornblower, J. (1981). *Hieronymus of Cardia*. See also Fraser, *Alexandria*, 1.495 ff. Tait, 'Wisdom', thinks Diodoros himself also visited Egypt. The information is often accurate, as in Diodoros' description of the mortuary temple of Rameses II (Ozymandias), 1.47–49. But few of Diodoros' reports of Egyptian *nomoi* can be substantiated by pharaonic period evidence, so at best they are suggestive only of practices during the early Hellenistic or perhaps the Late period: Murray, 'Review'.

157 Later *Aigyptiaka* by Hellanikos of Lesbos and Aristagoras of Miletos do not seem to have diverged much from Herodotos' content. The dramatists, notably in Aiskhylos' *Suppliants* and Phrynikhos' *Egyptians*, utilized similar material. Sophokles mentioned mummies and several writers, including Aristophanes, reference animal worship: *Birds* 504–506. For Greek literature on Egypt: Vasunia, P. (2001). *The Gift of the Nile*.

158 *The malice of Herodotos* 12 (*Moralia* 854e–874c). Translation and commentary: Bowen, A. (2002).

159 Cf. Harrison, T.H. 'Upside Down and Back to Front: Herodotus and the Greek Encounter with Egypt', in Matthews, R. and C. Roemer. (2003). *Ancient Perspectives on Egypt*, 153.

outdated.[160] Both of these responses are clearly visible in the Greek portrayal of Egyptian medicine.

1.4.2. *Greeks and Egyptian Medicine*

The topic of medicine is a microcosm of the Greek discourse of Egypt. In the *Odyssey*, the country provides a wonder drug:[161]

> Into the mixing bowl from which they drank their wine she slipped a drug, hearts-ease, dissolving anger, magic to make us all forget our pains ... So cunning the drugs that Zeus' daughter plied, potent gifts from Polydamna the wife of Thon, a woman of Egypt, land where the teeming soil bears the richest yield of herbs in all the world: many health itself when mixed in the wine, and many deadly poison. Every man is a healer there, more skilled than any other men on earth—Egyptians born of the healing god himself.

In Herodotean ethnography Egyptian medicine consisted of a series of distinctive features different in either degree or kind to Greek healing practice and practitioners: specialization, unchangingness, and obsessive purgation. Herodotos described these in his best 'neutral observer' manner in book 2. Yet at 3.125–137 he portrayed the Greek medical marvel Demokedes as having outperformed the Egyptian doctors at the Persian court, even though the latter were supposed to be the best in the world (see 4.4, pp. 192–193). Demokedes' pre-eminence asserted the superiority of sixth and fifth century Greek medicine over that of medicine's traditional exemplars. A dismissive fifth century attitude towards Egyptian medicine was also implied by its appearances in comedy. Aristophanes mocked the traditional description of Egypt in terms of the Nile by juxtaposing it with Egyptians' stereotypical obsession with laxatives:[162]

> These are the fair-maidened currents of the Nile, who in lieu of heavenly distilment floods the flats of bright Egypt for a people much given to laxatives (*melanosurmaiai*).

As I discuss in chapter 3, especially section 3.2.1, while these references tell us a good deal about Greek cultural attitudes, their use as information about Egyptian medicine is considerably more problematic.

---

160 E.g. Plato *Republic* 435e–436a: the Greeks love knowledge, the Phoenicians and Egyptians money.

161 *Odyssey* 4.219–234, and lines 241–260 in the translation by Fagles, R. (1996).

162 *Women at the Thesmophoria* 855–857, cf. *Peace* 1253–1254. The passage is discussed more fully in 4.2.2.1, p. 161.

1.5. *Ethnicity and Medicine*

The translation of Egypt into a Hellenistic kingdom with a sizable new immigrant population represented a political shift unusual in degree, if not in kind. For the majority of the non-Hellenic inhabitants of Egypt, the demands of the elite and the presence of Greeks must have represented an important, sometime difficult, but not unprecedented set of circumstances. The small literate elite meanwhile adapted Greek linguistic and cultural expectations as part of a new political reality. In turn, the Ptolemaic administration negotiated an identity for itself that was presentable and performed in terms of Egyptian elite ideology.

Acculturation and intermarriage produced a sub-set of individuals who could switch with apparent ease between the Hellenic identity advantageous in certain official contexts and that appropriate to Egyptian traditions and language. For many in this group, ethnocultural identity was not a single and exclusive declaration, but a continuing process of choice and context. For others, such as most peasant farmers, social status was relatively restricted, and strongly correlated with ethnic descent.

Facility with the Greek language was crucial, but whether other kinds of behavior regularly comprised part of the performance of Greekness is less clear. Certainly cultural institutions and activities that were strongly associated with being Greek, and not with being Egyptian, were supported and relatively widespread within urban centers and at least some parts of the chora. Gymnasia were built in new and older settlements in the Fayum; the government granted tax benefits to winners of athletic contests and the *technitai* of Dionysos. Wine, previously produced in small quantities in Egypt from native grapes, but primarily affordable only for the elite, benefited from the agricultural reforms and seems to have achieved widespread penetration into home markets among both immigrant and non-immigrant families, partly replacing beer as the everyday drink of Egypt; wheat also became more widely produced, used, and exported (see pp. 7–8). Meanwhile, syncretic or Egyptianizing pottery, burial practices, and patronage of local gods and temples indicate that for many a Greek identity was not compromised by the adoption of certain 'barbarian' forms.

In what follows, I shall investigate whether medicine was understood as part of ethnocultural identity, and whether either patients or practitioners viewed systems of healing as exclusive, interchangeable, or closely related. It is not uncommon for people in ethnoculturally pluralist societies like the modern United States to believe at one and the same time in ideas from two or more medical systems (e.g. classical Chinese medicine and biomedicine), and either consult practitioners from both at much the same time ('dual use') or in a series defined by relative specialization or perceived authority ('hierarchy of resort').[163] People may reject or be at best highly suspicious of one system in preference to another, rejecting either biomedicine, the health beliefs of the dominant sociocultural/ethnic group, for other traditions, or vice versa. The disease environment of Egypt outlined above is our understanding of what its inhabitants faced; but their perceptions of illness and healing were similarly conditioned by culturally derived understandings. The availability of certain healers, techniques or drugs, cultural chauvinism, exoticism, stereotypes, personal experience and preference, and the demonstration or perception of group and individual identity are all factors which might influence what people did and thought about illnesses. One such mode—perhaps the most widespread and frequently employed—are understandings of healing and illness which involve the gods.

[163] Chrisman, N.J. 'Transcultural care', in Zschoche, D. (1986). *Mosby's Comprehensive Review of Critical Care.*

CHAPTER TWO

MEDICINE AND THE GODS

This chapter is about ways in which people sought assistance from the gods on medical matters in Egypt. In particular, it focuses on oracular and medical practices at religious sanctuaries available to visiting pilgrims. In classical scholarship the usual shorthand for this category is 'temple medicine'. Many cult officials at Egyptian sanctuaries acted as healers, and the sanctuaries served as centers and producers of medical training and written knowledge. These aspects are discussed more fully in chapters five and three, respectively. Thus healing experts formed part of the medical resources of at least important sanctuaries. But the best attested form of medical assistance at temples is the oracle of the god, offering answers, advice or even a direct cure.

In what follows, we shall examine, in detail, the textual and archaeological evidence for Ptolemaic-period temple medicine. Much of this material comes from only a few major sanctuaries, in particular the Sarapieon of Memphis and the sanctuary of Imhotep and Amenhotep on the Theban west bank. In the fifth century BCE, Herodotos described oracles at Egyptian temples as variform (*Histories* 2.174; see p. 47 below), and a close reading of later texts suggests that this was the case for Ptolemaic temple medicine also. Third century Greek immigration and Hellenism's advantageous sociocultural profile seem to have increased the already notable diversity and flexibility of oracular and medical provision in Egypt.

Therefore, although we can set out clearly a broad outline of what was on offer to those seeking medical assistance from a sanctuary and from the gods, it is also evident that, within this outline, there was considerable diversity. Much secondary literature, which has dealt with temple medicine in Egypt only incidentally, as a subset of religious, archeological or medical analysis, has emphasized a particular form of medical assistance, the dream oracle or cure achieved through sleeping in a sacred place (incubation). In what follows I argue that this interpretation of the evidence has often been over-generalized and is in any case too broad a term, effectively concealing a more subtle picture. 'Incubation' can represent any one of a complex and varied set of procedures and expectations: who dreams, where, with what if any institutional support, and in expectation of what kind of response? How flexible is it, or how formulaic, and how much is it affected by cultural or linguistic factors? Our familiarity with relatively well-documented Asklepieian incubation risks obscuring differences, some sharp and some subtle, in the use and prevalence of medical incubation in the sanctuaries of Ptolemaic Egypt. A close reading of the surviving texts suggests incubation had unique advantages in certain circumstances, but was used primarily by those individuals who had access to sacred space and used dream interpretation to achieve religious status.

In addition, many other means of obtaining medical assistance were available. The assumption of incubation as the dominant mode often obscures these elements. They include the possible provision of long-term care at sanctuaries, the advice of cult officials, the use of other forms of oracular medical instructions, and the use of artifacts and substances impregnated with divine power through images and words. All of these can also show us something of the ways in which peoples of differing experience, expectations and preferences understood and sought the gods' assistance against illness; how their needs and desires were met by providers of medicine in the temples, and the role played by the interplay of Greek and Egyptian ideas about the gods and about medicine.

2.1.1. *Medical Oracles in Context*

A well-known form of oracle in Ptolemaic and Roman Egypt involved a question written on papyrus and submitted to the god's sanctuary. In fact, two questions were submitted to the god, through a cult official, that described alternative outcomes of the same situation. The cult official tore the papyrus and returned the correct alternative as selected by the god.[1] Examples in both Greek and demotic Egyptian are known from the Ptolemaic and especially the Roman periods.[2] Whatever the language, these post-

---

[1] Egyptian oracles: see Černy, J. 'Ancient Egyptian Oracles', in Parker, R.A. (1962). *A Saite Oracle Papyrus from Thebes*, 47. Kakosy, L. 'Orakel', *LÄ* 4, 600–606. For Roman Egypt see Frankfurter, D. (1998). 'Mutations of the Egyptian Oracle', chapter 4 in *Religion in Roman Egypt*, 145–197. For Greek oracle questions, see the comprehensive list, bibliography and discussion by Brashear, W. 'The Greek medical papyri', in Haase, W. (1995). *ANRW* 2.18.5, 3380–3684, especially 3448–3456.

[2] Listed by Brashear, *ANRW*, 3453–3454. Four are Ptolemaic in date (p. 3453): *P.Mil.Vogl.* III 127, TM 78533 (3rd–2nd BCE); *SB* XVI 14, TM 4142 (2nd BCE); *Atti del XVII Congresso Internazionale di Papyriologia*, 14 (2nd–1st BCE); *P.Tebt.* II 284, TM 42987 (1st BCE), a letter referring to an oracle's answer.

pharaonic questions are far more similar in structure and style to each other than they are to those from earlier in Egyptian history. They may have been the work of a small number of specialist professional scribes. They are extant primarily from the Fayum region, especially from Tebtynis and Soknopaiou Nesos, or from Oxyrhynkhos, and commonly involve forms of the crocodile god Sobek.[3]

Other modes of seeking divine assistance take a different form to the Greek and demotic double-questions and may not have involved a reply, or at least not in the same way. They do, however, also include medical examples. Both self-dedication of a person to a god, in return for protection against illness and other difficulties, and written demands for medical or other protection, deposited in a sanctuary, are Ptolemaic-period practices which appear to go back to the pharaonic era.[4] They survive only in demotic examples, unlike the double-answer oracle questions, but their existence emphasizes that there was far more than one way, in the Ptolemaic Fayum, to appeal to a god for medical help.

Herodotos said that oracles were a common practice at sanctuaries in fifth-century Egypt, but that the way of giving advice varied from temple to temple (2.174).[5] The oldest and most widespread form was the 'movement'

[3] The crocodile god Sobek, in various local forms, was the principal deity in the Fayum: Arnold, D. 'Fayjjum', *LÄ* 2, 87–93. Brovarski, E. 'Sobek', *LÄ* 5, 995–1031.

[4] Self-dedication: Thompson, H. (1940). 'Two demotic self-dedications', *JEA* 26, 68–78: 37 papyri contain ca. 50 self-dedications. Written demand: Ray, J.D. (1975). 'Papyrus Carlsberg 67: A healing-prayer from the Fayum', *JEA* 61, 181–188. (Brashear, *ANRW*, 4453 n. 365 lists this as an oracle question). Pharaonic examples of this genre, with medical subject matter: Djutmose, the author of several extant letters under Rameses XI (1098–1070), tells the letter's recipient, 'you shall tell Amun to remove this illness which is in me' (*P. Leiden* I 370 = Černy, J. (1939). *Late Ramesside Letters* 11 (no. 5), l. 16. Translation Wente, E. (1967). *Late Ramesside Letters*, 31). *P. Strassburg* 21 published by Spiegelberg, W. (1917). 'Briefe der 21. Dynastie aus El-Hibe (mit 16 Abbildungen und Tafel I–VII)', *ZÄS* 53, 13–14 (no. III.6) and plates 5–6 = Wente, E. (1990). *Letters from Ancient Egypt*, 208 (no. 337). Černy, 'Oracles', 46 reads a hieratic petition to Amun as a letter to the god rather than his priest '… saying: "Save him, cure him, chase away any illness which is in him"'; for a contrary view see Posener, G. (1982). 'Un papyrus d'El Hibeh', *JEA* 68, 134–138. Such depositions continued into the Roman period: e.g. Ammianus Marcellinus *Res Gestae* 19.12.3; Schubart, W. (1931). 'Orakelfragen', *ZÄS* 67, 113–114.

[5] The selection of the correct answer from one or more alternatives seems to be a characteristic of almost all oracle procedures in Egypt: Černy, 'Oracles', 47. At Memphis, hollow statuettes of Osiris or Horus (as falcon), buried on the sacred animal necropolis in the Late Period, probably contained written petitions or questions that were laid before the god's statue by a cult official, and then returned to the petitioner before being discarded or buried: Smith, H.S. (1974). *A Visit to Ancient Egypt* 34, 56; Sadek, A.I. (1988). *Popular Religion in Egypt during the New Kingdom*, 275. For an example of another possible method see e.g. McDowell, A.G. (1999). *Village Life in Ancient Egypt*, 107 ff. Cf. folded lead strips containing

oracle, used at festivals and important occasions, when the cult statue was carried out from the inner shrine to the relatively public areas of the outer sanctuary or beyond.[6]

A recurrent concern of those asking for oracular or other forms of divine assistance was defense against illness. In 132 BCE, officials of the cult of the crocodile gods Soknopaios and Isis Nephorses, at the village of Soknopaiou Nesos in the Fayum—the provenance of several later Greek and demotic oracle questions—wrote to the government official Apollonios, strategos and overseer of the revenues:

> Since, therefore, your life has been saved in sickness by the great god Soknopaios and Isis Nephorses the most great goddess and the associated gods, we entreat you ...[7]

They do not explain the circumstances of this healing, but a Greek letter of the mid-third century is more specific about a similar event. It refers to a medical instruction by 'the god' given as an oracle.[8] Given the context, the god in this case was probably Sarapis of Memphis. Another oracular communication probably lies behind the granite monument, dedicated in hieroglyphics by Ptolemy II and Arsinoe II, to a form of the Theban god Khonsu, in thanks for the salvation of Philadelphos from illness.[9]

---

questions for the oracle at Dodona in north-west Greece, which were answerable by yes or no: Parke, H.W. (1967). *The Oracles of Zeus*, 259–273. 'Voice' oracles, in which a cult official spoke as the god through a secret passage, are attested for the Roman period and may be earlier: J. Černy, 'Oracles', 43. Frankfurter, *Religion*, 150–152.

[6] Strabo 17.1.43 (C 814) and Diodoros Sikelos 17.50.6–7 (using the lost work of Kallisthenes). The movement oracle is attested since the New Kingdom but might well be older: Baines, J. and R.B. Parkinson. 'An Old Kingdom record of an oracle? Sinai inscription 13', in van Dijk, J. (1997). *Essays on Ancient Egypt in Honour of Herman Te Velde*, 9–27.

[7] *P.Amh.* II 35.31–35 (132), TM 8621: ἐπεὶ οὖν σέσωσαι ἐν τῆι ἀρρωστίαι ὑπὸ τοῦ Σοκνοπαῖος θεοῦ μεγάλου καὶ Ἴσιος {σ}Νεφορσῆτος θεᾶς μεγίστης καὶ τῶν συννάων θεῶν ἀξιοῦμεν ....

[8] *P.Cair.Zen.* III 59426, TM 1066 (263–229 BCE). See Edgar, C.C. (1928). *Catalogue général des antiquités égyptiennes du musée du Caire nos. 59298–59531. Zenon papyri* III, 156. Cf. below, 2.3.2, pp. 71–72.

[9] Daressy, G. (1894) in *Recueil de Travaux* 16, 43–44 (no. 93) = *Urk.* II 108 (no. 22). In Karnak, Khonsu Neferhotep was frequently identified with the production of oracles, in particular oracular amuletic decrees—declarations by a god that an oracle will be fulfilled, known mainly from the Third Intermediate period: Edwards, I.E.S. (1960). *Hieratic Papyri in the British Museum, Fourth Series: Oracular Amuletic Decrees of the Late New Kingdom*; Bohleke, B. (1997). 'An oracular decree of Khonsu in the Cleveland Museum of Art', *JEA* 83, 155–167. Khons was often identified with the oracular god Thoth: Brunner, H. 'Chons', *LÄ* 1, 960–963.

2.1.2. *Dreams*

In most of the examples above, oracular interaction between god and petitioner was mediated through institutional practice and cult personnel. In contrast, contact with a god through the medium of a dream is a direct contact between god and dreamer, in which institutional involvement, though common, is not required. A dream might be instigated by the god, and was considerably more free form in its delivery of meaning than other kinds of oracle.

In Ptolemaic Egypt, dream-oracles and epiphanic cures are described by Strabo for the temple of Sarapis at Kanobos or Kanopos, a coastal town about 15 km east of Alexandria.[10] Plutarch refers to this as the oracle in Kanopos: τὸ χηρστήριον ἐν Κανώβῳ ....[11] It therefore seems clear that incubation formed part of temple medicine in Ptolemaic Egypt, certainly in the first century BCE, and almost certainly before. This raises certain questions, including whether this should be seen as a common practice of Egyptian as well as Greek medical tradition, as a case of cultural influence, or as a relatively limited oracular mode.

The use of bowels of water, of mediums, and of dreams in obtaining assistance from the gods are all attested in Egypt before the pharaonic period, but as Brashear. 'Greek magical papyri', 3449 points out, almost all such evidence is from literary materials. 'Dream-books' catalogued images seen during sleep as good or bad omens, accompanying this classification with a brief summary of the symbol's meaning. Several demotic dream-catalogues are known from the Late and Greco-Roman era.[12] The dreams are never explicitly described as messages from the gods. Possibly that was simply taken for granted, but it might be a parallel for the common Greek division of dreams into those that are god-sent (an oracular dream) and those that lack any kind of agency and are simply signs of events.[13]

---

[10] Strabo 17.1.17 (C801): see below, 2.2.2, p. 65, cf. p. 65 n. 73.

[11] Plutarch *Isis and Osiris* 27 (*Moralia* 361e–f).

[12] For dreams (*rsw.t, qd*) in pharaonic Egypt see Szpakowska, K. (2003). *Behind Closed Eyes*; Vernus, P. 'Traum', *LÄ* 6, 746–750. Dream-catalogues: see references in Vernus, with later discoveries in Quack, J. 'A black cat from your right, and a scarab on your head', in Szpakowska, K. (2006). *Through A Glass Darkly*, 175–187. The only prior example is the New Kingdom's *Chester Beatty Papyrus* III. Dream-books probably evolved from calendars of lucky and unlucky days: Szpakowska, *Closed Eyes*, 71.

[13] Szpakowska, *Closed Eyes*, 135. For the Greeks on dreams and medical adaptations of this idea: von Staden, H. (1989). *Herophilus*, 306–310; Lloyd, G.E.R. (1987). 'Dreams', *The Revolutions of Wisdom*, 30–37.

In Egyptian thought, a dream was not an internal event but a vision; an open window onto the gods, dead and other inhabitants of the more dangerous world that co-existed with the waking one, but were not normally visible. Illness was often the result of night-time attacks by the otherworld's more malevolent denizens. Nightmares were literally dangerous.[14] On the other hand, dreams also provided a means for useful communication with beneficent deities, though before the Ptolemaic period the mortal protagonists of this rarely attested genre are almost invariably kings.[15]

The number of Egyptian texts that mention dreams is proportionately much greater during the Late and Greco-Roman periods than was previously the case. From the Late period onwards the dream-oracle appeared quite often in the kinds of literary-religious texts generated by the temple-based intellectual culture, and are extant in both Greek and Egyptian.[16] They have much in common, and in several instances Greek versions were based on demotic material, testifying to the production and diversification of the dream trope within elite Greco-Egyptian cultural discourse and literary production. Their collective existence suggests that the individual dream oracle had become a relatively common way to memorialize and narrate significant events. The power of a particular deity was played out in the autobiography of the dreamer; while the dreamer's account publicized and justified the god's cult. The sense of a negotiation guided both the interpretation of ill fortune and the expectation of profit, dramatizing the ideal of human-god reciprocity.

In the commonest dream-narrative form, the dream warns its recipient of neglect or danger to the god's cult; a reward follows the cult's formulation or renewal.[17] Several concern illness or healing. From either the Persian or

---

[14] Szpakowska, *Closed Eyes*, 16ff. The earliest references to dreams are in the 'letters to the dead' attested from the Old to the New Kingdoms: for two pleas for medical assistance in this form, by the living to their dead relatives, see Wente, E. (1990). *Letters from Ancient Egypt* nos. 349 (First Intermediate period) and 350 (Middle Kingdom).

[15] Non-royal individuals dream of deities in two extant New Kingdom hymns: Szpakowska, *Closed Eyes*, 135–141.

[16] Listed in Vernus, 'Traum', and Sauneron, S. (1959). *Les songes et leur interprétation dans l'Égypte ancienne*, 21–23; additional examples in Greco-Roman sources in Thissen, H.-J. (1966). *Studien zum Raphiadekret*, 52–53 (nos. 12–16).

[17] There is a fragmentary demotic tablet in which a king dreams in the burial vaults of the Memphis temple to Osiris-Apis, dated on paleographic grounds to the first half of the Ptolemaic period: Spiegelberg. W. (1912–1913). 'Zwei Kelksteinplatten mit demotischen Texten', *ZÄS* 50, 32–34 with 51, 137–138. Josephus attributes a story of Isis and Amenophis (Amenhotep) to the first century CE Greek-Egyptian philosopher Khairemon: *Against Apion* 1.32. The dream of Nektanebo (II) exists in both Greek (*UPZ* 81, pp. 369–374) and demotic

Ptolemaic period, the Bentresh stele found at Karnak told the story of the god Khons' mission (in the form of his cult statue) to a foreign kingdom in order to cure a sick daughter of its royal family; a scheme to prevent the god's departure failed after a threatening dream.[18] In 257 BCE, king Ptolemy Philadelphos' chief financial official, Apollonios, received a letter from a man he had recently met in Alexandria, Zoilos of Aspendos. Sarapis had apparently instructed Zoilos 'in [his] sleep' to tell Apollonios to build a sanctuary to the god 'in the Greek quarter by the harbor' of an unidentified town. Zoilos asserted that his initial reluctance to carry out this task caused Sarapis to make him very ill; only when he prayed to the god for a cure in exchange for fulfilling the commission did he recover quickly. If Apollonios also did his part, Zoilos added pointedly, he would not only be 'much greater and more honored in the eyes of the king' but also preserved by Sarapis 'in bodily health.'[19] A second century CE Greek text describing incubation in the temple of Imhotep at Memphis connected the delay in actual healing to its narrator's failure to advertise the god in a memorializing account;[20] three centuries earlier the funerary stele of the wife of the leading cult official of Ptah at Memphis recorded the exchange between her husband and Imhotep: a son in return for a building program.[21]

The dream-oracle evolved as a relatively private and free-form means of communication with gods, like the oracle questions and depositions discussed in 2.1.1, but was more flexible than these. It also deinstitutionalized oracles in favor of a personal claim to access and interaction with the divine, obtained through flexible and often informal means, or at the instigation of the god.

versions: Ryholt, K. (1998). 'A demotic version of Nectanebo's Dream (P. Carlsberg 562)', *ZPE* 122, 197–200.

18 Translation: Lichtheim, M. (1973). *Ancient Egyptian Literature* 3.90–94.

19 *P.Cair.Zen.* I 59034, TM 694 (257). Two other examples of dreams, without relation to medicine, appear in relation to the foundings of Sarapis cults. Soter's dream of the cult statue's location is known only from Roman sources but might have circulated as early as the mid-third century: Tacitus *Histories* 4.83–84; Plutarch *Isis and Osiris* 28.1–4; Clement *Exhortation to the Heathen* 4.48.1–3. Instructions on temple site and cult statue were given by Sarapis in dreams to his cult officials on Delos, founded by the Memphite cult official Apollonios: *IG* 11.4.1299 = *SIG*[3] II 644 = Roussel, P. (1916). *Les cultes égyptiens à Délos du IIIe au Ier siécle av. J.-C.*, 71–83, no. 1. Cf. Engelmann, H. (1975). *The Delian Aretalogy of Sarapis*; Fraser, P.M. (1972). *Ptolemaic Alexandria*, 1.253–254, 1.499–501.

20 *P.Oxy.* XI 1381 = TM 63689, LDAB 4898, MP3 2479, with additional bibliography. See further 2.4.1, pp. 86–87.

21 Taimhotep stele (BM 147). See further 2.3.6, pp. 81–82.

2.1.3. *Incubation*

A sub-group of dream oracles is those deliberately solicited, and a sub-group of solicited dreams are those solicited by means of sleeping in a sacred place. 'Incubation' is well known from the Greco-Roman world, and was very closely associated with healing cults, especially that of Asklepios.[22] In Egypt, incubation is not explicitly attested before the Ptolemaic period, in instances specific to certain circumstances that I discuss more fully below. Significant dreams as a group are rare before the Late period, and although dream-oracles are relatively common among Greco-Roman texts they again rarely mention incubation or even solicitation. If incubation was employed, the genre convention seems to have been to ignore this solicitative agency on the part of the dream recipient.

There are indications that sleeping in the vicinity of the god was commonly involved in the experience of an Egyptian dream-oracle. The future Thutmosis IV (ca. 14th century), for instance, fell asleep in the noonday shadow of the sphinx before seeing a god, though there is no indication that he did this with the aim of receiving a dream-message.[23] From the late New Kingdom, a hymn to Hathor mentioned the mountain-goddess Mertserger: 'I have spent the night in this forecourt. I have drunk the water ... My body has spent the night in the shadow of your face.'[24] According to Herodotos, the seventh century king Sethos (Shabataka) had a dream in the inner shrine of Ptah's temple at Memphis;[25] an account closely paralleled by the second tale in the demotic narrative of Setne Khamwas, extant on a Roman period papyrus. In this story within the story, the magician Horos son of Paneshe, experiencing problems with Nubian sorcerers, prayed to Thoth for advice in

---

[22] For Asklepios, see Wickkiser, B.L. (2008). *Asklepios, medicine, and the politics of healing in fifth century Greece.*

[23] Thutmosis IV Sphinx Stele (ll. 8–13), published by Zivie, C.M. (1976). *Giza au deuxième Millénaire*; translation Szpakowska, *Closed Eyes*, 189.

[24] BM stele 278 (Qenherkhopshef the younger). Bruyére, B. (1930). *Mert Seger à Deir el Médineh* and Marciniak, M. (1981). 'Un text inédit de Deir el-Bahari', *BIFAO* 88, 283–291, suggest this is incubation, cf. Quirke, S. (1992). *Ancient Egyptian Religion*, 136. Szpakowska, *Closed Eyes*, 145 points out that there is no reference to any divine communication, dream, or expectation of a dream.

[25] 2.141: τὸν δ' ἰρέα ἐς ἀπορίην ἀπειλημένον ἐσελθόντα ἐς τὸ μέγαρον πρὸς τὤγαλμα ἀποδύρεσθαι οἷα κινδυνεύει παθεῖν. ὀλοφυρόμενον δ' ἄρα μιν ἐπελθεῖν ὕπνον, καί οἱ δόξαι ἐν τῆι ὄψι ἐπιστάντα τὸν θεὸν θαρσύωειν ὡς οὐδὲν πείσεται ἄχαρι ἀντιάζων τὸν 'Αραβίων στρατόν. Spiegelberg, W. (1906.) 'Agyptologische Randglossen zu Herodot', *ZÄS* 43, 84–96.

the temple of Khnum. Having lain down to sleep in the temple, he received a vision of Thoth in his dreams.[26]

These accounts show that such direct encounters with the gods were perceived as particularly probable or significant when they occurred in as sacred a place as possible, usually a place of literal closeness to a god. The vocabulary of being in the god's shadow expressed not only this physical location but also its metaphorical extension, into a state of being under the protection and in the power of the god. This might have produced deliberate solicitation of visionary experience by sleeping in such places. Herodotos' account of Sethos' dream resembles incubation closely, but, given the usual problems with his sources, we cannot reconstruct an Egyptian interpretation of this event.[27] The difficulty is that sacred space is integral to all categories of dealings with the gods, and is always likely to be involved in experience of the divine, which is why pilgrims come to temples in the first place. How close one could get to the god—how far within their shadow—depended on whether an individual worked in temples or had the requisite purity and religious power. Most recipients of dream-oracles prior to the Late period (and many subsequent literary dreams) were kings, whose access to sacred space within a temple and importance to the otherworld was exceptional. The majority of the evidence for healing at Egyptian sanctuaries throughout the Late and Greco-Roman eras is for supplication and oracular function through diverse modes. The dream oracle solicited through incubation was probably largely a development of the Late and Ptolemaic eras; but nothing indicates it became the standard form of communication with the god, or of temple medicine.[28]

Our familiarity with the Asklepieian model is such that incubation is regarded as the default mode of temple medicine—often to the extent that it obscures other forms of Greek religious medicine, such as oracle cults, purifiers, root-cutters and domestic religion. Yet interpreting Egyptian

---

26 Setne II (*P. British Museum* 604); translation in Lichtheim, *Literature*, 3.138–151 esp. 146. Parallel noted by Griffith, F.Ll. (1900). *Stories of the High Priests of Memphis* 11, cf. Lloyd, A.B. (1976). *Herodotus, Book II: Commentary on 1–98*, 101.

27 For the debates on Herodotos' reliability and source material for Egypt, see 1.4.1, pp. 39–40 n. 155. Manetho (fr. 42 Waddell = Josephus *Against Apion* 1.14.73) is however revealing of an Egyptian view: 'Herodotos, out of ignorance, often lied about Egyptian history': ὅς καὶ πολλὰ τὸν Ἡρόδοτον ἐλέγχει τῶν Αἰγυπτιακῶν ὑπ' ἀγνοίας ἐψευσμένον.

28 It is important to note here the difference between the *possibility*, in certain circumstances, of a particular method, and that method's institutionalized dominance on either a sanctuary or national scale.

temple medicine through our understanding of Greek healing cults is methodologically problematic.

There were considerable structural, organizational and functional differences between Egyptian sanctuaries and Asklepieia. These are, in the first place, relevant to the question of whether incubation was an allowed-for possibility at Egyptian temples; but also to how we understand any such instances of dream oracles or solicitation within the spaces of an Egyptian sanctuary, which are both literally and functionally different from those of an Asklepieion. Evidence for oracular dreams and/or temple medicine is not in itself evidence for incubation, but the two have often been conflated.

2.1.4. *Asklepieia Contrasted with Egyptian Sanctuaries*

Asklepiean cult typically involved a sanctuary situated in a pleasant rural location, with water available for washing and purification.[29] A sacrifice, and probably an additional fee, were also necessary steps for the suppliant and visitor. Those seeking a dream slept in a structure, usually called an *abaton* (or *enkoimeterion*, as at Pergamon) and apparently limited to this purpose, within the small sacred space of the *temenos*. Purity regulations applied to this area. The *abaton* may have included a statue of the god as a stimulus to the dreamers and a means of invoking his presence. The cult statue itself, while not where the incubants slept, was accessible to visitors.

The focus on the dream experience produced a degree of unity in expectation, function and structure. At Epidauros, six steles within the sanctuary displayed narrative accounts of the visions and cures of pilgrims.[30] The monumental nature of the display reinforced the god's authority even for illiterate visitors (who would have understood or been told what the inscriptions represented). Compiled from narrative and pictorial votives and perhaps from oral traditions, these monuments reinforced not only expectations of the god's utility (only successful cures are recorded), but also of the nature of the experience itself. Such narrative accounts probably existed at other Asklepieia as well, collating the message of individual votives. An

---

[29] For Asklepieia see Graf, F. 'Heiligtum und Ritual. Das Beispiel der griechisch-römischen Asklepieia', in Reverdin, O. and B. Grange. (1992). *Le sanctuaire grec*, 159–204. The classic collection of Asklepieian materials remains Edelstein, L. and E. Edelstein. (1945). *Asclepius*. For Amphiaraos' incubatory healing at Oropos, see Pausanias 1.34–35; Dillon, M. (1997). *Pilgrims and Pilgrimage in Ancient Greece*, 157–160.

[30] *IG* IV^2 1, nos. 121–122. The most recent edition is LiDonnici, L.D. (1995). *The Epidaurian Miracle Inscriptions* = Edelstein and Edelstein, *Asclepius* no. 423, 221–238. Cf. Pausanias 2.27.3.

Asklepieion was all about healing. The cult had an unusually narrow focus and was strongly identified with a specific *modus operandi*.[31]

At a Greek temple *hiereis* were not normally providers of medical knowledge, although ancillary services were often available through private enterprise in the immediate locale. These might have included purifiers, physicians or drug-sellers. The priests' primary role was temple administration and organization, including the keeping of financial records and the arranging of votive decorations. On a daily basis they and the cult attendants divided up and ate the offerings of food and drink left for the god, guarded the sanctuary, and ensured that regulations as to purity and behavior were carried out. At Asklepieia their crucial role was to put out the lamp in the *abaton* and tell the incubants to go to sleep.[32] In later periods attendants sometimes offered opinions on treatment, but Aristides' experiences at Pergamon suggest that this was far from specialist advice. Aristides also consulted doctors for a second opinion, help with interpretation, or expert execution of the god's more technical instructions, but medical professionals and priests remained clearly separate categories.[33]

In Egypt—in sharp contrast to Greek society—cult officials were the medical experts.[34] Medical texts, like other technical and ritual works, were kept in the scriptorium attached to the sanctuary, the *pr ʿnḫ* (house of life).[35] Medicine was part of the knowledge of the literate elite, a group largely comprised by the upper personnel of the temples, army and court. It was delivered to the wider community by temple specialists, who also mediated between gods and ordinary mortals through funerary practices, defensive magic, and oracle-questions and petitions.

---

31 There are a few instances in which Asklepios' healing role is more broadly interpreted, including the restoration of a broken pot and a missing child in the Epidaurian *iamata*. Aelius Aristides interpreted many of his dreams as being about his rhetorical career or legal difficulties.

32 Aristophanes *Wealth* 660 and 676–681.

33 Aristides relied on himself, his friends, temple officials and physicians for help with interpreting or following the god's advice: Behr, C.A. (1968). *Aelius Aristides and the Sacred Tales*, 191–192. He consulted the famous physician Satyros in 147 (*Sacred Tales* 3.8–11, Behr 61). Physicians at Aristides' home and at Pergamon help him follow the god's instructions: 1.73 and references in Behr 44, nn. 11–12; as Behr, 31 n. 43 observes, 'It is most unclear whether the doctor Theodotus, whom Aristides frequently consulted in the temple, cf. II 34 and the dreams in I 13 and I 56, had any official position.'

34 In particular the lector priests, the priests of Sakhmet, and the priests of Serqet. See further 5.1.1, pp. 206–212.

35 Burkard, G. (1980). *Bibliotheken im alten Ägypten*, 79–115; Weber, M. 'Lebenshaus I', *LÄ* 3, 954–957; Gardiner, A. (1938). 'The House of Life', *JEA* 24, 157–179.

No structure or area in which dreams are regularly solicited or experienced within an Egyptian sanctuary—that is, a space with a functional equivalency to an *abaton* or *enkoimeterion*—is ever mentioned in the extant sources or identifiable from archeological remains.[36] The deity dwelt in a small open-fronted shrine hidden deep within the temple's complex of rooms. Cult officials moved relatively freely within the precinct as their level of purity allowed, but those with no official role were channeled to the outer, less sacred, spaces of the sanctuary, the long-established and institutionalized locations for contacting the gods and obtaining cures. A letter from Djehutmose, a scribe of the necropolis at Thebes around the beginning of the first millennium, to women in his household, asked that while he is away from the city:

> Please call upon Amun to bring me back, for I have been ill since I arrived north and am not in my normal state ... As soon as my letter reaches you, you shall go to the forecourt of Amun of the Thrones of the Two Lands [the mortuary temple of Rameses III] taking the little children along with you and coax him and tell him to keep me safe.[37]

The women did not have to go far: the mortuary temple was where the workmen were at this time living. The outer court(s) were the most sacred, nearest space to the god available to the general population—and evidently to both sexes and all ages. Crowds gathered in them at festival time for the god's semi-public appearances (the occasion for 'movement' oracles).[38] They contained statues of kings and other powerful men; these could be petitioned on their own account or as intermediaries. At Karnak, in the sanctuary complex of Amun, one such statue is inscribed (king) 'Rameses-who-hears-prayers'; several more depict the court official Amenhotep son of Hapy, whose mortuary cult developed, in the Ptolemaic period, into that of a well known oracular and healing god. These statues existed in such numbers that eventually they had to be buried below ground level to make way for new ones.[39] Prayers were to be made directly to the gods through shrines 'of the hearing ear', which in many temples were placed directly behind the sanctuary in the outer wall of the temple complex, and were thus also accessible to the non-purified. The simplest and most common form is a

---

[36] See further below, 2.3.4, pp. 77–78 and nn. 122–123, cf. p. 73 n. 108.

[37] Wente, *Letters*, no. 295.

[38] Called 'the hall of the multitude' in Ptolemaic times, where the lapwing hieroglyph *rḫyt* (people, subjects) on walls or columns probably marked where the crowds gathered.

[39] On Karnak, Blyth, E. (2006). *Karnak: Evolution of a Temple*. Statues: Sourouzian, H. 'Tempelstatuen', *LÄ* 6, 411–414.

niche with either a statue of the god or of their ear: a pictorial insistence on the shrine's function and power analogous to the *iamata* of Greek healing cult, but without the generic formulas of dream or focus on illness.[40]

All of this should make us wary of assuming that the Asklepieian model is the universal mode of temple medicine in Egypt—or even in Greece, where experience was more diverse, and methods of contacting the gods about medical problems more heterogenous, than the relatively standardized and idealized model of Asklepieian incubation to be found on the Epidaurian steles. The *iamata* of the latter are both revised and selective: designed to proselytize for Asklepios and to aid the mental readiness of incubants. Not all visitors to the sanctuaries came for the purpose of incubation; not all who did experienced a healing dream. LiDonnici, 49, points out that at Epidauros suppliants came from all over the Greek world, with 'each person perhaps bringing practices and expectations from very different local traditions.' Aristides' memoirs paint a more personal and much more confusing depiction of the unstructured and sometimes unsolicited medium of dream than do the Epidaurian *Iamata*, and although he had heard of the epiphanic dream cure, he had never experienced it.[41] The oracle sanctuaries of Dodona, Delphi and Asia Minor guaranteed a privileged—if expensive and relatively inaccessible—access to the gods through various non-incubatory modes. Medical problems were also treated by other kinds of ritualists, by root-cutters, and by doctors, all of whom were unaffiliated with the temples.

There are no surviving examples of Asklepieia in Egypt that are not Egyptian-form temples to Imhotep, the god with whom Asklepios was most commonly identified. The southern polis of Ptolemais Hermeiou contained a sanctuary to Asklepios, although none is attested for Alexandria (or Naukratis). The dedicatory inscription of Ptolemais' original third century temple also carried a variant on the traditional Erythraian hymn to Asklepios, making rather more of the holy waters of the Nile and the fame of Egypt than the original.[42] There are however no equivalents to the famous

---

[40] Blok, H.P. (1928). 'Remarques sur quelques stéles dites "a oreilles"', *Kemi* 1, 123–135; Sadek, *Popular Religion*, 245–267. Clement of Alexandria 5.7.43: 'The eyes and ears engraved on steles are a symbol—symbol of the deity who sees the acts of mortals and hears their conversations and prayers'.

[41] *Sacred Tales* 4.65, cf. 3.15 and 5.23. Such cures were still occurring: *IG* XIV no. 966 (T 438), *IG* IV^2 1 no. 127 (T 424), Oribasios *Medical Compilations* 45.30 (T 425).

[42] Baillet, J. (1889). 'La stèle de Menschieh', *RA* 13, 70–83; republished by É. Bernand (1969). *Inscriptions métriques*, no. 176. For Ptolemais Hermeiou (TM U08; Geo ID 2023) see Kessler, D. 'Ptolemais Hermiu', *LÄ* 4, 1183; Plaumann, G. (1910). *Ptolemais in Oberägypten*; Baines, J. and J. Malek. (2000). *Cultural Atlas of Ancient Egypt*, 109.

contemporary sanctuaries of Asklepios at Epidauros, Kos, Pergamon, Athens, and Rome, because powerful, well-established sanctuaries of deities strongly associated with healing already existed within Egypt.[43] The Egyptian temples of Osiris, Osiris-Apis and Imhotep were the Sarapiea and Asklepieia of the Greeks, and provide the overwhelming majority of the evidence for temple medicine in Ptolemaic Egypt. Worship of Asklepios' Greek form was relatively small scale, a matter of small local temples in areas and towns of concentrated Greek colonization. A rare example of what was probably such a Greek cult comes from the Zenon archive, which contains a letter from Philonides, a priest of Asklepios: Φιλωνίδης ὁ ἱερεὺς τοῦ Ἀσκληπιοῦ Ζήνωνι χ[αίρειν ...].[44]

Two gods closely associated with healing in the Greco-Roman period, as well as with the Ptolemaic dynasty, were Isis and the 'syncretic' Sarapis. In the next section, 2.2, I discuss the evolution of the relationship of these gods to healing and medical oracles within the Greco-Egyptian cultural environment.

2.2.1. *Reformulating Isis*

A sanctuary was defined by its relations with its local community, with other cults, and with the state administration. The upper ranks of Egyptian temple personnel, as part of the literate and socioeconomic elite of the country, were concerned with the use and acquisition of political, economic and cultural power through their relations with the king and the state. This dialectic continued under a Macedonian king and Hellenized administration, but often in adapted forms. Temple workers and officials had always produced innovative and individualized forms of worship and literature, which sometimes spread adaptively through region or country, but remained essentially locally driven rather than centrally directed. In this dynamic, Hellenism offered new modes of expression as a means of access to new and powerful audiences. The Greek elite participated in this process and co-opted it as part of their own understanding of Egypt and, in particular, of Egyptian gods.

This process can be clearly seen in the ways in which Isis is represented in Greco-Egyptian religious and literary materials. Certain aspects of the

---

[43] Philadelphos patronized a festival of Asklepios on Kos. *SEG* 12.368 (before 246). Sherwin-White, S. (1978). *Ancient Cos*, 99–100.

[44] *P.Zen.Pestm.* 42, *P.Col.Zen.* I 7, *PSI* VI 663, TM 1873 (257).

complicated layers of the Egyptian tradition became simplified, or at least de-emphasized, and among these was Isis' strong association with healing: a crucial feature of several myths and indeed of much medical practice. In older Egyptian texts, Isis was termed a physician (*swnw*), but the word does not appear in any Isean aretalogy, nor in the early Ptolemaic hymns composed for the decoration of her temple at Philae.[45] Later, more universalized understandings of Isis extracted her from the traditional mythic script and its specific medical context and content, subsuming the healer into the generalized features of a 'savior' god and emphasizing her royalty and power, an attribute important to her association with the Ptolemaic queens but as much an Egyptian interpretation as a Greek one.

Healing traits are occasionally, however, still visible in the Greek and demotic Egyptian 'magical' papyri, the *PDM* and *PGM*.[46] Like the Isean aretalogies and the *Hermetica*, these compilations developed out of the complex mutual re-imaginings and interactions of some elements of the Greek and Egyptian social elite.[47] Their content is that of syncretized, or universalized, gods and practices from Egyptian, Jewish, Greek and eventually Christian traditions into a pantheistic religious cosmos universally accessible to the learned—i.e. those with access to the sacred texts and their translations. This last requirement, in particular, articulated and maintained continuity with the pharaonic myth and ritual from which much of the material derived.[48]

The demotic texts, written by a single bilingual scribe, included both Greek and several forms of Egyptian, from contemporary language to older hieratic and Old Coptic glosses. The Greek papyri likewise frequently utilized passages or words of Egyptian in the form of *voces magicae*, many

---

[45] Zakbar, L.V. (1988). *Hymns to Isis in her temple at Philae*. See also n. 57 below, p. 62.

[46] Betz, H.D. (2nd ed., 1992). *The Greek Magical Papyri in Translation including the Demotic Spells*.

[47] Hymns of praise to Isis: Vanderlip, V.F. (1972). *The Four Greek Hymns of Isidorus and the Cult of Isis*. See also Heyob, S.J. (1975). *The Cult of Isis Among Woman in the Graeco-Roman World*; Charlesworth, J. (1994). *The Lord's Prayer and Other Prayer Texts from the Greco-Roman Era*, 243–244. The standard edition of the Hermetica is Nock, A.D. and A.J. Festugière. (1946–1954). For the *Corpus Hermeticum*: Copenhaver, B.P. (1992). *Hermetica: the Greek Corpus Hermeticum and the Latin Asclepius*.

[48] Derchain, P. (1962). 'L'authenticité de l'inspiration égyptienne dans le *Corpus Hermeticum*', *RHR* 161, 175–198. The non-technical *Hermetica* (2nd century CE), presented themselves as authentic Egyptian texts, demonstrating the 'naturalization of philosophy' into an Egyptian tradition: Preus, A. 'Greek philosophy in Egypt', in Coleman, J.E. and C.A. Walz. (1997). *Greeks and Barbarians*, 155–174. Cf. Fowden, G. (1986). *The Egyptian Hermes* 1–4, 140–141, 161–213.

of which were probably derived from Egyptian cultic ritual. Some appear purely Egyptian in origin. Many have elements very similar to much older examples of ritual practices, and contain little or no re-envisioning in terms of Greek and Judaic gods and concepts. *PGM* LI 1–27, for instance, was a necromantic request that follows the format of the classic 'letter to the dead', known from about 15 very early examples.[49]

The healing prescriptions in the *PGM* and *PDM* are generally brief recipes with little in the way of mythological or magical apparatus, but there are a few exceptions that utilized the myths of Isis and Horus in traditional healing fashion. For example, the demotic xiv. 1219–1227 featured a feverish and headachy Horus, son of Isis, finding the rest of the gods eating the produce of the Nile. Horus is the analogue of the patient, who rhetorically asks: 'Does Isis [stop] making magic? Does Nephthys stop curing?' Similarly *PGM* CXXII 1–55, reliably dated to the time of Augustus, was a love spell that utilized both Greek imagery of Aphrodite, and Isis' association with Osiris. It has an additional clause in which Osiris', Ammon's, Isis' and Nephthys' headaches will last until they have cured the sufferer. Threatening the gods, like the shared state of gods and patient, is characteristic of Egyptian ritual.[50] Finally, *PGM* XXVIIIa.1–7, b.1–9 and c.1–11 offered three incantations against the 'scorpion of Artemisos' using *voces magicae* which seem to contain the name of Horus.

So there is evidence that traditional Egyptian forms of healing ritual involving the creative causal roles of the gods sometimes survived in Hellenizing translation. More often, however, Isis' expanding identity in Hellenistic contexts reduced her dependence on the more distinctive aspects of pharaonic religion.[51] Her healing power was invoked in a manner continuous with her pharaonic self but less tied to specific mythic elements and traditional medical formulae, in line with an emphasis on her general attributes of care and protection, so that, unlike Sarapis or Imhotep-Asklepios, she was rarely presented in a specifically medical context.

For the majority of Egyptians, however, there is no reason to postulate a discontinuity in their relations with Isis and other gods through small village shrines, usually the most powerful available settings for appeals

---

[49] Mainly of the Old Kingdom and First Intermediate period (2686–2055); none are later than ca. 1069. See Wente, *Letters*, 212–219; Gardiner, A.G. and K. Sethe. (1928). *Egyptian Letters to the Dead*.

[50] Ritner, R.K. 'The religious, social and legal parameters of traditional Egyptian magic', in Meyer, M. and P. Mirecki. (1995). *Ancient Magic and Ritual Power*, 49. For the use of such 'spells' in medicine see 4.3.1, 185–187.

[51] Cf. Fowler, *Egyptian Hermes*, 66; Frankfurter, *Religion*, 100.

to the gods by people of low status and income, including appeals for healing or protection from illness. Deities of local shrines were necessarily generalists. A second-century BCE letter from an Egyptian farmer, of the village Kerkeosiris, incidentally revealed that its author had been to the local sanctuary of Isis in search of healing:

> To Menkhes, komogrammateus of Kerkeosiris, from Haryotes son of Phaësis, cultivator of crown land and an inhabitant of the said village. While I was in the great temple of Isis here for devotional purposes on account of the sickness from which I am suffering, on the 23rd of Pachon in the 3rd year, Horus son of Haryotes, a resident (*katochos*) in the aforesaid temple of Isis, picked a quarrel with me ...[52]

It is not entirely clear how Haryotes planned to appeal to or gain assistance from Isis' sanctuary, or how long he stayed there. The fact that his attacker was a *katochos* shows that, even in a small local sanctuary, people could remain within the precinct for reasons of their personal relationship with the god.[53] Priests may have been present at least some of the time; evidence from the Roman period shows them making the rounds of small village shrines.[54]

One or more such local cults might have emphasized Isis as a healer, preserving aspects that have faded from the extant literary-religious tradition. Among such particularized cults in the Roman period, probably derived from earlier tradition, were the oracular Isis of Menouthis (near Kanopos) and the agricultural Isis at the southern oasis site of Kysis (Kharga).[55] The most important and powerful temple of Isis to survive, on the southern island of Philae, seems nonetheless to have had little to do with healing.[56]

---

[52] *P.Tebt.* I 44, TM 3680 (114): Μεγχεῖ κωμογραμματεῖ Κερκεοσίρεως παρὰ Ἁρυώτου τοῦ Φαήσιος βασιλικοῦ γεωργοῦ τῶν ἐκ τῆς αὐτῆς. ὄντος μου ἐπὶ θεραπείαι ἐν τῶι αὐτόθι μεγάλωι Ἰσιείωι χάριν τῆς περιεχούσης με ἀρρωστίας, τῆι δὲ κγ τοῦ Παχῶν τοῦ γ (ἔτους) Ὧρος Ἁρυώτου τῶν κατοικούντων ἐν [τ]ῶι δεδηλωμένωι Ἰσ[ιεί]ωι συστησάμενός [μοι μά]χην ... For 2nd century BCE Kerkeosiris: Crawford, D. (1971). *Kerkeosiris*, 86–93. Menkhes: Verhoogt, A. (1998). *Menches, komogrammateus of Kerkeosiris.*

[53] For the dreams of the *katochos* Ptolemaios of the Memphis Sarapieon, see 2.3.5, pp. 79–80. For the (disputed) meaning of the term, see e.g. Kessler, D. (1989). *Die heilige Tiere und der König*, 139–142.

[54] Frankfurter, *Religion*, 100: officials in one 2nd century CE town make the rounds for rituals at shrines which lack permanent staff. Priests could be borrowed from other temples: Evans, J.A.S. (1961). 'A social and economic history of an Egyptian temple in the Greco-Roman Period', *YCls* 17, 205–206.

[55] Menouthis: Frankfurter, *Religion*, 163 (Roman period). Kysis: Frankfurter, *Religion*, 47, with bibliography.

[56] Of the six or seven known Isieia built in Greco-Roman Egypt, all except the Sarapiea of Alexandria are of Roman date: listed in Wild, R.A. (1981). *Water in the Cultic Worship of Isis and*

The textual decoration and official inscriptions of the temple suggests that this was very much a site of the royal and cosmic Isis.[57] This is supported by Andre Bernand's study of the Greek graffiti, which concluded that they served chiefly as declarations of loyalty to these qualities and their manifestations in current politics, trading on Isis' dynastic affiliations and her traditional role in providing cosmic protection for the pharaoh.[58] Griffith thought that the unusually large number of demotic inscriptions at Philae were left by mainly local visitors, which would be in keeping with the provenance of religious graffiti from the pharaonic period. There is very little evidence for non-local pilgrimage by Egyptians.[59]

Although only a small minority of visitors left inscriptions, and many of those do not explain their purpose, comparison with other sites suggests that examples of medical appeals would survive if the sanctuary was a well-known healing destination. At Abydos, Greek inscriptions, by visitors to the deserted Osirieion there, included several references to healing by Sarapis.[60] At Philae, however, none of the inscriptions involved such appeals; nor did they seek assistance with childbirth or fertility. The nearest is a Roman demotic inscription, by Pakhom son of Lucius, which described him as having come with his family, who were 'all in misery together.' He asked Isis to be reconciled to him.[61] Appeals with similar content are known from

Sarapis, 208 n. 9, who also includes the Sarapieon of Kanopos in this group. Fifteen earlier Isieia in Egypt and Nubia (Wild, *Water*, 208 n. 10) were mainly small in scale and importance. See also the evidence for the worship of Isis, Osiris and Sarapis in Fayum villages and towns of the period: Zecchi, M. (2001). *Geografia Reliogiosa del Fayyum*, esp. appendix 2 and for Greek evidence, Rübsam, W. (1974). *Götter und Kulte in Faijum während der griechisch-römisch-byzantinischen Zeit.*

[57] Haeny, G. (1985). 'A short architectural history of Philae', *BIFAO* 85, 197–223; Vassilika, E. (1989). *Ptolemaic Philae*; Dietze, G. (1994). 'Philae und die Dodekaschoinus in ptolemäische Zeit', *AncSoc* 25, 68–72. For the ideological framework of Isis' cult at Philae see Zakbar, L.V. (1988). *Hymns to Isis in her temple at Philae.*

[58] Greek inscriptions: Bernand, A. (1969). *Les inscriptions grecques et latines de Philae*; declarations of loyalty, 1.55. See also Rutherford, I. 'Island of the extremity: space, language and power in the pilgrimage tradition of Philae', in Frankfurter, D. (1988). *Pilgrimage and Holy Space in Late Antique Egypt*, 229–256. Demotic graffiti published by Griffith, F.Ll. (1937). *Catalogue of the Demotic Graffiti of the Dodekaschoenus.* For *proskynemata* generally: Geraci, G. (1971). 'Ricerche sul Proskynema', *Aegyptus* 51, 3–211.

[59] Beinlich, H. 'Wallfahrt', *LÄ* 6, 1145–1146; Yoyotte, J. (1960). 'Les pèlerinages dans l' Égypte ancienne', 55.

[60] Perdrizet, P. and G. Lefebvre. (1919). *Les graffites grecs du Memnion d'Abydos*, nos. 8, 368, 390, 414.

[61] Griffith, *Catalogue*, no. 449. Translation from Rutherford, 'Island of the extremity', 240–241.

the New Kingdom, but there is not enough evidence to decide of what this 'misery' might have consisted, or whether, at Philae, such appeals were exceptional, or relatively common but unrecorded.[62]

Two other buildings at Philae might also have been used by those appealing for healing, health or fertility. A 'birth house' adjoined the Isis temple. Birth houses are a standard feature of the Ptolemaic era (the first examples are from the Late period).[63] They are decorated with the scenes and story of the birth of the young god in a divine triad; at Philae the triad is that of Horus-the-child, Isis, and Osiris. Because these smaller structures, linked to but separate from the sacred, restricted spaces of the principal temple, offer a celebratory evocation of fertility and maternal success, it seems plausible that people came to them to appeal for just those outcomes. No direct evidence, however, survives for this at Philae or at birth houses elsewhere. In the former, the decorative program again affirmed Isis' royal genealogy and protection of the king, rather than any invocation of her fertility or maternal nature. As for the island's small, unfinished temple to Imhotep-Asklepios, it might not have been in use after the reign of its founder, Ptolemy V, and there is no evidence of its being commonly visited for healing purposes.[64] In conclusion, it seems that Philae's ideological orientation was not that of a healing sanctuary.[65]

2.2.2. *The Sanctuaries and Roles of Sarapis*

In the Ptolemaic period, Sarapis appeared often as a healing god in both Greek literary materials and in connection with several sanctuaries of Osiris, in particular at Kanopos and Memphis.

The name Sarapis is a Hellenized form for the 'osiris' of Apis, the sacred bull of Memphis after its death and, hence, a form of Osiris, king of the afterworld and elder king of Egypt.[66] In the early Hellenistic period the Greek

---

62 For New Kingdom evidence, Sadek, *Popular Religion*, 237–238.

63 Daumas, F. 'Geburthaus', *LÄ* 2, 462–475.

64 Bernand, *Inscriptions*, 99–109, esp. 102 (no. 8); Wildung, D. (1977). *Imhotep und Amenhotep*, 153–162 (nos. 101–109). A reused block of stone supplies a fragment of a dedication to Asklepios, but little more than half the god's name can be read and the dating, on stylographic grounds, can be dated no more precisely than to the Hellenistic era: Bernand, *Inscriptions*, 385 (no. 127).

65 *Pace* Bernand, who views Philae as a healing sanctuary, and in agreement with Rutherford, 'Island of the extremity', 253: 'There is no sign that Isis or any other deity at Philae was approached as a healing deity.'

66 For Sarapis and Osiris-Apis: Hölbl, G. 'Serapis', *LÄ* 5, 870–874; Kessler, D. 'Das Hel-

cults of Sarapis, his sister-wife Isis, and their son Harpokrates, were patronized by, and strongly associated with, the ruling family. The association conferred legitimacy on Soter and his descendants in terms of Egyptian royal and religious ideology, by maintaining continuity with this Egyptian royal triad (Osiris, Isis and Horus-the-child). It also rendered participation in Sarapis' cult a declaration of loyalty to the governing ideology, especially in the first decades of Ptolemaic rule.[67]

In Egyptian myth and ritual, Osiris is the saved, not the savior; the self-determining process and state of renewal, not the third party agent of its coming to be for others. The mythic spine of the cult was his murder and dismemberment by the usurper Seth and subsequent restoration by Isis.[68]

This triumph over death ensured the continuation of rightful royal power, the renewal of agricultural and animal life in the Nile valley each year, and survival in the afterworld. The Greco-dynastic imagining of Osiris retained the focus on his roles of king and progenitor, with strong chthonic and solar associations. As Sarapis, however, he was represented in an active, bearded form, in keeping with Greek expectations about ruling male deities, even though Greeks perceived Sarapis as an Egyptian god.[69] His regenerative, beneficent and chthonic powers were similarly interpreted along interventionist Greek lines, and his healing activities emphasized, although he was never exclusively a god of healing in the way that Asklepios was. He seems also to have been associated with dreams; in Greece dream oracles were traditionally sent by Zeus, who was often identified with Osiris (Sarapis). Zeus Sarapis was a well-established identity by the later first century CE (although attestations in the Hellenistic period are rare, and none are from Egypt).[70]

The Athenian politician and one-time Peripatetic Demetrios of Phaleron was a high-ranking official in the early days of Ptolemaic rule, about 307–

lenistische Serapeum in Alexandria und Ägypten in Ägyptologischer sicht', in Görg, M. and G. Hölbl. (2000). *Ägypten und der östliche Mittelmeerraum im 1. Jahrtausend v. Chr.*, 163–230.

[67] For the Ptolemaic Greek cult see Stambaugh, J.E. (1972). *Sarapis under the Early Ptolemies.* Fraser, P.M. (1960). 'Two Studies on the Cult of Serapis', *OAth* 3, 3–54.

[68] Griffiths, J.G. 'Osiris', *LÄ* 4, 623–633. Allusively referred to in ritual and writings from the Pyramid texts onwards, the fullest version to survive is that of a 2nd century CE Greek author living in Boeotia: Plutarch, *Isis and Osiris.*

[69] An Egyptian god: e.g. Aelius Aristides *Oration* 2.68; Plutarch *Isis and Osiris* 362d.

[70] See Stambaugh, *Sarapis*, 82–83 with references. Two Hellenistic inscriptions: *CE* 126 (Delos, 112/111) and *SEG* XV 426 (Byzantion, 1st century). Roman era references: Tacitus *Histories* 4.84.5; Achilles Tatius *Leucippus and Clitophon* 5.2.1; *P.Oxy.* XI 1382, TM 63699 (2nd century CE).

280. According to Artemidoros' second century CE work on dream interpretation, Demetrios was the author of five books which consisted entirely or largely of records of dream 'orders and cures' provided by Sarapis.[71] A fragment of Diogenes Laertios' third century CE biography also linked Demetrios to a healing cult of Sarapis: 'He is said to have lost his eyesight in Alexandria and to have retrieved it from Sarapis, which is how he came to compose those paeans which are still sung today.'[72] Both claims might be apocryphal; they date from long after Demetrios lived and do not appear in other writers' accounts of his activities. They do attest, however, to an earlier tradition connecting Sarapis to healing, and in particular healing through dreams, which might go back to the early third century BCE, when Zoilos' dream also represented Sarapis in terms of illness and cure (see 2.1.2, p. 51).

Strabo's description of the visitors to the Sarapieon of Kanopos, seeking cures and dreams, implies that its reputation was greater than that of the contemporary Sarapieon at Alexandria.

> Kanobos has the sanctuary of Sarapis, which is honored with great reverence, and brings about cures, so that even men of the highest repute believe in it and sleep in the sanctuary on either their own account or on behalf of others. Some record the cures there, and others the wonders of its pronouncements.[73]

This may be due to a more general decline in the Alexandrian Sarapieon's popularity by the late first century.

The town of Kanopos, meanwhile, was a popular religious resort for Alexandrian tourists.[74] The dedicatory inscription of the Ptolemaic temple enclosure there has survived: it was founded under Ptolemy III and Berenike I 'to Osiris' (Ὀσίρει), possibly on the site of an earlier shrine. Apart from this, however, Kanopos has gone largely unexcavated and virtually

---

[71] 2.44 (*Bibliotheca Teubner* ed. R. Pack 171.11–18); translation from Fortenbaugh, W.W. and E. Schütrumpf. (2000). *Demetrius of Phalerum*, T86: ... συνταγὰς καὶ θεραπείας τὰς Σαράπιδος δοθείας.

[72] Diogenes Laertios *Lives of the Philosophers* 5.76. Translation: Fortenbaugh & Schütrumpf, *Demetrius*, T1, 19–21.

[73] Strabo 17.1.17 (C801): Κάνωβος ... ἔχουσα τὸ τοῦ Σαράπιδος ἱερὸν πολλῇ ἁγιστείᾳ τιμώμενον καὶ θεραπείας ἐκφέρον, ὥστε καὶ τοὺς ἐλλογιμωτάτους ἄνδρας πιστεύειν καὶ ἐγκοιμᾶσθαι αὐτοὺς ὑπὲρ ἑαυτῶν ἢ ἑτέρους. συγγράφουσι δέ τινες καὶ τὰς θεραπείας, ἄλλοι δὲ ἀρετὰς τῶν ἐνταῦθα λογίων. For Kanopos (modern Abuqir), see Thissen, H.-J. 'Kanopus', *LÄ* 3, 320–321. Breccia, E. (1926). 'Le rovine e i monumenti di Canopo', *Monuments de l'Égypte gréco-romaine* 1.35–50. Cf. p. 49 n. 10.

[74] Strabo 17.1.10 implies that the area of the Alexandrian Sarapieon was by then somewhat abandoned, but the grammar leaves it unclear if Strabo is including the Sarapieon itself.

nothing is known of the site beyond its description in the literary sources.[75] Strabo differentiates clearly between the issuance of oracles (τῶν ... λογίων) and cures (τὰς θεραπείας) there, though the vocabulary of incubation that he uses (ἐγκοιμᾶσθαι) might apply to both.

Archaeological remains do survive from the contemporary temple to Sarapis at Alexandria, also founded by Ptolemy III, that replaced a small earlier shrine to Isis and Sarapis.[76] A monumental approach featuring obelisks and (probably) Egyptian statuary exoticized a basically Greek architectural plan[77]—a reversal of the Sarapieon in Memphis, where Greek statues and decoration reinscribed the approach to the already existing Egyptian sanctuary of Osiris-Apis.[78] In Alexandria, dedicatory plaques placed in the Sarapieon's foundations, in accordance with Egyptian ritual, were written in both Greek and hieroglyphics.[79] One of the statues found on the site depicted an Egyptian priest, Pa-shere-en-ptah: although no Egyptian statuary is definitely attested for the Ptolemaic era temple, priests with Egyptian names are known for Sarapiea and Isea elsewhere within Egypt.[80] That at least some of the cult there accorded with traditional Egyptian ritual is suggested by the presence of a Nilometer. A hidden passage between two other buildings within the sanctuary could have been used for rituals unsuitable for general view, as at Edfu and Dendera, or possibly for a voice oracle.[81] The dedicating inscription for the small shrine of Harpokrates within the inner

---

75 *SB* V 8296 = Bernand, A. (1970). *Le Delta égyptien d'après les textes grecs*, 1.236–237 = Dunand, F. (1973). *Le culte d'Isis* 1.112–113. In the fourth century CE Rufinus identified depictions of a human-headed vase as the local cult variant, the so-called Osiris Kanopos (*Ecclesiastical history* 11.26), but other gods are known in this form and not all examples are from the region of Kanopos itself. See Panofsky, E. (1961). '"Canopus Deus". The iconography of a non-existent god', *Gazette des Beaux-Arts* 57, 193–216. For non-Osirian Canopic forms see Kayser, F. (1991) 'Oreilles et couronnes à propos des cultes de Canope', *BIFAO* 91, 215.

76 Tacitus *Histories* 4.84.

77 Rowe, A. (1946). *Discovery of the famous temple and enclosure of Serapis at Alexandria*; McKenzie, J. et al. (2004). 'Reconstructing the Serapeum in Alexandria from the archaeological evidence', *JRS* 94, 81 ff. Cf. the Greek design with Egyptian elements for Sarapiea and Isieia outside Egypt: e.g. Wild, *Water*, 209 n. 10.

78 For references see 2.6, p. 98 n. 189.

79 Rowe, *Discovery*, 13–14; McKenzie, 'Reconstructing', 82; Letellier, B. 'Grundungszeremonien', *LÄ* 2, 912–913.

80 Breccia, E. (1922). *Alexandria ad Aegyptum*, 44; Rowe, *Discovery*, 60–61; cf. Fraser, *Alexandria*, 1.266. Egyptian statues on site are attested for the Roman period and might have been present in the Ptolemaic temple also: McKenzie, 'Reconstructing', 100–101. Fraser, 'Two studies', 18 n. 4: an Egyptian priest of Sarapis at Philae (see p. 71 n. 102).

81 McKenzie, 'Reconstructing', 89. The function of the extensive underground passages known from the Roman period temple is unclear, but sacred animal burials are a possibility: Wild, *Water*, 99.

court says that it was founded by Ptolemy IV in accordance with the orders of Sarapis and Isis: another example, as in many of the dream narratives, of the role of oracular divine instruction in the foundation story of a cult. It may have functioned as an Egyptian 'birth house'.[82]

The practice of incubation is not well attested at sanctuaries of Sarapis and Isis outside Egypt, and even within the country the Kanopos Sarapieon's reputation for incubatory healing marked it as special.[83] This seems likely to have been the result of contingent circumstances, including the town's proximity to Alexandria in the early years of Macedonian rule. Perhaps Greek visitors at the beginning of Ptolemaic rule understood the original sanctuary of Osiris as an oracular site of a powerful god, who was already closely linked to the dynastic house. The site's reputation would have snowballed rapidly at the expense of its nearest rival, encouraging its use as an incubatory oracle, and by Strabo's time this had become a regular feature of the newer sanctuary. Such circumstances were not necessarily replicated elsewhere. In the next section, 2.3, we shall examine closely the archaeological and textual evidence for a site often identified, in both ancient and secondary literature, as one of the principal locations for temple healing in Ptolemaic Egypt.

2.3.1. *Healing and the Sacred Animal Necropolis at Saqqara*

The city of Memphis, a former capital of Egypt and the first residence of Ptolemy I, was located on the west bank of the Nile just north of the Fayum, a region of intensive Greek settlement.[84] The leading god of Memphis itself was the craftsman god Ptah; but the divine Apis bull—not a species sacred to a god, but an individual—also had a stall and sanctuary within the city.[85] A large population included several originally immigrant communities,

---

[82] Rowe, *Discovery*, 55. Birth house: Arnold, D. (1999). *Temples of the Last Pharaohs*, 285–286. Cf. Vespasian's vision in the Roman era temple: Tacitus *Histories* 4.81–82. The tradition of kings experiencing epiphanic visions of gods has several pharaonic precedents: kings were natural recipients of important messages from the gods and had access, as chief official of all cults, to their most sacred rooms.

[83] Renberg, G.H. (2003). 'Was incubation practiced in the Latin West?', *Archiv für Religionsgeschichte* 8, 105–147 found no evidence for incubation at western sanctuaries. Wild, *Water*, 2–3: water features at Sarapiea and Isieia linked to purification, not incubation.

[84] Herodotos 2.99.4; Strabo 17.1.31–32.

[85] Apis: Herodotos 3.28.3; Diodoros 1.84.4–85.5; Strabo 7.1.22, 27, 31; Pomponius Mela 1.9.58; Plutarch *Isis and Osiris* 43 and *Moralia* 718b; Aelian *Nature of Animals* 11.10. Winter,

such as Phoenicians, Jews, and the descendants of Greek and Carian mercenaries and settlers, in separate quarters of the city.[86]

The modern village of Saqqara occupies the separate site of the sacred animal necropolis, and included temples to gods strongly associated with both healing and oracles: Imhotep (Asklepios) and Osiris-Apis (Sarapis). The necropolis was situated on the high ground to the north of the city and inhabited by numerous permanent residents working in the temples and the associated trades, as well as a floating population of transients. The career of Ptolemaios son of Glaukias gives some idea of the pluralistic nature of the area and the complexity of ethnocultural identity possible.[87] The son of a Macedonian soldier and, probably, an Egyptian mother, he spent at least 20 years as a recluse or detainee (*katochos*) in the temple of the Syrian goddess Astarte on the Memphite necropolis, while writing letters and autobiographical texts in reasonably literate Greek. In a complaint to the Greek administration of the area, Ptolemaios claimed to have been twice beaten up for being Greek.[88] He was certainly bilingual, however, and most of his friends and acquaintances have Egyptian names.[89]

The principal buildings of the sacred animal necropolis had been constructed between the early and middle fourth century under the last indigenous kings, although the area had been used since the Old Kingdom for burials of important officials.[90] The most important of these sanctuaries, which Greeks called the Sarapieon, was that of the 'osiris' of Apis. The bodies of the dead bulls, carried up from Memphis, were entombed in the catacombs in great granite sarcophagi. The site of the temple of Imhotep, the great Asklepieion (House of Imhotep, *Pr-' Ỉj-m-htp*), is uncertain, as is the loca-

E. (1983). *Der Apiskult im alten Ägypten*; Kater-Sibbes, G.J.F. and M.J. Vermaseren. (1975). *Apis*; Kessler, 'Das Serapeum'.

86 Strabo 17.1.32. Thompson, D.J. (1988). *Memphis under the Ptolemies*, 82–105.

87 Wilcken, U. (1927). *Urkunden der Ptolemäerzeit* 1; Thompson, *Memphis*, 217–219.

88 παρὰ τὸ Ἕλληνά με εἶναι: *UPZ* I 7.21–22 (163), TM 3398 and *UPZ* I 8.14 (161), TM 3399 (ἐμέ τε παρὰ τὸ Ἕλληνα εἶναι). See further 2.3.3, pp. 74–75 and 1.3.1, p. 31 n. 124; and for his dreams, 2.3.5, pp. 79–80.

89 Cf. the bilingual dream of his friend Nektembis: *UPZ* I 79 (159), TM 3470; also *P.Cair.Goodsp.* 30.7–9, TM 10308 (after CE 192), where the author proposes in Greek to record his dream in Egyptian.

90 For the animal necropolis, see the excavation reports of W.B. Emery in *JEA* 1965, 1966, 1969, 1970, 1971; Guilmot, M. (1962). 'Le Sarapeion de Memphis', *CdÉ* 37, 359–381. Martin, G.T. (1981). *The Sacred Animal Necropolis at North Saqqara: the southern dependencies of the main temple complex*; Smith, H.S. and S. Davies. 'Sacred animal temples at Saqqara', in Quirke, S. (1997). *The Temple in Ancient Egypt*, 112–131.

tion of his actual tomb.[91] Elsewhere on the necropolis were the catacombs and temples of jackals (sacred to Anubis), cats (Bastet), falcons (Horus), ibises (Thoth), baboons (Thoth), and the Isis cows, mothers of the Apis bulls. In addition to Sarapis and Imhotep/Asklepios, Thoth, Horus and Isis were also gods strongly associated with medical knowledge. Healing was not, of course, exclusive to any cult.

2.3.2. *The Sarapieon of Memphis: The Greek Dream Interpreter*

Around the year 200 BCE, a small inscribed stone stele was erected in the precinct of the Memphis Sarapieon. It displayed a clearly recognizable color painting of the Apis bull standing beside an altar. Two women with abaci on their heads frame the scene. The iambic inscription read: 'I interpret dreams, having instructions from the god, with good fortune. This interpreter is Kres.'[92]

Kres[93] offered a Greek language service for pilgrims or inhabitants who had experienced a dream oracle, probably in the necropolis or at the outer limits of the Sarapieon precinct itself. A major sanctuary was a place where one naturally found authoritative dream interpretation: visitors might come specifically for that or make use of the opportunity while there on other business. The dreams might have been experienced through incubation, but we cannot reliably identify a location for this activity. (Some buildings in the necropolis area have been proposed as possible sites for incubation, apparently on the grounds that no evidence particularly suggests any other activity).[94]

The concept of interpreting symbolic dreams was common to both Egyptians and Greeks of the Ptolemaic era.[95] In both cultures it was a service

---

91 Smith, H.S. 'Saqqara. Late Period', *LÄ* 5, 412–428, surveys possible candidates for the temple site.

92 *SB* I 685, TM 6574: Ἐνύπνια κρίνω τοῦ θεοῦ πρόσταγμα ἔχων, τύχ' ἀγαθᾶι. Κρής ἐστιν ὁ κρίνων τάδε. Among the various publications, for the stele as a whole, see especially Edgar, C.C. (1903). *Catalogue Général des Antiquités Égyptiennes du Musée du Caire: Greek Sculpture* (CGC) 53, no. 27567. Cf. Roeder, G. (1960). *Kulte und Orakel im alten Ägypten*, 192–194, pl. 14; Winter, E. (1983). *Der Apiskult im alten Ägypten*, 34, and fig. 10; Kater-Sibbes and Vermaseren. (1975). *Apis I*, 10, no. 25 (with bibliography).

93 Κρής as personal name: Fraser, P.M. and E. Matthews. (1987). *A Lexicon of Greek Personal Names*. Or, 'of Crete', as e.g. in La'da, C.A. (2002). *Foreign Ethnics in Hellenistic Egypt*, 133, no. E1102.

94 See further 2.3.4, pp. 77–78 and 2.3.3, p. 73 n. 108.

95 The earliest explicit evidence for interpretation of a god-sent dream in Egypt is from

one would expect to find near a sanctuary, but the personnel involved were somewhat different. Even in the Ptolemaic period, when Egyptian dream interpretation was probably a routine activity of the *pr ʿnḫ* (the archive-scriptorium of a temple), it was not a specialist skill. Interpreters consulted dream books of this and earlier periods, which summarized dreams and categorized them as 'favorable' or 'unfavorable'. John Ray has argued that the temple staff involved were the *pastophoroi.* This Greek term (meaning carriers of sacred objects) specified one of the functions of temporary or minor cult officials, who underwent purification for various cultic roles.[96] Thus dream-interpreters attached to Egyptian temples were not usually high-ranking officials. Their status reflects, however, not the status of dream interpretation in itself, but the status of those making the inquiry. Dream interpretation was practiced authoritatively and in difficult cases by important temple officials, as the second-century BCE archive of Hor reveals (below, 2.3.5, pp. 78–81).[97] But the Greco-Roman *oneiropolos*, a specialist explainer of cryptic dreams, was essentially a freelance profession; one of the businesses that flourished around a sanctuary without being officially a part of them.[98] In fourth century Greece one Lysimakhos apparently scratched a 'very poor' living in a manner very similar to that of Kres, 'from a kind of tablet for interpreting dreams, while sitting next to what is called the Iakkheion ...'.[99] This tablet may be an early dream interpretation handbook; 'Antiphon' is said to have written a book about dream interpretation at around the same time.[100] The only such work to survive is Artemidoros' second century *Oneirokritika.*

As for content, extant demotic dream-books and the *Oneirokritika* contain many examples of illness-related dreams, predicting onset or recovery, but not offering medical advice. A god-sent dream might be more expansive, but professional interpretation was not a crucial element of the dream-

---

the seventh century BCE: the 'Dream Stele' of king Tanutamani (664–656): Szpakowska, *Closed Eyes*, 54–57.

96 Ray, J.D. 'Phrases used in dream-texts', in Vleeming, S.P. (1987). *Aspects of Demotic Lexicography*, 89–91. *UPZ* I 84.79: ἐνυπνιοκριτής.

97 Cf. king Tanutamani's highly symbolic dream in the seventh century BCE (above, n. 95), which was interpreted in politically useful terms, probably by the leading priest of the principal god of the period: the first servant (*ḥm nṯr tpy*, high priest, first seer) of Amun-Ra in Thebes.

98 For the earliest mention see Akhilleus at *Iliad* 1.43ff.: 'Come, let us enquire about some *mantis* or *hiereus* or interpreter of dreams (*oneiropolos*), for dreams come to us from Zeus ...'.

99 *SOD* T104 = Plutarch *Aristides* 27.3–5, quoting Demetrios of Phaleron's lost *Sokrates.*

100 Diels, H. and W. Kranz. (1964). *Die Fragmente der Vorsokratiker*, B78–81a, cf. A1–2, but in fact this author is probably not Antiphon the sophist.

oracle, even at a temple, and interpretation was not very standardized between or within either tradition. Asklepieian dreams were usually non-symbolic and self-explanatory. Aristides' were sometimes puzzled over by himself, friends, fellow-incubants and family, but were generally explained by events. He seems never to have consulted a professional dream interpreter or handbook.

Some bilingual *pastophoroi* might have offered dream interpretation to private clients.[101] Kres might have been one of them. People with Greek names working as temple staff occur from both the Late and Ptolemaic periods, occasionally even holding high level positions in Egyptian cults.[102] Other dream-interpreters (ἐνυπνιοκριταί) capable of working in Greek are attested for the Memphis Sarapieon. He might also have been working on a strictly private basis.

The Zenon archive contains an example of the kind of divine instructions that Kres might have had to interpret, or produce. Several decades before Kres' advertising stele was erected at the Sarapieon, the Greek estate manager received a letter requesting medical supplies:

> Dromon to Zenon, greetings ... As you are about to sail up in good health, instruct someone in your employ to procure a *kotyla* of Attic honey. For I have need of it for my eyes, according to the instructions of the god.[103]

Dromon's letter uses the standard Greek formula for divine instruction, *kata prostagma tou theou*, a phrasing almost identical to that of the Kres stele. Zenon is plainly in Alexandria, but Dromon himself is up river and quite possibly in Memphis. In this context, 'the god' may be Asklepios, but Sarapis is more probable. Honey is a common ingredient in both Greek and Egyptian medical prescriptions, but that it should be from Attica in particular

---

101 Such (unspecified) private commissions are attested for at least the Roman period, according to the Gnomon of the Idios Logos (*BGU* V 1210, TM 3475). This forms part of a much larger text, itself datable to after CE 149. See Rowlandson, J. (1998). *Women and Society in Greek and Roman Egypt*, 174–177.

102 Ray, J.D. 'Jews and other immigrants in Late Period Egypt', in Johnson, J.H. (1992). *Life in a Multi-Cultural Society*, 273: a fourth century carer for the sacred ibises with the name of Ariston. Eraton, the 2nd century high priest of Isis at Philae: Bernand, *Inscriptions*, no. 14 (142) and no. 23 (114) = *PP* 3.5385. Cf. Syron, a priest of Sarapis and Isis who also left an inscription (of uncertain date) at Philae: Bernand, *Inscriptions*, no. 85, and Ptolemaios, of Macedonian male descent and a resident in the Astartieion of Memphis (cf. 1.3.1, p. 31 and 2.3.3, pp. 74–75; for his dreams 2.3.5, pp. 79–80).

103 *P.Cair.Zen.* III 59426, TM 1066 (263–229 BCE): cf. 2.1.1, p. 48. Δρώμον Ζήνωνι χαίρειν ... ὡς δ' ἂν ἀναπλέηις ὑγιαίνων, σύνταξόν τινι τῶν παρὰ σοῦ ἀγοράσαι μέλιτος Ἀττικοῦ κοτύλην, χρεῖαν γὰρ ἔχω πρὸς τοὺς ὀφθαλμοὺς κατὰ πρόσταγμα τοῦ θεοῦ. (ll. 1, 5–7).

implies that at some stage those *prostagma tou theou* were understood in terms of Greek medicine. A parallel can be found in another third century Greek letter to Zenon, whose writer is also seeking medical ingredients of Greek origin—wine from Lesbos or Khios, and honey (variety unspecified).

> If we had found for sale in the the market-place anything of what is written below, in accordance with the doctors' prescriptions, we should not have troubled you; but as it is we write to you of what it is that we have need, as Apollonios thinks necessary. So if it is convenient for you, send to us a jar of wine from Lesbos or Khios, as sweet as possible, and in particular a khous-measure of honey; and if not, as much as you can get: also arrange that a jar is filled full of salted fish for us. For they judge there is much need of both these. If then we should be healthy and go abroad to Byzantion, we will bring you back excellent salted fish.[104]

In this case, however, the instruction comes not from a god but from physicians (*iatroi*). The god's command to Dromon is therefore roughly in line with contemporary Greek medical practice.

2.3.3. *The Sarapieon of Memphis: The Greek Medical Text*

The letters to Zenon above demonstrate a typical feature of ancient medicine across cultures. Most healing involved the use of pharmaceutical substances (including foodstuffs), generally in combination with ritual oral formulae. Pharmaceutical treatments were a long-standing area of cross-cultural interaction and an important part of international trading relations.[105] Most Greek healers combined oral formulae with more material substances; the treatments of the extant Egyptian medical papyri and healing spells employ similar techniques. New drug formulations multiplied within healing traditions and the lists of alternative ingredients could be adapted to different botany and biology, or according to criteria such as expense, making foreign pharmaceutics just another option subject to avail-

---

104 *PSI* IV 413, TM 2096 (third century): ... εἰ μὲν ἦν τι τῶν ὑπογεγραμμένων̣ π̣ράσιμον λαβεῖν ἐκ τοῦ ἐμπορίου, καθάπερ οἱ ἰα[τ]ροι συντάσσουσιν, οὐκ ἂν ἐνωχλοῦμεν ὑμᾶς: νυνὶ δὲ γεγράφαμέν σοι ὧν χρείαν ἔχομεν, καθάπερ Ἀπολλώνιος ᾤιετο δεῖν. εἰ οὖν παράκειταί σοι ἀπόστειλον ἡμῖν ο[ἴνο]υ τε ἢ Λεσβίου ἢ Χίου κεράμιον ὡς ἡδίστου, καὶ μέλιτος μάλιστα μὲν χοῦν, εἰ δὲ μή, ὅσον ἂν ἐνδέχηται: καὶ ταρίχου τὸ σταμνίον σύνταξ[ο]ν ἡμῖν ἐμπλῆσαι. τούτων γὰρ ἀμφοτέρων πλείστην χρείαν νομίζουσιν εἶναι. ἐὰν γὰρ ὑγιάνωμεν καὶ εἰς Βυζάντιον ἀποδημήσωμεν, ἄξομεν ὑμῖν πάλιν σπουδαῖον τάριχον.

105 Guralnick, E. 'The Egyptian-Greek connection in the 8th to 6th centuries BC: an overview', in Coleman, J.E. and C.A. Walz. (1997). *Greeks and Barbarians*, 127–154; Totelin, L. (2009). *Hippocratic Recipes*.

ability and the authority of the source advising them. Trade offered access to special ingredients—such as Egyptian exotica in classical Greek pharmaceutics. The transmission of information and ingredients went both ways: late Ptolemaic and Roman demotic papyri on medicine included substances from Greek and Roman parts of the world;[106] in the second century CE Galen attributed several pharmaceutical innovations to the sanctuary of Hephaistos (Ptah) in Memphis.[107]

Memphis' location near the trade route of the Nile, its close relations with the régime, and its large and diverse population was ideally suited to such adaptive interchange. Fragmentary books of Egyptian medical recipes and incantations have been found in two rubbish dumps near the northern part (Hepnebes) of the sacred animal necropolis.[108] A demotic accounts list mentioning 'the sick' was found in the same sector.[109] Further away, within the main Sarapieon precinct, an unpublished papyrus contained 'a piece of a Greek medical text'. E.G. Turner, in his preliminary report, dated the papyrus to the fourth or third century; he was unable to identify the Greek treatise on it with any other known work.[110]

The presence of medical texts in the temple sanctuaries is in itself not surprising. Technical materials, including medicine, were regularly part of the attached libraries, reflecting the temples' distinctively Egyptian function as centers of expertise and learning. Variant and sometimes conflicting versions of many texts—including medical papyri, demotic dream-books, narrative fictions and myths—accumulated; while some were no doubt better known or more authoritative than others, there was no canon that automatically excluded other works. They were kept not only as culturally valued texts, but also as materials used regularly by the cult officials. The Greek

---

106 E.g. Reymond, E.A.E. (1976). *A Medical Book from Crocodilopolis*. See further 3.4, pp. 135–136, nn. 127, 130; 4.2.3, p. 167, n. 107.

107 Galen *The compounding of drugs according to kind* 5.2 (13.778 Kühn).

108 Martin, *Sacred Animal Necropolis at North Saqqara*. Both dumps are in sector 7, the area south of the principal sanctuaries of the northern sacred animal necropolis (Hepnebes, containing the baboon, falcon and mothers of Apis temples). The South Dump (part 9: 57–61) contained demotic fragments; the West Dump (part 10: 62–68) fragments of a hieratic medical text. Martin suggested that the adjacent building, Block 5, might have been an 'incubation centre': see p. 77 and n. 122.

109 Davies, S. and H.S. Smith. 'Sacred animal temples at Saqqara', in Quirke, S. (1997). *The Temple in Ancient Egypt*, 124.

110 Preliminary description: Turner, E.G. (1975). 'The Greek papyri from Saqqara', *Proceedings of the XIV International Congress of Papyrologists, Oxford, 24–31 July 1974*, 250. The text was never published and the photographs of it have since disappeared. I am grateful to Professor John Tait for his help on this matter.

name for the *ḫry-ḥbt*, 'lector priest' (lit. he who is with the book), shows how religious authority in Egypt was derived from access to the exclusive, reliable information and the instantiated magical power of writing. The lector priest carried (literally, in the form of the rolled-up papyrus scroll) the ritual functions of the temple into the community; lector priests read the set incantations during funerary preparations and used the medical papyri in their role as healers.[111] The subject matter of the text found in the Sarapieon is unfortunately lost, but Turner's remarks suggest that it was not simply a list of recipes.

We know that Greek and demotic texts were copied for or collected by cult officials even at small village shrines in the Fayum, supporting the possibility that medical works in Greek and other languages might have been collected, copied, and perhaps used by cult officials at Egyptian sanctuaries.[112] Many Egyptians who dealt regularly or officially with Greeks were bilingual, while the reverse was much less common, and at Memphis temple staff were in regular contact with the local and Alexandrian military and civil administration. Cults competed both economically and for cultural-political influence with other shrines and places. Such competition motivated cult officials, artisans and providers of related services to adapt to the expectations of their visitors.

So while the Greek medical text may have been in private hands or in use only among people of primarily Greek linguistic and medical habits, it may be evidence of cultural interchange of this type, perhaps as providers extended their pharmacological range or adjusted to the assumptions or preferences of clients. If so, it was, like the demotic pharmaceutical compendia, probably utilized by doctors resident in the necropolis, and possibly by Osiris-Apis' own cult officials. The *katochos* Ptolemaios, writing a complaint in Greek, mentions the *iatroklystes* Harkhebis. This individual was one of a number of necropolis residents who attacked Ptolemaios for reasons that are not entirely clear; an event that places Harkhebis in a social circle of temple cleaners, water carriers, bread makers, a cloak seller, and so on.[113]

---

[111] Eberhard, O. 'Cheriheb', *LÄ* 1, 940. For lector priests and other cult officials as healers see 5.1.1, pp. 206–212.

[112] Minnen, P. van. (1998). 'Boorish or Bookish? Literature in Egyptian villages in the Fayum in the Graeco-Roman Period', *Journal of Juristic Papyrology* 28, 99–184. See further 2.6, p. 100; 3.3, p. 129 and especially 5.2.1, pp. 221–222. A private copy might belong to the family of such an official, doctor or other literate individual.

[113] *UPZ* I 8.34, TM 3399 (161), l. 34: Ἁρχῆβ[ις]..[ἰατρο]κλυστής. In *UPZ* I 7 (163), TM 3398, line 11, the same individual appears as Ἁρχήβιος ἰατροῦ. Cf. 1.3.1, p. 31, n. 124; 2.3.1, p. 68, n. 88; 2.3.5, pp. 79–80.

He was not one of the medical experts of the upper cult hierarchy, but was probably identified in demotic texts as a *swnw* (physician), albeit one of relatively limited status and authority, or possibly as an 'amulet man' (*s3w*). In any case, he demonstrates that the long-term and temporary population of the sacred animal necropolis was sufficient to sustain specialized medical experts.

2.3.4. *The Asklepieion of Memphis: The Greek Patient*

A fragmentary letter in Greek, dating to the mid or later third century, refers to someone who was ill and—apparently as a consequence—in a temple of the Memphite necropolis: '... know that Satyros is sick in Memphis and spending his time in the Asklepieion ...'.[114] The sanctuary in question was not the Sarapieon but the Asklepieion, that is, the temple of the deified official Imhotep.

It was not unusual for the chronically ill to remain at Asklepieia in the Greek world for long periods. An epigram by the early 4th century orator Aiskhines, inscribed in the Epidaurian sanctuary as a dedication, says that he was cured of an head wound after spending three months in an Asklepieion.[115] In the second century CE the wealthy Aelius Aristides remained a regular incubant at the Pergamon Asklepieion for two years. He was not, however, a resident in the abaton or sanctuary itself, but stayed in the house of his friend the priest.[116] Incubants from further afield, especially those who stayed for any length of time, were relatively wealthy individuals.[117] The other principal category of those seeking cures or treatment at temples was the local area resident.

As mentioned above, (p. 73, n. 109) a demotic accounts list discovered on the necropolis makes frequent reference to a category of 'the sick'. It could be a list of medical pilgrims staying on the site, perhaps as incubants. The casualness of the references of the letters from the Zenon archive to the

---

114 *P.Petr.* III 42.H(4) = P. *Petr.* I 30, TM 7670 (third century BCE): ... γίνωσκε δε] [Σάτ]υρον ὄντα ἐν Μέμφει ἀρρωστοῦντα καὶ τ[ὰς δ]ιατρ[ιβὰς ποιούμενον ἐν] [τ]ῶι Ασκληπιείωι ...

115 *Palatine Anthology* 6.330.

116 For his 2 years as incubant: *Sacred Tales* 2.35, 46, with 2.78 and 4.106–107. Behr, 30 note 39: 'IV 89–90 must refer only to a brief visit, as does IV 83.' In 5.28, Aristides stays at an inn.

117 Cf. Dillon, M. (1997). *Pilgrims and Pilgrimage in Ancient Greece*, 80, for the tendency of the major healing sanctuaries to attract the upper socioeconomic groups; a point also emphasized by Behr, 42, with regard to Aristides' social circle at sanatoria.

Asklepieion of Memphis and 'the god' who prescribed for Dromon (pp. 71–72) demonstrated a familiarity with healing at the site among Greeks living or traveling in the region.[118]

The list might also have referred to a category of those off work through sickness, as in the accounts from the workmen's village of Deir el-Medina, during the New Kingdom, or the Roman period records for quarrying at Mons Claudianus.[119] The Deir el-Medina records refer to some of these injured or ill workers being treated by the village's medical experts.

Among the large numbers of dedicatory offerings found on the sacred necropolis are some plaster casts in the shapes of human body parts, mingled with other votives in the upper baboon gallery or in a large cache nearby, where they were buried in sand in front of the entrance to an Old Kingdom tomb. They are cast in the shapes of hair, torsos, legs, hands and feet, and two male faces, one with the eyes covered by a lump of plaster. There were also casts of wigs, a beardless king wearing the double crown, a hawk, and the left side of a child's head with the features obscure and the ear in high relief.

Some of these may have originated as practice casts during the making of statuary in the local workshops.[120] The ear relief on the child's head probably references a god's 'hearing ear'; this kind of votive was common in the pharaonic era (above, 2.1.4, p. 56). Ears were also dedicated at Asklepieia but similarly imply not the deafness of the pilgrim but the attentiveness of the god. The majority of these casts, however, are probably anatomical ex votos that depict the part of the body involved, as their original excavator, W.B. Emery, thought. As no parallels are known from Egypt, Emery argued chiefly on the basis of comparative votives at Greco-Roman Asklepieia from outside Egypt. Terracotta versions have been found at the

---

[118] Much of the evidence for the cult of Sarapis and healing at Memphis derives from the protagonists of the Zenon papyri. As Fraser, *Two Studies*, 7 points out, these are a significant but atypical minority of the (Greek) population. It is also among this sometimes bilingual class of administrators and agents that the cult of Sarapis was at its most popular.

[119] Janssen, J. (1980). 'Absence from work by the necropolis workmen of Thebes', *SAK* 8, 127–152. Examples from Roman Mons Claudianus: e.g. *O.Claud* II 191–210, TM 23961–23980 (ca. CE 138-ca. 154) and *O.Claud.* II 211, TM 23981 (ca. CE 138-ca. 154). See also the summary of these texts by Cuvigny, H. 'La mort et la maladie', in Bingen, J. et al. (1992–2000). *Mons Claudianus, Ostraca Graeca et Latina* 2.19–21.

[120] Emery, *JEA* 1970, 5–11. Davies and Smith, 'Sacred animal temples' 123 n. 67, suggest that the example with the covered eyes and a few others mimic the condition relieved by the god. They also argue that the single detached limbs would not have been useful as models. But many of the casts were not so detached. Similar votives were found in the settlement of the Anubieion: see Jeffreys, D.G. and H.S. Smith. (1988). *The Anubieion at Saqqâra* 1.63, n. 3.

sanctuaries of Corinth and Rome, while the inventories of the Athenian Asklepieia list many dedications, often of gold or silver, in the shape of body parts.[121]

The lack of parallels from pre-Roman Egypt is a problem, but the few examples of dedications in thanks for healing that have survived suggest that such votives were—as in the Greco-Roman world—diverse and rather free form, being largely at the discretion of the giver and chiefly concerned with the particular circumstances of the case. Anatomical votives could have developed within the Egyptian tradition; alternatively they originated or were popularized in response to demand from Greek pilgrims. Votive makers offered customers a skilled rendition in suitable materials of the customer's own sense of what was an appropriate dedication.

So far the evidence indicates that Greek pilgrims from the Fayum and further afield joined local inhabitants of the Memphis area in seeking the help of the necropolis gods. Experts in medicine and dream interpretation were available among cult officials or on a private basis. Medical texts in both languages were collected and used by medical practitioners associated with the temples; pharmaceutical recipes and perhaps incantatory formulae—to judge from the *PDM* and *PGM*—were borrowed or adapted between linguistic and medical traditions. Some sick people remained on site, possibly in the precinct of the temple of Imhotep. The cache of anatomical probable ex votos, the only known example of this type of votives in Egypt, is support for the idea of Saqqara and Memphis as a center of healing pilgrimage.

An ancillary building in the Hepnebes area (p. 73 n. 108), originally identified as a small temple but with puzzling features, might have been an 'incubation center.'[122] The fragmentary medical papyri found in rubbish dumps near this building, including the accounts list for the sick, remain the only positive evidence for a sanatorium or incubation center for healing (the former does not necessarily include the latter function). Other excavators have suggested that an area of the Anubieion, some distance away at the western entrance, constituted quarters used by incubants; some view the

121 Athens: Aleshire, S. (1989). *The Athenian Asklepieion*, 4–5 and especially van Straten, F. 'Gifts for the gods', in Versnel, H.S. (1981). *Faith, Hope and Worship*, 105–149. Corinth: Roebuck, C. (1951). *The Asklepieion and Lerna*, 114–128, pls. 33–45. Cf. at a sanctuary of Demeter in Thrace: Vavritsa (1973). *Praktika tes en Athenais Archaiologikes Hetaireias* 77, 79 with pls. 93, 95.

122 Martin, *Sacred Animal Necropolis*, part VI: 34–51, 'Block 5', esp. p. 35 (cf. p. 73 n. 108 above).

Bes chambers, also within the Anubieion, as having an actual incubatory function (along the lines sometimes suggested for birth houses).[123] They contained groups in which Bes was flanked by naked female figures, so would have been for fertility rather than other kinds of illness. 'Incubation' in this context might mean either communication with the divine through a dream; or a response from a god in the form of a more direct intervention, i.e. a cure.

All these suggestions beg the question of whether Memphite incubation was a regular feature of any cult for which provision for visitors needed to be made. The clients of Kres, or of those *wꜥb* (pure) temple personnel who had access to dream books, may or may not have experienced their dreams on site. The anatomical casts, if indeed they are ex votos, indicate that appeals for healing were being made, but not that such appeals regularly took the form of incubation. Dromon's letter to Zenon could be a non-dream oracle, a category for which there is also evidence from the sacred animal necropolis; or it might refer to a dream experienced elsewhere, such as at home, as with the dream of the Egyptian priest of Sarapis on Delos (2.1.2, p. 51 n. 19).

The best evidence for incubation, including incubation for medical problems, at the sacred animal necropolis does not relate to provision for pilgrims, but comes from individuals within the temple community itself. The texts in question are the archive of Hor, an Egyptian cultic attendant of the Ptolemaic era; and the funeral stele of Taimhotep, the wife of Memphis's high priest at the end of Greek rule in Egypt. Their evidence, discussed below in 2.3.5 and 2.3.6, demonstrates the fact of incubation and other dream-oracles at Ptolemaic Saqqara. From the greater extent and detail of these texts, moreover, we can draw out some tentative ideas about the procedures and context of dream-related healing at Saqqara, and about the people and goals involved.

2.3.5. *Hor*

In the years between 1965 and 1972, a cache of demotic ostraka was excavated from the Memphite necropolis. It contained a series of autobiographical drafts by Hor of Sebennytos, mainly concerning his dreams and their

123 Davies and Smith, 'Sacred animal temples', 114, 124; Thompson, *Memphis*, 25–26; Frankfurter, *Religion*, 171–172, who notes that Bes is not attested as an oracle until the Roman era.

relation to events in his life. He was experiencing dreams at Memphis by 171, and from the mid-160s was a permanent resident there, as a minor cult official of Thoth's ibis-cult.[124]

Some dreams were particularly cryptic. These required expert interpretation by high-level officials in several major cults, such as the lector priest of Imhotep, a specialist in such technical knowledge.[125] Several concern personal and administrative tensions among officials; and occasionally Hor's dreams became items of national political importance, gaining him high level contacts within the administration and, on one occasion, an audience with the king and queen. It is therefore not surprising that one dream involved Isis supplying, via Hor, a 'remedy' (*pẖrt*) for the queen.[126] Egyptian medical recipes included both an incantation and a material component. Hor's dream demonstrates that by the second century, this kind of detailed medical instruction could be part of the dream experience among Egyptians. Finally, the dream of *O.Hor* 13 was achieved through incubation: the solicitation of a significant dream in a sacred place. In lines 1–7, the suppliant prays to the gods for a visitation in the ibis-galleries; on the third day he seems to have obtained a vision, described in the more fragmentary remainder of the text, from line 8.[127]

This ostrakon is strong support for incubation as a regular part of necropolis temple activities, and as the precursor to interpretative services like those provided by Kres. At around the same time, the personal archive of Ptolemaios son of Glaukias, the Sarapieon *katochos*, also testified to the importance of dreams as a mode of access to the gods. His brother Apollonios eventually despaired of his family's trust in dreams, accusing the gods of having misled them.[128] Yet nothing written by Ptolemaios about his dreams or those of his friends and family mentions solicitation, though an incubatory setting is arguably built into his permanent location as a

---

124 Ray, J.D. (1976). *The Archive of Hor (O.Hor)*, with 3 other texts and ibid. (1978). 'Observations on the archive of Hor', *JEA* 64, 113–120. For the few associated Greek ostraka see Ray, *Archive*, 1–3. All translations by Ray.

125 In the pseudo-epigraphic Ptolemaic-era inscription often referred to as the 'famine stele', Imhotep interpreted the dream of king Djoser (= Netjerkhet, ca. 2668–2600 BCE), see Lichtheim, *Literature*, 3.94–103. For the oracular power of Imhotep as a god in the Ptolemaic era see section 2.4.1 below.

126 *O.Hor* 28, possibly also *O.Hor* 32; see Ray, *Archive*, 134.

127 Ray, *Archive*, 6–7 nn. a-m ad loc., especially b, c, f. The date was probably 10 March 155. Ray also views *O.Hor* 12 as an example of incubation; and invocations of *O.Hor* 10 (to Isis) and 18 as soliciting dreams: 131–132.

128 *UPZ* I 70, TM 3461 (152). For Ptolemaios see also 1.3.1, p. 31; 2.3.1, p. 68; 2.3.3, pp. 74–75.

detainee within the Sarapieon enclosure. (He had small, shared living quarters in the temple to Astarte).[129]

Given that proximity to sacred space, a doorway between the mortal and the otherworld, a precise, fixed location is equally unimportant for Hor's incubatory modus operandi. In *O.Hor* 13, one of the gods he prays to is Osiris-Mnevis, the dead sacred bull of Heliopolis, who has no cult or place on the sacred animal necropolis of Memphis. The supplications to this god and to Osiris-Apis are made neither in Heliopolis nor in the Memphite Sarapieon, but 'before the house of rest of the ibis'; that is, the catacombs of the ibises sacred to the god Thoth. Thus incubation practiced by Hor utilized the semi-sacred spaces of the sacred animal necropolis available to him as a minor cult official of the ibis cult, but within those limits the actual location of his dreams appears to have been both variable and irrelevant.[130] An *abaton* was not required.

Ptolemaios, as far as we know, did not take his dreams to any cult official or other interpreter, in spite of their frequent opacity. He also failed to translate his visions into high level political access, again unlike Hor. Hor is in fact not typical of many of the city's residents, whatever their cultural and linguistic background. His official status within the cult of the ibis was apparently lowly, only a little higher than that of Ptolemaios, yet it is clear from the archive as a whole that he was fully integrated into the powerful religious and civil networks of Lower Egypt in the middle decades of the second century.[131] His use of dreams should be seen in this context. It is partly a continuation of the long tradition within Egypt of the use of oracles in literary and especially biographical constructions justifying events and actions. But Hor has successfully extended personal meaning into political power, a more recent development in which the potential of dreams to bypass institutional structures—such as other kinds of oracle—is fully utilized. This use of dreams to authenticate authoritative and important knowledge obtained by a member of a lower elite—as a literate individual Hor remains within a very small minority of the Egyptian population—seems to be a development of the Late and Ptolemaic periods. Oracles had conferred legitimacy on kings since the New Kingdom; Hor invents himself as a personal oracle. Nonetheless he still operated within the political-

---

[129] Clarysse, W. (1986). '*UPZ* 6a, a reconstruction by Revillout', *Enchoria* 14, 43–49; Ray, J.D. 'The dreams of the twins in St. Petersburg', in Szpakowska, *Through A Glass Darkly*, 189–203.

[130] Cf. Ray, *Archive*, 56 note d.

[131] Ray, *Archive*, 117–124. Ptolemaios was also on the temple payroll, under the direction of the *pastophoroi*: Thompson, *Memphis*, 218–219.

religious structures and networks of the temple and administration: the lector priests of the cults interpreted his dreams.

Thus Hor's incubation(s) and Ptolemaios' dreams are significant evidence for the developing use and importance of dreams within the community of a sanctuary complex with political connections. They are however not representative of the experiences of visitors to the sanctuaries. They do not show that incubation was a routine, expected part of an oracular or healing event. The same applies to the last instance of a significant dream experienced in Ptolemaic Memphis and frequently cited as an example of incubation.

2.3.6. *Taimhotep*

Dating from the late first century, the funeral stele of Taimhotep, wife of Psentais III, the first servant of god of Ptah, displays her autobiography, including her inability to produce a son.

> ... I was pregnant by him three times but did not bear a male child, only three daughters. I prayed together with the high priest to the majesty of the god great in wonders, effective in deeds, who gives a son to him who has none: Imhotep son of Ptah. He heard our pleas, he hearkened to our prayers. The majesty of this god came to the head of the high priest in a revelation of truth (*m wp mꜣʿt*). He said: "Let a great work be done in the holy of holies of Ankhtawi, the place where my body is hidden. As reward for it I shall give you a male child." When he awakened from this he kissed the ground to the august god. He gave the orders to the prophets, the initiates, the priests, and to the sculptors of the gold-house also. They did as he had said. He performed the opening of the mouth for the august god. He rewarded the sculptors on behalf of the god. He gladdened their heart with all good things. In return he (the god) made me conceive a male child. He was born in year 6 [38 BCE], day 15 of Epiphi, in the 8th hour of the day, under the majesty of the queen, the lady of the Two Lands, Cleopatra, life-prosperity-health. It was on the offering-feast of the august god Imhotep son of Ptah. His (the child's) appearance was like that of the Son of South-of-his-wall. There was jubilation over him by the people of Memphis. He was given the name Imouthes (Imhotep) and was also called Pedibast. Everyone rejoiced over him ...[132]

It is unclear whether this vision was solicited, where it occurred, or whether a dream was expected as the form of the response to the high priest's prayers. In other words, Taimhotep's stele is not reliable evidence for

[132] BM 147. Lichtheim, *Literature* 3.59–65. Wildung, *Imhotep*, 68–70 (no. 45).

incubation either, but does indicate continuity within the Egyptian tradition for appeals to the gods and the terms used to describe the ways by which they reveal their wishes and presence. The phrase translated here a 'revelation of truth' (*m wp mꜣ't*) is used for such an epiphany in a much earlier parallel, *The Instruction of Amenemhat*. There is disagreement over whether the phrase necessarily signifies a dream, but night-time visions, described in Greek texts of the Ptolemaic period, followed a similar pattern.[133] In exchange for some public display advertising the god's power, usually a building, the dreamer is saved or rewarded, and the genre is common to Egyptian and Greek texts. In the Greek examples, Zoilos and certainly the Delian priest Apollonios situate their unsolicited dreams as taking place in their own homes; narratives of Soter's dream also fail to specify any sacred space or an incubatory context (2.1.2, p. 51 n. 19).

The funeral stele of Taimhotep—our main medical example—advertised the power of a Memphite god and the successful efforts of her husband on Imhotep's behalf. The experience is described using a language of revelation that has long-standing antecedents; it does not imply (or exclude) incubation as the mode of solicitation. Hor constructed his biography by utilizing the intimacy of a dream relationship with a god to its full extent; this might have been a relatively new development in Egyptian oneiromancy. The self-identified Greek recluse Ptolemaios, meanwhile, sought a similar understanding through dreams, but could not find a similarly transformative meaning. Kres was more successful. At least as biculturally fluent as Ptolemaios, he offered a service that suggested a significant number of clients preferred a speaker of Greek as well as Egyptian, albeit one of low cultic status.

In conclusion, this evidence indicates that in the Ptolemaic period (as earlier) dreaming was a mode of contact with the gods employed in Egyptian cultic contexts. Such dreams were often solicited, sometimes by sleeping in a sacred place. Looking more closely at the narratives of Hor and Taimhotep, and the way in which they used dreams to construct their social

---

133 Gunn, B. (1941). 'Notes on Ammenemes I', *JEA* 2, 2–3, thought it meant 'revelation in a dream', the meaning also favored by Lichtheim (who translates as 'revelation'). The standard Egyptian term for 'dream' is *rsw.t* or *ḳd*. In the *Instruction of Amenemhat*, the same phrase is employed for the king's appearance to his son in a vision. Anthes, R. (1957). 'The legal aspect of the Instruction of Amenemhat', *JNES* 16, 176–191, argued that *m wp mꜣ't* should be translated 'determination of right' and means Imhotep is the one who reveals truth to her husband. Szpakowska, *Closed Eyes*, 10, takes a similar line for the *Instruction* with the translation 'revelation of truth'.

and biographical identity, we can see that significant dreaming offered a personal and flexible relationship with the gods, which Hor and others were able to transmute into authority and status within both a cultic context and the larger political-religious world. But this is evidence about a particular and quite specialized group of people. It tells us nothing about the practice of dreaming and its relationship to medicine for other groups of people, such as visitors to a sanctuary.

Such visitors left traces of their presence at the joint sanctuary of the healing-oracular cults of Imhotep-Asklepios and Amenhotep, at Deir el-Bahari on the Theban west bank. In the following section, 2.4, we examine both this evidence and, firstly, the evolving roles and representations of Imhotep and Amenhotep in Greco-Egyptian culture.

2.4.1. *Imhotep (Asklepios) and Amenhotep (Amenothes): The Pre-Ptolemaic Background*

The god Imhotep appeared in the lives of Hor and Taimhotep even though both were more immediately connected with other divinities. Memphis' necropolis was the center of his cult, but he was represented in sanctuaries and votive offerings throughout Egypt during the Ptolemaic era, especially in the north. Worship of Imhotep originated in the mortuary cult of an Old Kingdom official, but since the Late Period Imhotep had been supplied with divine ancestry as the son of Ptah.[134] It is, as always, difficult to establish whether this secure authority among the elite was reflected in any 'popular' worship of the god. In the south he was usually depicted in conjunction with the similarly deified official Amenhotep son of Hapy, whose origin, iconography and functional attributes were very similar to those of Imhotep.[135] Amenhotep had also been a high-ranking official with a subsequent mortuary cult: the architect and 'director of all works' of king Amenhotep III in the fourteenth century.[136] One important aspect of his position was to

---

[134] In general, Wildung, *Imhotep*. For the acquisition of divine status by Imhotep and Amenhotep, and what it signifies, see the discussion by Laskowska-Kusztal, E. (1984). *Le sanctuaire ptolémaïque de Deir el-Bahari*, 89–104. Amenhotep is first attested as a god in a private Greek text of the third century, followed slightly later in demotic sources: Lajtar, A. (2006). *Deir el-Bahari in the Hellenistic and Roman Period*, 24–25; Wildung, *Imhotep*, 153–162 and 189–192 (nos. 101–109, 131–132).

[135] Wildung, *Imhotep*, 201–220, 241–244 (nos. 142, 153).

[136] Amenhotep, son of Hapy: Helck, W. 'Amenophis', *LÄ* 1, 219–221; Wildung, *Imhotep*, 201ff.; Sadek, *Popular Religion*, 278–280; Varille, A. (1968). *Inscriptions concernant l'architecte Amenhotep fils de Hapou.*

mediate between the king and those requiring the king's favor; statues of Amenhotep son of Hapy erected in Thebes, both during and after his lifetime, were employed for this mediation between mortals and divinities, and advertised this role for Amenhotep. By the Late Period his reputation as an oracle and a healer was well established. A votive stele dedicated in 628/627 by a daughter of the royal household made preemptive thanks for the cure of her eye problem: '... May you cause that I be healthy at once. I have made this as recompense for it'.[137]

Imhotep and Amenhotep were gods closely associated with the healing of illness and infertility, as numerous inscriptions from temple decorative programs show. At Philae, the birth house contained decoration, carried out under Ptolemy VIII, which declared Imhotep to be: 'Master of life, giving life, lord of health, bringer of life to the dead ...'.[138] In the hymn inscribed on the southern doorpost of Ptah's sanctuary at Karnak, composed under the Roman emperor Tiberius, Imhotep protected Egypt, drove out diseases, granted life and health, cured sterility, and prolonged life, a 'helpful god, coming to the one who calls upon him, granting life to all men.'[139] The Vatican's 30th dynasty statue of Psentais, probably from Memphis, carries two inscriptions: 'An offering which the king gives to Imhotep, son of Ptah, who heals illness, who cures the limbs', and '... from the lord of life who gives a son to him who asks for a son, a woman to him who prays for her, and heals every suffering child.'[140] An official inscription from the mid-first century CE, on the pronaos façade of the temple to Hathor at Dendera, offered an inclusive list in which Imhotep was said to cure infertility, protect pregnant women and children, rejuvenate the elderly, and mitigate illness.[141] A list of his titles and powers at Deir el-Bahari included the phrase '... who gives air for the closed throat without breath ...', implying scorpion bite.[142]

---

137 *P.Choix* 15 (TM 46114); Malinine, M. (1953). *Choix de textes juridiques en hiératique anormal et en démotique* 1, 102–106.

138 Wildung, *Imhotep*, 166 (no. 116); *PM* VI 222 (194).

139 Lichtheim, *Literature*, 3.104–107, with earlier bibliography; Wildung, *Imhotep*, 206–209 (no. 143.1); PM II^2 197 (4c). A matching hymn to Amenhotep on the north doorpost is now badly damaged: Wildung, *Imhotep*, 209–211 (no. 143.2).

140 Vatican 163–164; Wildung, *Imhotep*, 42–44 (no. 20); Ritner, R.K. (1984) 'Review of Wildung *Imhotep und Amenhotep*', *JNES* 43.4, 354 translates the last phrase as 'gives ... health during every painful suffering'. *PP* III no. 5891: the statue may be Ptolemaic in date.

141 Wildung, *Imhotep*, 139 (no. 94b).

142 Laskowska-Kusztal, *Le sanctuaire*, 32–33 (no. 23). The name of the scorpion goddess Serqet means 'That one who makes the throat to breathe': von Kanel, F. (1984). *Les Prêtres-ouâb de Sekhmet et les conjurateurs de Serket*, 285. For priests of Serqet as healers, see 5.1.1., p. 208; 5.1.2, pp. 212–213.

At Edfu a caption dated to the reign of Ptolemy VI declares 'At his order all come to life, he cures all the illnesses in Egypt.'[143] At the small Ptolemaic temple to Imhotep, Amenhotep, and Thoth at Qasr el-Aguz, built in the later Ptolemaic period to the south of Medinet Habu, Amenhotep says to the king that he, 'drives out all the illnesses from limbs.'[144] Amenhotep was asserted to cure infertility in a demotic letter from the end of the third century.[145] Some of the many children at Memphis named for Imhotep—or, in Greek, for Asklepios—probably reference their parents' appeals for sons.[146] His shrine at Philae was dedicated by Ptolemy V and Cleopatra I with their son Philometor.

> ΒΑΣΙΛΕΥΣ ΠΤΟΛΕΜΑΙΟΣ ΚΑΙ ΒΑΣΙΛΙΣΣΑ ΚΛΕΟΠΑ[ΤΡΑ] ΘΕΟΙ ΕΠΙΦΑΝΕΙΣ ΚΑΙ ΠΤΟΛΕΜΑΙΟΣ Ο ΥΙΟΣ ΑΣΚΛΗ[ΠΙΩΙ]

Philometor was born in 186, after they had been married for seven years without a child, and it is tempting to see their dedication of the temple as a thank-offering for Imhotep's assistance.[147] Difficulties surrounding pregnancy and childbirth were common concerns in both Egypt and Greece. Fourteen percent of the inscriptions from the Asklepieion at Epidauros concerned infertility and pregnancy; only the blind were more frequent visitors. In Egypt, earlier medical texts testify to reproduction as a particularly common or important set of dangers, where amulets and other objects protected young infants from diseases and other evils.[148]

It is easy to see why Imhotep was identified as Asklepios, the Greek healer par excellence and another case of a mortal who became a god through his capacity to benefit humankind through knowledge. The identification was unusually exclusive: Imhotep is never identified as any other Greek god.[149]

---

143 Wildung, *Imhotep*, 141–142 (no. 96); *PM* VI, 140 (141a); Laskowska-Kusztal, *Le sanctuaire*, 110.

144 Wildung, *Imhotep*, 238 (no. 151.2). The temple was built in the time of Ptolemy VIII. For an oracular cult of ibis-headed Thoth, Imhotep and Amenhotep son of Hapy here see Quaegebeur, J. (1975). 'Tëephibis, dieu oraculaire?', *Enchoria* 5, 19–24; against this interpretation see Volokhine, Y. (2002). 'Le dieu Thot au Qasr el-Agoüz, *ḏd-hr-pj-hb, ḏhwty-stmd*', *BIFAO* 102, 405–423.

145 See below, 2.4.2, p. 91.

146 Thompson, *Memphis*, 209 (Imouthes, Peteimouthes, Asklepiades, Asklepios).

147 Bernand, *Inscriptions*, 99–102 (no. 8). For the temple see Wildung, *Imhotep*, nos. 101–110. In thanks for Philometor's birth, cf. Bernand 102; Arnold, D. (1999). *Temples of the Last Pharaohs*, 181; Lajtar, *Deir el-Bahari*, 12.

148 Baines, J. (1987). 'Practical Religion and Piety', *JEA* 73, 79–98.

149 Although Asklepios could be identified with Sarapis: the earliest example extant is Tacitus *Histories* 4.84.5. Amenhotep was not identified with any Greek equivalent; Greek texts simply transliterated his name as Amenothes.

The similarities, however, should not be overstated. The above formulae emphasized healing from amongst Imhotep's and Amenhotep's characterization as providers and guarantors of life, breath and health to the king, the sick, the dead, and the universe in general.[150] They knew the movements of the stars and were experts in ritual knowledge, in some inscriptions carrying the title *ḫry-ḥbt* (lector priest). Artistic representations of Imhotep and Amenhotep son of Hapy show each as a 'scribe' (*sẖ*), usually holding unrolled papyrus rolls.[151] Their divine nature was an extension of their mortal roles as these literate officials, whose elite position and religious function in Egyptian society derived from the understanding of written texts, an understanding closely connected to control of the creative or effective power *ḥkꜣ*. This kind of knowledge was applicable to all forms of maintaining, manipulating and strengthening forces of order and life in the universe, whether in terms of funerary architecture, the use of magic and writing, or the exercise of healing.

There are hints that Hellenizing identifications of Imhotep produced counter-reactions that reframed Imhotep as Egyptian and explicitly distanced him from Asklepios. In a later Ptolemaic or Roman Greek-language spell, 'Asklepios [who is worshipped] in Memphis' was addressed as 'MENOPHRI (he from Memphis)' and the magicians asked for 'the true Asklepios, not some deceitful daimon instead of the god.' Jacco Dieleman has argued that this shows a distinction was being drawn between Greek and Egyptian versions of Asklepios.[152] A similar approach is visible in a Greek text extant from the second century CE, *P.Oxy.* XI 1381 (TM 63689), which is also notable as a rare, though late, example of a dream-cure involving Imhotep.[153] It displays considerable continuity with earlier dream oracles, as it is a classic example of the genre of legitimizing a particular cult through the narration of a favor exchange between god and mortal, accomplished through the medium of dreams.

---

[150] See formulae quoted on p. 84 above, e.g. 'bringer of life to the dead'.

[151] Iconography: Wildung, *Imhotep*, 33 ff. For recent bibliography on statues of Amenhotep see Collombert, P. (2002). 'Une statue thébaine d'Amenhotep fils de Hapou trouvée à Esna', *BIFAO* 102, 137–142. Amenhotep more commonly wore an apron from breast to ankle; Imhotep a kilt, with the navel exposed: Teeter, E. (1995). 'Amenhotep son of Hapu at Medinet Habu', *JEA* 81, 234–235.

[152] *PGM* vii. 628–642. Dieleman, J. (2005). *Priests, Tongues, and Rites. The London-Leiden Magical Manuscripts and Translation in Egyptian Ritual (100–300 CE)*, 150 note 47.

[153] Wildung, *Imhotep*, 93–98 (no. 60) with Ritner, R.K. (1984). Review of Wildung 1977, *JNES* 44.4, 384.

The explanatory introduction of how the text came to be written has an unnamed first person narrator, whose mother had been ill for three years. The narrator and his mother therefore appealed to Imouthes (Imhotep), who duly appeared to her in dreams, prescribing simple remedies. When the narrator himself fell ill he saw the god in his dreams simultaneously with the waking vision of his mother: he was instantly cured. However their future requests for aid met with no response, and the god repeatedly told them, through his priest (ll. 85–86), that he was not satisfied by their expressions of gratitude. At last the narrator realized that a textual tribute was required. The ease and succinctness with which his book praising Imouthes-Asklepios was achieved convinced him he was right, just as the speed with which the Delian temple was constructed was attributed to Sarapis' involvement by Apollonios the priest, and just as Zoilos described himself as having been convinced by illness to get a move on with the same god's temple (2.1.2, p. 51 and n. 19). Events proved the dreams reliable.

In this work the god was addressed by both his Egyptian and Greek names, but seemed to be envisaged in Imhotep's traditional form: a temple scribe in Egyptian dress carrying a rolled papyrus in his left hand. He was taller than mortal and shone brightly, a characteristic sign of Egyptian divinity. The author characterized his aim in ethnolinguistic terms, seeking to co-opt the market reach of Greek culture in the service of the local Imhotep (ll. 198–202): Ἑλλην[ὶ]ς δὲ π[ᾶ]σα γλῶσσα τὴν σὴν λαλ[ή] [...]σε[ι] ἱστορίαν ḳ[αὶ] πᾶς Ἕλ[λ]ην ἀνὴρ τὸν ṭ[ο]ῦ̣ Φθᾶ σεβήσεται Ἰμοῦ[θ]ην. ('Every Greek tongue will tell your story, and every Greek man will worship the son of Ptah, Imouthes').

2.4.2. *Imhotep and Amenhotep at Deir el-Bahari*

The disappearance of Imhotep's temple and tomb at Memphis makes it difficult to establish much about the nature of healing practices there, but the southern site of Deir el-Bahari, with its dual cult of Amenhotep and Imhotep, is more informative.

Around 300 BCE, a shrine for Amenhotep became established in the abandoned funerary sanctuary of the female king Hatshepsut. It took over the upper terrance, and probably the rock-cut rooms behind it at the far western end. A less important cult of Imhotep was also installed there at some point between 300 and the later second century, around 124–117 BCE, when new building work was carried out.[154] Hieroglyphs on the north wall

[154] A portico with six columns, erected in front of the terrace, contains cartouches of

of this shrine name Amenhotep as 'the good doctor (*swnw nfr*) who protects the people of his city (Thebes)'.[155]

The first evidence for the cult is a Greek ostrakon of 261–260.

> Under the King Ptolemaios son of Ptolemaios, and Ptolemaios the son, in the 25th year, in the month Khoiak, Polyaratos set up this in order to make known the *aretê* of Amenothes [Amenhotep]. I became the victim of a serious and dangerous illness that lasted for eight years. [[Starting with the glands, my muscles were constricted along the whole body and I was paralyzed and I suffered pains that were difficult to withstand]]. I thought about salvation for a long time, but without result [---]. I had also recourse to physicians, but they were unable to make me healthy. Since I have heard from many people that Amenothes has accomplished numerous *aretai*, that he is merciful and that many desperate people have found salvation through him, so I [---], also being desperate, came, fleeing for protection, as a suppliant to the sanctuary of Amenothes [[with the supplication of which I have written a copy]]. Amenothes appeared to me and I was cured by him manifestly and I have been healthy. For that reason I would like to praise him and the gods worshipped together with him on the same altars and in the same temple, making known their *aretê* in the form of an inscription for all those who, affected by an illness, come to the sacred precinct of Amenothes in order that [[they know the power of the god who appeared manifestly]] they know [---] manifestly by the god who [---].[156]

Polyaratos' ostrakon is probably a draft of a more permanent record. This might be a stone inscription, as with other aretalogies and Asklepios' cures at Epidauros. Or it might be a textual archive in the keeping of the cult officials, to be shown to visitors. As with the much later papyrus narrative found at Oxyrhynkhos, *P.Oxy*. XI 1381 (pp. 86–87), the sufferer was ill for many years and exhausted other recourses before his eventual cure; the same motifs of baffled doctors and incurable, mysterious, chronic disease are present in Aelius Aristides' tributes to Asklepios and Sarapis in the second century CE.

In total, there are 320 Greek and about 180 demotic inscriptions extant from the sanctuary; as well as two bilingual examples and a small number

---

Ptolemy VIII Euergetes II. The decorative reliefs of Amenhotep and Imhotep were almost certainly added at the same time. Lajtar, *Deir el-Bahari*, 35.

[155] PM II² 368 (147) = Wildung, *Imhotep*, 223–224 (no. 143.4). Greek hymn: Lajtar, *Deir el-Bahari*, 22–46 (no. 219).

[156] Cairo Museum 67300. Entire text first published by Bataille, A. (1937). 'Nouveau fragment d'un ostracon concernant Aménothès fils de Hapou', *Études de papyrologie* 4, 125–131. Text according to Lajtar, *Deir el-Bahari*, 395–396, 'Reading text'. Translation by Lajtar, 396, slightly adapted.

of hieroglyphs.[157] Dating is difficult and usually relies upon paleographical considerations, but about 55 of the Greek and bilingual inscriptions are or might be from the Ptolemaic period; most but not all of the Greek inscriptions were written by people using Greek rather than Egyptian names. Most, especially the demotic inscriptions, employ stereotypical formulae and contain little information besides the visitor's name and sometimes occupation. Some of the Greek inscriptions were by the casual visitor, but the majority were *proskynemata* or used similar formulae. As Adam Lajtar, in his comprehensive publication and analysis of the site, points out (p. 87), even after allowing for more inscriptions than are currently extant, the vast majority of visitors, many of whom must have been illiterate, did not leave a written memorial. Among the earliest are some Macedonian Greeks, often in small groups of apparently touring soldiers, but later visitors—whether they wrote in demotic or Greek—seem to have been mainly from the local area, judging by their nomenclature and the occasional place name. Those who specified their occupation were predominantly of low social status, unlike the VIPs who visited Philae.[158] Among the Greek names is Zoilos the physician.[159] Some came more than once. Most could have made the return trip to the sanctuary in a single day, but a few are recorded as having stayed the night.

Imhotep never appears in demotic graffiti, but only in the reliefs and hieroglyphs of official decoration dating from the second century BCE, and most visitors, whether Greek or Egyptian, would not have comprehended hieroglyphics. His Greek presence is not much more noticeable. Asklepios is named in a very small proportion (13 out of 322) of the Greek inscriptions—again, probably only after the official renovation of the sanctuary under Euergetes II.[160] This low profile is typical for Imhotep in the Thebaid region, where the Memphite god is often shown in officially sponsored decoration during the later Ptolemaic and Roman periods, but lost out among lower status inhabitants to the locally well-established Amenhotep.

157 Greek and bilingual inscriptions: Bataille, A. (1951). *Les inscriptions grecques du temple de Hatshepsout à Deir El-Bahari*; and now Lajtar, *Deir el-Bahari* (including graffiti previously unpublished). Demotic: see a preliminary study by Winnicki (below n. 168), 101, and the inscription published by Spiegelberg, W. (1932). *Die demotischen Denkmäler*, 3.1–2, no. 50032 = Wildung, *Imhotep*, 262 (no. 167).

158 Only three of the signed texts suggest authors from beyond Thebes, and even those are probably temporary residents in Diospolis or Memnonia: Bataille, *Inscriptions grecques*, X. Cf. Lajtar, *Deir el-Bahari*, 83–84.

159 Bataille, *Inscriptions grecques*, no. 16; Lajtar, *Deir el-Bahari*, no. 25; *PP* IV 16601. Third or second century. Cf. nos. 94, 165: Roman era physician-visitors.

160 Lajtar, *Deir el-Bahari*, no. 116 is a possible exception.

A second Greek ostrakon found at the site is a collection of ethical maxims under the title Ἀμενώτου ὑποθῆκαι, the Instructions of Amenot(h)es.[161] These are of Greek origin, but have been somewhat recast and attributed to Amenhotep as an Egyptian embodiment of wisdom. They would appear to be an effort to assimilate Amenhotep into Greek religious and ethical tradition with the aim of popularizing a cult with no direct Greek equivalent. The Oxyrhynkhos papyrus from the Roman period also presents Imouthes—rather than Asklepios—for a Greek audience, as a figure of oracular power and a healer who visited patients in dreams.[162] A fragment of Manetho suggests a similar approach, in which the god's knowledge and oracular status is described for the Greek readers of *Aigyptiaka*: Amenhotep was a 'wise and prophetic man.'[163]

Among the Greek inscriptions, two of Ptolemaic date concern illness and healing, as do three or four from the Roman period.[164] Andromakhos the Macedonian, who was probably employed in the region of the sanctuary, left two missives to posterity, the second and fuller of which is as follows:

> Andromakhos, Macedonian, came as a hired worker to Amenothes, a good god, and became sick and the god helped him on the same day. Farewell.[165]

The simplest explanation is that Andromakhos felt unwell and later recovered, quite possibly without formally consulting Amenhotep at all. Certainly the specification of the 'same day' seems to rule out overnight incubation. Similarly nothing about the following request to the god on behalf of a third party implies an oracular inquiry or even formal appeal:

> I would like that my son (?) quickly becomes healthy again (for) he is suffering. Well be the one who wrote (this).[166]

---

[161] Bataille, *Inscriptions grecques* 1, 13; Wildung, *Imhotep*, 258–259 (no. 161), with discussion; see Lajtar, *Deir el-Bahari*, 27.

[162] Above, pp. 86–87.

[163] Jacoby, *FGrHist* no. 609 F 10a; Waddell, *Manetho*, fr. 54; Josephus *Against Apion* 1.26.232–233.

[164] Roman era inscriptions relating to healing: Lajtar, *Deir el-Bahari*, nos. 112, 129, 208, (?) 322 (Bataille, *Inscriptions grecques*, nos. 74, 86, 128, 182).

[165] Ἀνδρόμαχος Μακεδὼν ἀφίκετο πρὸς Ἀμενώθην χρηστὸν θεὸν μισθοῦ ἐργαζόμενος καὶ ἐμαλακίσθη καὶ ὁ θεὸς αὐτῷ ἐβοήθησε αὐθημερί. ἔρρωσο. DB 373. Bataille, *Inscriptions grecques*, no. 48a, 48b, cf. 43.; Wildung, *Imhotep*, 229 (no. 43); Lajtar, *Deir el-Bahari*, no. 68, 68a cf. no. 60; La'da, *Foreign Ethnics*, 168, no. E1407. Bataille and Wildung both translate 'worker for hire' but see Lajtar, *Deir el-Bahari*, 156, note ad loc. All translations from Latjar.

[166] Lajtar, *Deir el-Bahari*, no. 50. Bataille, *Inscriptions grecques* (no. 36) had a slightly different reading (uncle, not son). Possibly from the later Ptolemaic period.

In addition to Polyaratos' ostrakon (above, p. 88), evidence for written appeals comes from two Ptolemaic era demotic sources, a letter on a wooden tablet from the late third century and two ostraka of the second. Although neither gives a location, both almost certainly refer to the Deir el-Bahari sanctuary. On the wooden tablet, Ouserwer, divine father and god's servant of Amonrasonter, king of gods, asks Amenhotep to cure his wife's infertility.[167]

> The voice of a servant, the divine father and prophet of Amenrasonter, Ouserwer, son of Hor, son of Ouserwer, (addresses himself) to his master, the royal scribe Amenhotep, son of Hapy, the great god: If it happens that Taipe, daughter of Peteamestous, becomes pregnant, I will give a (deben of) silver, or 5 stater of silver, or, then, a (deben of) silver. If it happens that she gives birth, I will give another (deben of) silver ... the day that you do what I say.

On an ostrakon, similarly, a woman named Senamunis asks 'the master, the royal scribe, Amenhotep son of Hapy', to heal sterility. This was found in the bark shrine room in the Hatshepsut complex, and dates to the second century, probably to the reign of either Epiphanes (204–181) or Philometor (180–145).[168]

Senamunis' and Ouserwer's 'letters to the gods' are examples of an Egyptian oracle and appeal genre (2.1.1, p. 47 n. 4; cf. p. 80). The narrative on Polyaratos' ostrakon also suggests the process of obtaining healing involved a written petition or query (ll. 23–26). The god's response may be simply the requested result—pregnancy, a perceived improvement in illness—but Polyaratos' miraculous cure apparently followed a vision, probably during sleep and possibly following incubatory solicitation. His aretalogy is much fuller and free in its form than the two demotic examples: less a request than an autobiography.

The content of another demotic ostrakon, from the second century, is not an appeal to but a response from the god. It is possible that the following was the interpretation of a dream; but a reply to an oracle petition is at least as likely:

> I asked the great god Amenhotep. He answered that a fever was in the body of Teos and three Syrian figs may be given to him, watered from the evening to the morning ... The liquid shall be poured in a vessel with broken bread and

[167] Malinine, M. (1962). 'Une lettre démotique à Aménothès, fils de Hapou', *RdÉ* 14, 37–43 and plate 2; Wildung, *Imhotep*, 255–256 (no. 158); *PP* IX 5669d. Probably from the reign of Ptolemy IV: 221–205 BCE.

[168] Winnicki, J.K. (1983). 'Amenhotep son of Hapu and Imhotep at Deir el-Bahari—Some Reconsiderations', *MDAIK* 39, 93–105.

> mixed well. He shall drink this and shall continue for four days ... The god gave him a ... snake of iron, in order to tie it on his arm. There is no failure in it.[169]

The last line here is reminiscent of the assertions of effectiveness made for certain recipes in Egyptian medical papyri.[170]

All this evidence certainly implies the existence of an oracle at the sanctuary, one of a type that included the provision of detailed healing formulae rather than a simple yes-no answer. The iconography and titles employed in the hieroglyphic decoration, as analyzed by Ewa Laskowska-Kusztal, also indicate that Amenhotep and Imhotep had a strongly oracular identity at Deir el-Bahari. On yet another demotic ostrakon of around the same period (paleography suggests a date in the middle of the Ptolemaic era), the author reported dream content in need of interpretation, apparently experienced in a *mr* (sanctuary?)[171] of Amenhotep, with a strong implication of deliberate solicitation or at least expectation.[172]

> (A communication from) ... [] *hb* the chief of deliveries (?). I make salutations for you before the royal scribe Amen[hotep the] great [god] great of love who creates all good fortune for you. I came to this m[r] sanctuary of the royal scribe Amenhotep. Here are the dreams which I saw, specifically on the night of the 23rd through to the 24th. It was [a d]og (?) that I saw, which was running after an ibis, so that (I) said 'I shall need to [look] after it; rescue (?) it from him. [[But I could not (release) it]] from [his] mouth (?). The second ... The third (dream) [...

The listing formula ('The first dream ... the second dream ... the third dream ...') is characteristic of this demotic incubatory genre. The same organization can be seen in the archive of Hor, for example in *O.Hor* 8, as can the need for interpretation of such dreams.

The author might have come to the sanctuary only to gain interpretation for dreams he had elsewhere, as his approximate contemporary Hor

---

169 Thompson, H. (1931). 'A demotic ostracon', *Proceedings of the Royal Society of Biblical Archaeology* 35, 95–96 with plate 27; Wildung, *Imhotep*, 263–234 (no. 169).

170 E.g. Ebers 131: 'Truly effective a million times'.

171 For *mr*, meaning at Deir el-Bahari probably the temple of Amenhotep, see Lajtar, *Deir el-Bahari*, 20, 28–31.

172 Ostracon Nicholson Museum Sydney R. 98. Published by Ray, J.D. 'Dreams before a wise man', in Leary, A. and J. Tait. (1999). *Studies on Ancient Egypt in Honour of H.S. Smith*, 241–247. Figs are a common medicinal substance, with 50 mentions in the Ebers. The snake-form of the arm-ring may be a reference to Mertseger, goddess of the local sacred mountain area. She was identified with Hathor, to whom earlier visitors to Deir el-Bahari had appealed for healing.

went to the lector priest of Imhotep.[173] It is however easier to read the text as Ray did subsequently (Ray, 'Dreams'): the sanctuary is visited for the purpose of experiencing significant dreams, just as Hor certainly solicited some of his visions. But rather than deduce from a single ostrakon that visitors to Deir el-Bahari routinely sought dreams and had them interpreted, the parallels with the writings of Hor imply a similar category of inquirer: someone closely involved with religious activities in the area for whom access to sanctuaries could translate into close and personal access to the gods. This might represent a personal religiosity or concern with dream-meanings on the part of the dreamer, but, as with Hor, it also suggests that this person used dreams to assert his status and access to the otherworld of the gods. In previous eras, such access to the gods—like that of Amenhotep son of Hapy as a mortal—was very closely associated with having an official position within an institutional framework. Dreams, however, were a means of communicating with the otherworld that potentially bypassed such institutions.

The remaining piece of evidence for incubation at this site is from the second century CE. In a fascinating but sadly fragmentary text the soldier Athenodoros describes himself praying and invoking Asklepios, Amenothes and Hygieia, and then as having heard the god's voice and seen him 'in the night.' Athenodoros then opened the door of the god's sanctuary, stood in front of the god's image and seems to have asked for help, though the text is by now very broken. Subsequent lines mention illness, possibly as reprisal for invading the god's inner sanctum, and then cure. A voice oracle may be part of the explanation of this unique account, from a cult official normally hidden behind the door that separated the more public rooms of the cult from the inner sanctuary. Alternatively, all or part of this experience may be psychological, possibly—since it happened 'in the night'—even a dream.[174]

2.5. *Medical Modes at Healing Sanctuaries*

The evidence suggests that the inhabitants of the Thebaid perceived the sanctuary of Amenhotep at Deir el-Bahari as a significant sacred site. Visitors included Greco-Macedonian immigrants, as well as Egyptians and

[173] *O.Hor* 10.

[174] Lajtar, *Deir el-Bahari*, 60–61, 293–298 (no. 208); Bataille, *Inscriptions grecques*, 22–24 (no. 126). Other bibliography: see Lajtar, 293.

Greco-Egyptians literate in demotic. The sanctuary was however multifunctional. Firstly, it served its original purpose as the site of Amenhotep's mortuary cult. Secondly, the traditional understanding of Amenhotep and Imhotep as oracular and beneficent intermediaries was expressed in the reliefs and texts of the official redevelopment of the cult in the later second century, part of which role was the curing of illness and in particular infertility. The Greek and demotic ostraka, as well as a few inscriptions, testify to their healing functions and also to their oracular ones, from very early in the cult's history to at least the visit of Athenodoros in the second century CE. This kind of activity is not very different from that of an earlier stage in Deir el-Bahari's history, when Ramesside Egyptians applied to the houses of Amun and Hathor.[175]

Since most of the surviving inscriptional evidence is not related to healing or other prayers, there is very limited evidence from which to draw any general conclusions, negative or otherwise. There is however no reason to think that incubation was the only or the commonest method of obtaining the god's help at Deir el-Bahari, to the exclusion of other oracular methods. As reported by Strabo for Kanopos, both 'cures' and *prostagmata* may well have occurred at Deir el-Bahari. Moreover, some of those cures, like Andromakhos' (p. 90), might have occurred without incubation or epiphanic appearance. A basic difficulty with assuming incubation to have been a common practice is just how few texts mention dreams or sleep, as Malinine noted in his commentary on the Ouserwer text.[176] It is a difficulty that applies to healing sanctuaries in Egypt generally. Parallel texts on Asklepieian incubation, in contrast, use formulae that insist on sleep and vision, that is, e.g. compounds of verbs meaning 'sleep in a special place', such as ἐγκαθεύδω and ἐγκατακοιμάομαι, ἐγκοιμάομαι. Epiphanic vision is

---

[175] Graffiti from the 20th dynasty, with some from the 19th. One hundred forty-two such texts were published by Marciniak, M. (1974). *Deir el-Bahari* 1: *Les inscriptions hiératiques du Temple de Thoutmosis III*. For translation and brief commentaries see Sadek, A. I (1984). 'An attempt to translate the corpus of the Deir el-Bahari hieratic inscriptions', *GM* 71 and 72, 67–91 and 65–84.

[176] Cf. Sauneron, *Les songes*, 48: 'Il n'est pas certain que le songe ait été, en ce point d'Égypte, la méthode thérapeutique couramment appliquée: les textes sont muets sur ce détail'. Oppenheim, A.L. (1956). *The Interpretation of Dreams in the Near East*, 188: 'As to Egypt, it should be understood that, notwithstanding all statements in popular and semi-popular presentations, actual incubation dreams are not mentioned in pre-Ptolemaic texts and that the pertinent evidence even in the latter is very slim'. Grapow, H. (1956). *Grundriss der Medizin* 3.140: 'Heilungen durch Träume sind aus dem alten Ägypten nicht bekannt. Sie entsprechen griechischem Glaubem'. These remarks all predate the discovery of the archive of Hor and the demotic ostrakon quoted on p. 92 (cf. n. 172), but the overall picture has not changed much since.

indicated by ὄψις or ἐνύπνιον. Cures occurred, in the Epidaurian *iamata*, during sleep (ὕπνον; καθ' ὕπνον).[177]

I am not claiming, on the basis of an argument from silence, that incubation was definitely not a regular part of the process at Deir el-Bahari, or anywhere else. Most of the graffiti are devotional formulae and some consist only of a name: any number and variety of experiences at the shrine may lie behind these bare assertions of presence. But as G.H. Renberg argued in an article reassessing the evidence for incubation in the Latin West, 'the burden of proof must always be on those proposing that a site be recognized as an incubatory sanctuary'.[178] It is not enough to say with Lajtar (*Deir el-Bahari*, 52): 'One can presume that the major role in the healing process was played by incubation ...'. To assume that healing involving a god is synonymous with incubation is to rule out other, arguably more plausible alternatives on the supposition that all healing oracles worked in precisely the same way, whatever their god, history, or visitors. Such an assumption cannot be made even for Greco-Roman healing sites. References to dreams in the primary sources, which often lack any description of an institutional apparatus, are taken in the secondary literature as references to incubation. The support offered for this assumption is circular: either other noncommittal primary sources, or other unsubstantiated assumptions in secondary literature.[179]

At Karnak, a chapel of the Late period (664–332) in the precinct of Mut (another oracular god) contained three internal walls covered with 'healing' texts written in hieroglyphs.[180] These detailed the story of Isis' salvation of her young son Horus from the poisonous attacks of creatures associated with their enemy Seth.[181] The words of this significant myth of protection were, when activated, powerful against dangers, especially against toxic bites and (probably) other forms of illness. They appear also on the stone monuments (*cippi*), common from the Late Period onwards,

177 LiDonnici, L.R. (1995). *The Epidaurian Miracle Inscriptions*, 85 with n. 6, 46–47.

178 Renberg, G.H. (2003). 'Was incubation practiced in the Latin West?', *Archiv für Religionsgeschichte* 8, 105–147: 40.

179 Cf. Malinine, 'Une lettre', 41, disposing of his own suggestion (on the grounds of a parallel with Memphis), that incubation took place at Deir el-Bahari: 'Bien au contraire, des documents attestent formellement l'existence à Thèbes d'une practique differente conduisant à la guerison, fondée sur la consultation directe de la divinité.'

180 Traunecker, C. (1983). 'Une chapelle de magie guérisseuse sur le parvis du temple de Mout à Karnak', *JEA* 20, 65–92.

181 Isis is assisted by the gods Nephthys, Selket, and the powerful oracular-medical god Thoth.

that carried images and texts relevant to Horus' triumph over crocodiles and other chaotic beings. When water had flowed over this image, or over the powerful formulae often also inscribed on the stone, the water had the same power to protect and heal as did the words.[182] The preserved text at Karnak is a match (with some lacunae) for lines 168–204 of the largest and best known healing *cippus*, the Metternich stele.[183] The chapel might also have contained a healing statue. While some smaller *cippi* were probably for domestic use, larger examples stood in temple forecourts, places of relatively public access. Two are known from elsewhere in the Karnak complex.[184] François Daumas argued, in a classic article of 1957, that part of the sanctuary complex of Hathor at Dendera, a large mud-brick building erected early in the first century CE, was similarly a building designed for healing: a *cippus* on a larger scale. Water that had flowed over a large inscribed granite block (found in situ) would have run along the central corridor, to an area that contained a number of differently sized architectural features for bathing. Visitors literally soaked themselves in spells of protection.

Daumas also proposed, however, that the eleven rooms that opened off this corridor, each with a wall niche for a divine image, were for incubation during the healing process.[185] He cited in support J.S. Milne's belief that the references to healing in Deir el-Bahari graffiti involved incubation.[186] But a link between a *cippus* and visions of a god during sleep is otherwise unattested. The ancillary shrines at Dendera become incubatory only if we assume that incubation was a regular part of any medicine practiced at the temple of Dendera in the first century CE. Rather the Dendera building fits easily into the history of internal developments in Egyptian religious practice during the Late period and continuing into the Greco-Roman. The myth of Isis' salvation of Horus was of long-standing importance in Egyptian medical practice and protective 'magic.' By the Late period, the myth's power was available to local inhabitants in written form through the use of healing steles and statues situated in the outer, accessible, regions of

---

[182] Lacau, P. 1921–1922. 'Les statues 'guérisseuses' dans l'anciente Égypte', *Académie des inscriptions et belles-lettres, Commission de la fondation Piot, Monuments et Mémoires* 25, 189–209. For the use of water in this fashion see also Ritner, R.K. (1993). *The Mechanics of Egyptian Magical Practice*, 106–110. See 4.3.3, pp. 190–192.

[183] Republished by Allen, J. (2005). *The Art of Medicine in Ancient Egypt*.

[184] Frankfurter, *Religion*, 48; Traunecker, 'Une chapelle', 75.

[185] Daumas, F. (1957). 'Le sanatorium de Dendera', *BIFAO* 56, 35–57.

[186] Milne, J.S. (1914). 'The sanatorium of Deir el-Bahri', *JEA* 1, 96–98.

important temple precincts. More complex forms included immersion in water or being otherwise surrounded by its power, as in the Karnak chapel. As such, it complemented prayers to intermediary statues or 'hearing ear' shrines and provided the same ongoing protection as the obtaining of an oracular decree.

In contrast, incubatory healing is more closely associated with Greek pilgrims until well into the Roman period. We might thus allow incubation healing as possible for early Roman Dendera, especially for its Greek or Hellenizing visitors, on the basis of comparison with other sites at the end of the Ptolemaic and the Roman period—at Strabo's Kanopos, for example. At around the same time, southern Egypt contains another site that hints at incubation for the cult of Imhotep-Asklepios among Egyptian visitors. At Athribis a small rock-cut temple is dedicated to ΑΣΚΛΗΠΙΩΙ; behind the door are a forecourt, two rooms and a cult niche excavated into the hill.[187] Among the thirty-seven demotic depinti in the interior is one that lists twenty-three persons by name and says, according to the excavators' summary, that these people had spent the night there for reasons of their health. There are no photographs of the demotic graffiti, only of the dedicatory Greek text, and I have been unable as yet to discover the exact phrasing of the inscription. It could be incubation: the experiencing of significant dreams. It might also represent the kind of activity engaged in by the younger Qenherkhopshef in the Theban area centuries previously, when he spent the night in the shadow of the mountain goddess, but without any indication of a dream.[188] Proximity to a god is a significant act and experience in itself.

At Deir el-Bahari, the cheapest way to gain the god's help for those who needed it would have consisted of a small votive offering, or an inscription—probably in need of official approval—left on the sanctuary walls. Written petitions with detailed rescripts, as in the cases of Polyaratos and Teos, were more expensive. Speculatively, incubation was the preserve of either the wealthy or something akin to the professional visionary, as with the demotic dreamer in the *mr* of the ostrakon now in Australia, and perhaps Polyaratos as well. His account, in its complexity and length, is as much a story about his own dramatic journey to salvation, as it is about the

[187] El-Farag, R., U. Kaplony-Heckel, et al. (1985). 'Recent archaeological explorations at Athribis (Hw.t Rpjj.t)', *MDAIK* 41, 1–8. Modern Wannina, south of Sohag. The excavators date the shrine on paleographic grounds, to the late Ptolemaic or early Roman period (most of the dateable inscriptions are early Roman).

[188] 2.1.3 above, p. 52, n. 24 (BM stele 278).

power of the god. But for the majority of those seeking aid, older forms of access and response, mediated by official personnel, were usually sufficient.

2.6. *Conclusions*

Temple medicine in Ptolemaic Egypt can be divided into two types of activity, with some conceptual overlap. The first is that of healing procedures accessible at temples, and the second, a subset of oracular consultations with gods. Healing *cippi*, the presence of Egyptian experts in technical medical and protective materials, and direct epiphanic cures experienced through visions of the god are examples of the former. It is also probable that some supplicants had access to places inscribed with significant texts and images, which induced healing, fertility or protection: as in the Late period Karnak chapel, the Bes room at Saqqara, and possibly birth houses. These were not methods restricted exclusively to the sanctuaries, but were closely associated with them, especially in terms of the relative authority and power available.

In the second category were procedures for obtaining advice, guarantees or cures from the god through the submission of oral or written prayers.

These procedures were all embedded within the physical, organizational and conceptual space of a sanctuary precinct. In the best-known, high-status examples, from which most of our evidence derives, these conformed to the functionality and decorum of Egyptian religion. Additions or new temples built under Ptolemaic reign only rarely involved Hellenistic imagery or language, and then, as at the sacred animal necropolis of Memphis, only on the peripheries of sacred ground and as an expression of, not an alternative to, the Late period cults established there.[189] Greek immigrants of the third century and their descendants utilized these temples, and many if not all such visitors came for what we might term religious purposes. A degree of Greek religious chauvinism is attested in some Greco-Roman literary sources from outside Egypt itself, but if any immigrants preferred to avoid Egyptian temples or sacred animals entirely, they are a silent group, and appear to be a minority.

---

[189] E.g. the juxtaposition of sphinxes, statues of Greek intellectuals, and Dionysiac-Osirian imagery on the approach route to the Memphis Sarapieon, which aroused the disapproval of Mariette, A. (published posthumously by G. Maspero, 1882). *Le Sérapeum de Memphis par Auguste Mariette Pacha*, 16: 'Toutes sont d'un pitoyable style et plupart des têtes manquent'. See also Lauer, J.-Ph. and Ch. Picard. (1955). *Les statues ptolémaïques du Sarapeion de Memphis*, esp. 108–118.

The degree to which visitors interacted with the institutional apparatus of a temple varied. Oracular petitions that required a response must have involved cult officials, and probably often the service of professional writers on private commission. Dedications had to be organized, and the services of local providers and artisans employed. If people with chronic conditions did stay within or near a sanctuary, there must have been provision for their requirements—shelter, food, water, purification. Any such long-term users of alleged 'sanatoria'—a word with unfortunate associations with Victorian spas—must have either maintained themselves in some way, along the lines of the *katochos* Ptolemaios' business activities, or been significantly wealthy, and therefore often Greek. Visits lasting less than a few days are more likely, but would restrict visitors to those living near a particular shrine and to sites on the Nile, especially those attractive to traders. At large and readily accessible sanctuaries, like that of Memphis, many users of the temples must have been the artisans, merchants, temple personnel and others whose livelihoods were based upon the economy of the sanctuary or in the villages and towns nearby.

Speakers of Greek navigated this terrain. Some were bilingual, like Ptolemaios: their Greek identity dominant in some contexts but not in others. Egyptians who lived in the cities, or who dealt regularly with a Greek-speaking administration, learned to speak some Greek, although only those with socio-political ambitions felt the need to learn to write in it. First generation Greek immigrants, however, and those from large Greek communities, had little need to learn to speak the Egyptian language. They obtained oracle petitions written in Greek but in accordance with contemporary Egyptian form; had their dreams interpreted by Kres—most probably a descendent of earlier immigrants to Memphis; left graffiti at Amenhotep's rock-cut temple in acceptance of the locally recognized god of healing. They do not seem to have engaged in petition deposits or self-dedication in large numbers; at least not under their Greek identities.

The numbers of speakers of Greek in several parts of the country, combined with the Hellenistic identity of most of the ruling administration, made some degree of adaptation advantageous to cult officials and other providers of services or materials as a group. Egyptian temple culture also emphasized the collection and improvement of the written word; higher-ranking cult officials formed a hereditary socioeconomic elite for which literacy was a definitive marker. The distinctive world of Greco-Egyptian literary-religious culture evolved through their interactions with Greek language speakers and texts; and possibly also practices. The language—actual and metaphorical—of Hellenism extended Egyptian modes into Greek and eventually Roman discourses; Greek interest and ideas were a factor—among others—in play in internal religious, technical and artistic developments within Egyptian temple culture, including medicine. There is no direct evidence that Greek-speakers frequently consulted the temples' medical experts, since it seems that the relatively wealthy protagonists of private letters preferred Greek pharmaceuticals, but the fact that temple libraries added or incorporated Greek medical materials within their own collections might imply an interest in Greek clients.[190] Incubation is linked to epiphanic cure in the contexts of Greek suppliants at medical cults, notably Kanopos, Deir el-Bahari, and perhaps the Memphis Sarapieon. But it also appears to have emerged among cultic personnel as a de-institutionalized form of oracle, in a development of Late period trends that might well be solely internal to Egypt. Egyptian gods and myths were through the processes of translation exoticized, appropriated and sometimes transformed, while there is some evidence for resistance and attempts at re-appropriation for Imhotep (Asklepios).

---

[190] See the Greek texts, including medical examples, from temple archives in Tebtynis in the south-west Fayum: published in Andorlini, I. and R. Flemming. (2001–2009). *Greek Medical Papyri*, 2 vols. Cf. Minnen, P. van. (1998). 'Boorish or Bookish? Literature in Egyptian villages in the Fayum in the Graeco-Roman Period', *Journal of Juristic Papyrology* 28, 99–184; Hanson, A.E. 'Greek medical papyri from the Fayum village of Tebtunis: patient involvement in a local health-care system?' in van der Eijk, Ph. (2005). *Hippocrates in Context*, 387–402. See also 3.3, p. 129; 5.2.1, pp. 221–222.

CHAPTER THREE

THEORETICAL PERSPECTIVES

'Illness is identified with the perspective of the popular or folk sectors of the health care system and thus to the patient; disease is tied to the perspective of the professional sector and its practitioners.'[1] A theory of the nature and causes of illness forms the basis for diagnosis, prognosis and, if there is treatment, therapy. It justifies the healing response and situates the healer within a particular intellectual and social context. In this way the explanation and understanding of disease claimed by the healer is a very important part of their claim to authority as a healer. Patients and society at large, however, also impute meanings to their experience and have a causal understanding of the world of illness. The disease theory or theories of any 'professional sector' elaborate, develop, and sometimes diverge from the beliefs of patients, but the understanding of disease utilized by specialist or expert healers is closely related to broader views on the nature of illness.[2] In antiquity, evidence for the stance of the patient rather than the professional, and evidence for beliefs about illness causation operative within society more widely, consist primarily of inscriptional evidence and private communications between individuals, such as letters on papyrus, together with references in non-technical works. In this chapter I am concerned mainly with the more detailed, and thus more distinctive, concepts utilized by professionals and technical literature.

Our knowledge of medical theories in Greece and Egypt is almost entirely dependent upon extant written sources produced, in each society, by a group of unusually literate individuals. In Egypt, medicine is part of the domain of elite knowledge for which written authority is paramount.[3] Medical texts, like other works of technical ritual, represented the most reliable

---

[1] Kleinman, A. (1980). *Patients and Healers in the Context of Culture.*

[2] Kleinman, A., L. Eisenberg and B. Good. (1978). 'Culture, illness and care: clinical lessons from anthropologic and cross-cultural research', *Annals of Internal Medicine* 88, 251, for an example of how non-specialists can (mis-)understand a medical model they ostensibly subscribe to: the patient believed that angina pectoris and coronary thrombosis were mutually exclusive. Since he had the former, he could not suffer from the latter.

[3] See Baines, J. (1983). 'Literacy and ancient Egyptian society', *Man* 18.3, 580 ff.

and authoritative access to the knowledge and power of the gods; they were written to be used and used because they were written. Temple libraries and scriptoria contained and produced such works, but private copies were made or acquired by the families of scribes and other temple officials. The professional healers of Egypt were drawn from this group: modern distinctions between 'scribe', 'physician' and 'priest' are largely anachronistic.[4]

Practicing physicians were also often the authors of Greek and Latin works on disease theory, but theoretical medicine was also, in the classical and later periods, part of a liberal education and a form of competitive intellectual display.

In both societies the relationship of these texts and their authors and audiences to other and perhaps more broadly held views on illness is difficult to establish. Nor can we be sure how representative is the surviving material across time periods or geographical region. In Egypt, twelve or so extant papyri and fragments containing medical content date to between about 1850 BCE and the 3rd century CE, a period of over 2000 years. Even in those copied towards the end of this time span there is content dating back to the second millennium BCE.[5] Several are fragmented or damaged to the extent of being difficult to read and reconstruct. The only text concerning traumatic injury, the Edwin Smith, is extremely truncated. The lengthiest, the Ebers, is a long roll made up of more than 100 sheets of papyrus. It is a compilation of several otherwise unknown but apparently more specialized texts. The number of close parallels—often down to identical wording—between the surviving texts suggests a degree of internal coherence and long-term stability for theory and therapy within the literary tradition, but the compiler-copyists sorted, excluded, and added material from various sources to produce the texts as we have them.[6] They also provided numerous glosses in order to explain compressed, unfamiliar or otherwise cryptic

[4] Allen, J. (2005). *The Art of Medicine in Ancient Egypt* views the priests of Sakhmet as co-extensive with *swnw* (physician); from the late first millennium this term is also interchangeable with lector priest and embalmer: Quirke, S. (1992). *Ancient Egyptian Religion*, 152. See further chapter 5.1.1, pp. 206–212.

[5] The earliest of the extant texts are the Kahun gynecological and veterinary papyri, from around 1850 BCE, though Bardinet, T. (1995). *Papyrus médicaux de l'Égypte pharaonique*, 18–19, argues that the Ramesseum medical papyri date to slightly earlier than this. The extant texts were often based on earlier material: see the summary by Nunn, J. (1996). *Ancient Egyptian Medicine*, 28 and for the Ebers, Bardinet, ibid., 17. For a detailed description of the papyri and their contents, as well as medical ostraka, see Westendorf, W. (1999). *Handbuch der Altägyptischen Medizin*, 6–64.

[6] For this structure in the Ebers, for example, see Bardinet, *Papyrus médicaux*, 160.

information and instructions. There are also traces of disagreement or rival traditions. Two paragraphs in the Ebers papyrus have two different totals for the numbers of vessels (*mtw*) in the body (52 and 12, with the latter probably a scribal error for 22).[7]

Assessing both similarity and difference is complicated by the considerable difficulty of translation and interpretation. There is considerable disagreement amongst Egyptologists and other specialists on medically relevant items, especially plant names. Most of the surviving material consists of instructions and ingredients for remedies, though the preservation of some diagnostic formulae tells us a little about nosology and about doctors' interactions with patients.[8] Explicit references to physiological and pathological ideas are present but rare, and theory is not discussed in detail in any extant work. Many of the terms used—whether for disease, disease causes, bodily organs, symptoms, or ingredients in remedies—do not occur outside the medical texts and are of uncertain and possibly multiple meanings that depended heavily on a contextual understanding, one that we have great difficulty recovering.

We are better off in regard to the Greco-Roman evidence. The earliest expository medical works in Greek society are those later selected as comprising the 'Hippocratic corpus', though fragmentary speculations of Pre-Socratic thinkers also survive. All are, of course, far later than the majority of the Egyptian material. The selection during the Hellenistic era of some sixty works as by Hippokrates ensured their survival but also produced chronic confusion about their authorship, interpretation, and interrelations.[9] Thanks to the chance survival of part of a fourth-century doxography within the Anonymus Londinensis papyrus, describing physicians and theories that would otherwise be entirely unknown to us, it is also clear that the corpus is not entirely representative of even elite medicine of the relatively well documented classical period. As for the period of Greek Egypt itself, the work of even its most famous physicians survives in a state of fragmentation.[10] Almost everything we have on Greek medicine of the Ptolemaic period is refracted through the lenses of Celsus, Rufus, Soranos and,

---

[7] See Nunn, *Egyptian Medicine*, 48.

[8] See especially the recurrent phrase of the Smith papyrus 'then you say about him … (diagnosis, prognosis).' Translation Allen, *Art of Medicine*.

[9] A brief overview is Nutton, V. (2004). *Ancient Medicine*, 60–62.

[10] The fragments of Herophilos and known Herophileans are collected, translated and analyzed in Staden, H. von. (1989). *Herophilus: the Art of Medicine in Hellenistic Alexandria*. Those of Erasistratos were collected by Garofalo, I. (1988). *Erasistrati fragmenta*.

overwhelmingly, Galen; all of them writing some three to five centuries after the Alexandrian anatomists. Their theoretical innovations, moreover, are unlikely to have penetrated into medical training and practice beyond the urban environment, or even beyond the court circle and upper socioeconomic strata with which Herophileans, Erasistrateans and Empiricists are associated.

The direct evidence for theoretical interchange between Greek and Egyptian practitioners and theorists of medicine is extremely limited, both before and during the Hellenistic period. Even in the Roman era, when authors such as Pliny and Rufus of Ephesos mention 'Egyptian physicians', they seem to be referring to Greek physicians working in Egypt (Alexandria). This chapter highlights situations in which interactions over theoretical matters between practitioners in Ptolemaic Egypt may have occurred. In section 3.1, I discuss points of comparison between the most prominent surviving theories of Egyptian and Greek medicine, using evidence from all periods where it seems reasonable that these were continuous with views also current in the Ptolemaic period. I want to establish an arena for possible interaction between nosology and methodology, in which 'interaction' includes rejection of views considered different or inferior, as well as perceptions of acceptability and usefulness that provoked adoption or adaption of an underpinning theoretical construct. Several such cases, based upon apparent similarity or distinction, have been proposed for the classical Greek period (the fifth and fourth centuries BCE) from the point of view of modern observers: I discuss these in section 3.2. Section 3.3 considers the evidence for whether and how medical theory and therapy was perceived in ethnocultural terms in antiquity, such as Herodotos' description of 'Egyptian' medicine as compared to 'Greek', and of what these perceptions consisted. Finally, in 3.4, we examine the limited direct evidence for the transmission of nosological and pharmaceutical terminology and conceptualization during the Greco-Roman era.

3.1.1. *Nosological Concepts: Gods and the Greek Understanding of Disease*

In his 1995 translation of the Egyptian medical papyri, Thierry Bardinet observed that the central theory of Egyptian medicine, throughout its 2500 years or so of recorded history, was that of divine intervention.[11] Divine

[11] Bardinet, *Papyrus médicaux*, 60: 'L'idée centrale, parfois sous-jacente, parfois exprimée

power was responsible for the creation, maintenance and order of life, including that of the living person, the second life of the justified dead, and the living statue of the god's image. Gods and other denizens of the other-world could disrupt or alter the internal order of the unviolated body, producing illness and death. Such beliefs are evident in inscriptional and archeological evidence from a wide social range. Several steles dedicated by the necropolis workers of Thebes, in the late second millennium, are appeals to gods to cease their punishment. Neferabu says he swore falsely by Ptah, and Ptah caused him to see 'darkness by day'. Another man swore falsely by the moon, and had to ask the lunar god Thoth to turn away the resultant affliction.[12] Protective and curative amulets and statuettes attest indirectly to similar conceptions among the population at large, and some of the written material was probably written by professionals on behalf of illiterate individuals. The professional healers of Egypt were all experts in intercession and the appeasement of otherworld powers, and many remedies invoked helpful deities or defended against malevolent forces.[13] The medical papyri also offered a much more detailed and complex picture of disease in terms of anatomical-physiological entities and processes, but the substances and causes involved are conceptualized as divine or demonic, and are usually of an external and hostile origin.

The gods are also central to the Greek understanding of disease, in spite of the implicit and in one case explicit rejection of them in this role among most classical period writers on medicine and philosophy. The depiction of medicine in the 8th century Homeric poems—the earliest written sources for Greek medicine—is that of a craft-based system of knowledge,[14] but aristocrats, heroes and gods also demonstrated medical expertise: their healing prowess expressed their ability to act in the divine world.[15] Gods appear in the *Iliad* and *Odyssey* as the causes of illness,

sans équivoque, mais constamment présente dans toute la documentation, est celle de l'intervention divine directe.'

12 BM stele 589 (on reverse); Turin stele 284: see Sadek, I.A. (1988). *Popular Religion in Egypt*, 236 ff.

13 Prominent healers were cult officials of Sakhmet, the 'amulet men' (*s3w*), and less often 'lector priests', cult officials of Heka, and others. The *ḫrp šrḳt*, officials of Serqet specialized in bites and stings. For the *swnw*, 'physicians', 5.1.1, pp. 206–212.

14 *Odyssey* 17.383–386.

15 Notably Asklepios' sons Makhaon and Podalirios: *Iliad* 11.518, 506. Other heroes also treat their friends, including Akhilles, who had learnt from the centaur Khiron, 'wise in drugs.' Apollo treats other gods at *Iliad* 5. 401, 901. When the epidemic that begins the poem strikes the Greek army, they require the prophet Kalkhas: epidemics are from gods.

psychological states, and even traumatic injuries; medical experts such as Makhaon used incantations as well as topical ingredients and bandaging techniques.[16] Expertise in medicine was necessarily expertise in interaction with gods. Traces of a view in which diseases are themselves hostile entities are also still visible in early sources; such pestilences roam the landscape in Hesiod's *Works and Days*.[17] Illness can be ascribed to the assault of a daimon, according to the *Odyssey* (5.394–398). This view of illness as god-dependent or even demon-caused is eclipsed in the written sources of the classical era and sometimes explicitly attacked, as in *The sacred disease*,[18] but it remained a mainstream view. An enormous amount of evidence attests to the general prevalence of religion and prophecy as a guide and justification to thought and action in Greek society, amongst both individuals and states. 'Whenever people have a dream or see a vision', said Plato, 'they put up altars and shrines in every home and village.'

Salesmen at the door offered to write curse tablets or raise the dead against their customers' enemies (also according to Plato).[19] The rapid expansion and popularity of the healing cult of Asklepios demonstrated widespread and continuing acceptance of gods' and heroes' power for healing.[20] Even the author of *The sacred disease* did not deny that the gods provide medical aid, although he sought to restrict their sphere of action to the established pieties of temple cult.[21] The author of *Dreams* allowed that some dream-messages and omens were sent by the gods, but he left their interpretation to a field other than medicine. In third century Alexandria, Herophilos also included god-sent messages in his tripartite categorization of dreams.[22] Root-cutters, shepherds, and other collectors and makers of

---

16 *Iliad* 4.193–218. For gods and the physical body see Holmes, B. (2010). *The Symptom and the Subject. The emergence of the physical body in ancient Greece.*

17 1004; 238–245. For this interpretation see Nutton, *Ancient Medicine*, 39–40.

18 *The sacred disease.* For discussion and modern reinterpretations of this text and its views on gods and disease, e.g. Lloyd, G.E.R. (1979). *Magic, Reason and Experience*, 15ff.; Laskaris, J. (2002) *The Art is Long*; van der Eijk, P.J. 'On the 'theology' of the Hippocratic treatise *On the sacred disease*', reprinted in ibid. (2005) *Medicine and Philosophy in Classical Antiquity*, 45–73; Jouanna, J. (2003). *La maladie sacrée.* For a very different reading see Longrigg, J. (1993). *Greek Rational Medicine*, 34–38.

19 Plato *Laws* 10.909e–910a; *Republic* 364b5–c5, cf. Johnston, S. (1999). *Restless Dead*, 119.

20 Wickkiser, B.L. (2008). *Asklepios, medicine, and the politics of healing in fifth century Greece.*

21 He points out failures of consistency in the claims of purifiers, but his overall objection to explaining illness as god-caused, or to private practice in divine healing, is largely theological. Gods are pure and good entities who work within the acceptable social conventions and pure spaces of temple sites and practice.

22 *Dreams* (*Regimen* 4) 4.86 (6.640 Littré); von Staden, *Herophilus*, 386–387 (T226). Aris-

medical materials, as well as the purifiers and 'magic-users' attacked in *The sacred disease*, were professional providers of medicine, expert pharmaceutical knowledge, and dietary and ritualistic advice. Their claims to authority and expertise were explicitly based in their understanding of divine and miraculous causation operative in the world and their ability to manipulate and manage its effects.[23]

According to the *The sacred disease*'s description of the purifiers' views, the god causing a specific form of the 'sacred disease' (epilepsy and conditions involving sudden seizure and loss of consciousness) is identified by the patient's symptomatology. There is not much information in that treatise as to why gods should cause this to happen, but elsewhere in Greek literature gods impose disease as a response to pollution and/or impiety. Herodotos often cited both 'naturalistic' explanations and more direct divine interventions for disasters, illness and, especially, madness.[24] In discussing the madness of the Persian king Kambyses, he is willing to allow a physical disease as the cause, but his understanding is also compatible with that of his sources (probably the cult officials of Apis), who attributed Kambyses' insanity to his killing of the Egyptian bull-god Apis: Καμβύσης δέ, ὡς λέγουσι Αἰγύπτιοι, αὐτίκα διὰ τοῦτο τὸ ἀδίκημα ἐμάνη, ἐὼν οὐδὲ πρότερον φρενήρης. (3.30.1).

There is also evidence in classical and later Greece for the role of the dead in disease. Many people thought that terrors and madness were caused by heroes, or by Hekate, sending the dead.[25] Madness and sterility were the forms of illness most commonly attributed to ghosts, but a fragment of Aristophanes implies that heroes, at least, could cause other diseases.[26] The murdered and otherwise angered dead were chiefly to be feared; experts in ghosts such as the *goes* or *psychopompos* could pacify the dead and release

---

totle excludes the gods as causes of dreams, except in the sense that all nature is divine: *Divination in sleep* 463b12 ff.

[23] For 'root-cutters' see Lloyd, G.E.R. (1983). *Science, Folklore and Ideology*, 119–134. The chief ancient source is Theophrastos, *Inquiry into plants* and *The causes of plants*.

[24] See e.g. Sophokles *Oedipus the King*; Aiskhylos *Eumenides*. The classic study of pollution is Parker, R.A. (1983 repr. 1990). *Miasma*. Herodotos' approach is discussed by Lloyd, *Magic, Reason and Experience*, 29 ff.; Thomas, R. (2000). *Herodotus in Context*, 28–74.

[25] *The sacred disease* 4.30–33, cf. Plato *Laws* 865d6–e6; Xenophon *Cyrus* 8.7.18–19. Johnston, *Restless Dead*, 145–146.

[26] Aristophanes fragment 322. Heroes also cause city-wide difficulties in the shape of epidemics, mass sterility, famine, etc. Johnston, *Restless Dead*, 155–156. Sterility: as early as Homer the Erinyes cause childlessness, *Iliad* 9.454. The *strix* embodies fears centered around reproduction: e.g. Plato *Republic* 381e1–6. For the relation of the Erinyes and other agents of retribution and its relation to 'pollution' (*miasma*) see Parker, *Miasma*.

their victims.[27] Sarah Iles Johnston argued that these effects of the dead upon the living are accomplished chiefly through their appearance rather than any innate strength or power of the dead: their victims go mad from horror and fear.[28]

3.1.2. *Invasion from Outside: Disease Conceptualization in Egypt*

The Ptolemaic era temple of Horus at Edfu lists *The book of appeasing Sakhmet* among its sacred texts. Epidemic disease was linked both to Sakhmet and to certain times of year, as in eight spells against 'annual epidemic' on the verso of the Edwin Smith papyrus, written around 1550 but with content probably dating back to ca. 2500. One of the Smith spells was for 'barring air of the bitterness of the night-demons, those of smallness, Sakhmet's messengers.' These are not different groups so much as a single causal agency described in various different ways. Similarly, in the *Book of the Last Day of the Year* more such messengers of Sakhmet shoot arrows of plague from their mouths.[29] All such imagery expressed an idea of causal transmission, in which the malignancy of disease is physically transferred from Sakhmet's rage, through subordinate agents of hostility (winds, breath, or arrows) to the sufferer, where it became a pathological state of the body. The arrow motif re-appeared in Greek iconography of Apollo, Artemis and Herakles; all epidemic and apotropaic gods. As Faraone remarks, 'The image of arrows showered down upon a group of people seems to be a common ancient explanation of the multiple appearance of fevers and epidemic plagues in an army or any other closely packed group of people.'[30]

A crucial element in Egyptian texts, and one generally absent from Greek references, is the notion of an invasive agent entering the body. The illness-causing messengers of Sakhmet are part of a more general category of external entities producing disorder in physiological function. In the Smith papyrus, the phrase 'something entering from outside', in case 8, was explained by a later copyist (gloss D) as referring to 'either the breath of a god, or death.' He was insistent upon the point: 'It is not an entering of

[27] Plato *Phaedrus* 244d5–245a1, with Burkert, W. (1992). *The Orientalizing Revolution*, 66; Johnston, *Restless Dead*, 108, 120.

[28] Johnston, *Restless Dead*, 145, 147.

[29] Goyon, J.-C. (1974). 'Sur les formule des rituels de conjuration des dangers de l'année', *BIFAO* 74, 79–83.

[30] Parker, *Miasma*, 35–56; Faraone, C.A. (1992) *Talismans and Trojan Horses*, 54–74, quote from p. 59. As killers, e.g. *Iliad* 24.605–606, *Odyssey* 15.407–411, Pindar *Pyth.* 3.31–37.

that which is created by his flesh'.[31] A passage in the Ebers explained that the breath of life enters a man by the 2 vessels (*mtw*) located in his right ear, and the breath of death via the matching 2 *mtw* of the left ear.[32] There are a total of 44 mentions in the medical papyri of a morbid condition associated with something called an ꜥꜣꜥ (*aâa*), a noun that does not appear outside the medical works.[33] The usual determinative of the ꜥꜣꜥ noun was a discharging phallus, and in non-medical texts, the verb ꜥꜣꜥ refers to the discharging of any fertile, creative liquid from the body of a god;[34] its use in medical contexts is closely connected to sexual violation by otherworld entities—gods, adversaries from the otherworld of gods and men (m. *ḏꜣj*, f. *ḏꜣt*), or the dead (collectively, these or their effects are often approximately translatable as 'demon'). Eight of the references qualify the ꜥꜣꜥ as that of a god, goddess, dead man or dead woman.[35]

Morbid kinds of ꜥꜣꜥ are thus identified with a kind of toxic semen, introduced into the body of a sleeping victim (most of the remedies against ꜥꜣꜥ are to be taken at night). Another word for semen, *mtwt*, also means poison, and this is used in the context of rape in the mythic narrative of the conflict between Horus and Seth, in which poisonous semen is inserted through the ear.[36] The medical texts indicate that such a malignant substance caused or became intestinal worms, hence Ebers 62: 'Another remedy ... to be eaten by a man who has *ḥrr.t*[-worm] in his body. It is the ꜥꜣꜥ which has made them ...'.[37] The term is accompanied by the determinative sign for worm or snake. Some intestinal worms, notably roundworms and tapeworms, are of a size to be empirically observed under the right conditions; the presence of smaller

31 *GdM* 5 (text), 311; 4/1 (translation), 178; 4/2 (notes), 142–143. Translation given here from Allen, *Art of Medicine*, 79. On this point Wilson, J. (1952). 'A note on the Edwin Smith Surgical Papyrus', *JNES* 11, 79–80; Nunn, *Egyptian Medicine*, 103–104.

32 Ebers 856g = Berlin 163g, cf. Ebers 854f.: *GdM* 5, 16 and 3; 4.1, 9 and 2. The breath of life occurs frequently in non-medical texts: Nunn, *Egyptian Medicine*, 55.

33 Counting 'other' prescriptions and parallel texts. There is a rare verb ꜥꜣꜥ with the same determinative. Deines, H. von and Westendorf, W. (1961). *GdM* 7/1, 129–133, esp. 132 argued that ꜥꜣꜥ was an etiological principle, not a specific disease; specifically, the toxic semen of a demon. Cf. Nunn, *Egyptian Medicine*, 63. This has replaced earlier suggestions, including that of hematuria: Grapow, H. *GdM* 3.60, 65.

34 Bardinet, *Papyrus médicaux*, 123.

35 Berlin 58, 189; Ebers 99, 168, 225, 229, 231, Hearst 83. Cf. Leiden I 348.

36 *Mtw.t* (as disease) in *GdM* 7/1, 412. See Te Velde, H. (1967). *Seth, god of confusion*, 37–39 for Sethian rape and illness, and on *mtw.t* as poisonous semen, 45.

37 *GdM* 7, 630. The dead include both the justified dead of the afterworld (m. *ꜣḫ*, f. *ꜣḫ.t*) and unjustified ghosts (*mt, mt.t.*). *GdM* 7/1, 11 (collective term for gods, ghosts and demons); 409 (dead); 7/2 993–994 (demons).

kinds might easily be extrapolated from signs of intestinal trouble or malnutrition.[38] Thus worms were easily understood as active agents of disorder within the body, and as the diagnostic sign of invasion by the equally corporeal ʿꜣʿ-semen, on the model of semen's role in reproductive fertilization, but with a malignant twist.

A worm-determinative was often used with the names of otherwise mysterious diseases.[39] The literal (probably) and the metaphysical here coincided: the serpent-form was commonly understood as an agent of dissolution and disorder in mythology and iconography.[40] Every night, the giant underworld constrictor Apophis attacked the barque of the sun god as it travels through the underworld, perpetually threatening a collapse of the cosmos into the unstructured, atemporal chaos of night. On a more local scale, the bite of poisonous snakes injected their fluids into the human body in the same manner as the assaults of the night-attacking demons. The Brooklyn medical papyrus, from the late sixth to early third century BCE, is almost entirely concerned with the bites of snakes and scorpions. Many of these animals are identified in the text as manifestations of a god: the species of chapter 18, for instance, is a manifestation of Sobek, chapter 21's, of Hathor; chapters 15 and 16 featured snakes linked to Apophis.

Worms and maggots were also visible in putrefying corpses, reinforcing the link between these creatures and the visible decay of illness. 'Such is he who is decayed; all the bones are decayed, the body is dismembered (*smꜣ*), the bones are softened, the *jwf* is made into an evil liquid. He smells, he rots, he becomes a mass of maggots, all maggoty.'[41]

This kind of invasive model of illness causation is more general than the use of the term ʿꜣʿ or the sign-determinative for serpent. In the Brooklyn magical papyrus, from the early Ptolemaic period, a spell offered protection against ghosts ejaculating in the victim's ear during sleep.[42] A demon in

---

38 Nunn, *Egyptian Medicine*, 71.

39 *GdM* 7: *pnd*-worms (pp. 267–268), *ḥ̣fꜣ.t* (pp. 594–595), *ʿnʿr.t* (p. 143), *fnṯ*- (p. 303), *sꜣ*- (p. 705), *sp*- (p. 741), *srf.t* (?) (p. 782); *ddf.t*- (p. 1018), cf. 1022.

40 Some snakes have positive meanings in Egyptian mythology and language, notably the protective power of the fire-spitting cobra, coiled ready to strike as the protective uraeus of royal iconography. The harvest goddess Renenutet, 'nurturer', is also shown as a snake, referencing predation of mice and rats and thus the protection of the wheat harvest.

41 Naville, E. (1886). *Das ägyptische Todtenbuch der XVIII. bis XX Dynastie*. I: 179 (no. 154) col. 4. Translation from Walker, J. (1996). *Studies in Ancient Egyptian Anatomical Terminology*, 49 with n. 61.

42 Sauneron, S. (1970). *Le Papyrus magique illustré de Brooklyn. Brooklyn Museum 47.218. 156*: 23–24 (col. 4^8 and 5^3), with discussion of parallels, 10–11.

bodily form (*ḏt*) intruding into someone's flesh (*jwf*) causes illness, according to the text of an unpublished papyrus now in Turin.[43] Commenting upon this phrase, van Dijk suggested *ḏt* should be translated as 'bodily manifestation of someone's personality'. A large number of conditions in the medical papyri are identified or linked with gods and 'demons', often conceptualized as material pathogenic entities within the body.[44]

The dead were also a common cause of such violations, whether these were the unburied or unjustified dead—denied a new life in the next world—or those with specific grudges against living individuals. Like other inhabitants of the otherworld, non-living persons were a very real presence. Sometimes they were 'seen' in sleep: in the few instances extant, the dreamer's reaction was often one of unease about what the dead might require of him. Slightly more numerous are the twenty or so 'letters to the dead' left in tombs, in which the living letter-writer sought the intercession of a dead individual personally known to them. The dead were asked to guarantee a healthy child, for assistance against living enemies (as in inheritance disputes), or for protection against attacks on the living by other dead spirits. Sometimes the dead addressee was the cause of disasters that have befallen those still living. The author of one letter is quite certain his late wife is behind his recent misfortunes: '... you have laid hands on me, although I had done nothing evil to you'.[45]

The catch-all phrase 'every dead man (*mt*) and every dead woman (*mtt*)', a formula commonly used in protective magic, referred to such hostile dead.[46] The Ebers medical papyrus opened with a similarly comprehensive spell:

> O Isis, great of magic, loose me, release me, from all things bad, evil and red; from the stroke of a god, and the stroke of a goddess; from a dead man or dead woman, from a male enemy or female enemy who may oppose himself to me.[47]

---

43 For this papyrus and the meaning of *ḏt* see van Dijk, J. (1979–1980). 'The birth of Horus according to the Ebers papyrus', *JEOL* 26, 19, with n. 71.

44 For disease demons see Westendorf, W. (1970). 'Beiträge aus und zu den medizinischen Texten' III, *ZÄS* 96, 145–151. A list of demon-terms and conditions is given by Borghouts, J.F. (1978). *Ancient Egyptian Magical Texts*, 117.

45 *P. Leiden* I 371 (from 1295–1186 BCE) = no. 352 in Wente, E. (1990). *Letters from Ancient Egypt*, 210–219, nos. 342, 345, 349, 350. The majority of such 'letters' are earlier than the New Kingdom.

46 Cf. many of the invocations in Borghouts, *Magical Texts*, e.g. no. 6.

47 Ebers 2 (1, 13–16): *GdM* 4/1, 309; 4/2, 232–233; 5, 532. Bardinet, *Papyrus médicaux*, 42.

The inclusive terminology served to defend the speaker against all possible attacks by any potentially hostile force. Only the gender and 'species' of the attacker—deity, dead spirit or any other kind of otherworldly or living enemy—needed to be specified to ensure completeness.

Numerous private, royal and temple ritual texts include spells for defense against otherworld entities, which were particularly common during the vulnerable night hours as Ra and his companions progressed through the underworld.[48] Medical works are contiguous with this defensive genre, but dealt with a specific subset of attacks: those which succeeded. They offered a specialized expertise for recognizing and eliminating the morbid substances that had been introduced into the body.

3.1.3. *Within the Body: Physiology and Pathology*

To sum up so far, the conceptualization of disease operating in the Egyptian medical papyri appears to be one of malign or at least chaotic entities, which are nonetheless physically substantive. The external triggers—the messengers of Sakhmet, the poisonous bite of a snake or scorpion, the ejections or invasions of 'demons' and dead people—are internalized as morbid bodily states and substances.

No explicit treatment of physiological or pathological theories is extant among the surviving texts. As Bardinet concludes in the introduction to his 1995 edition (p. 10):

> Nos textes, essentiellement techniques, ont été rédigés pour permettre à un médecin de reconnaître les maladies dans son exercice quotidien et de proposer un traitmente. Ce ne sont pas de traités théoriques au sens moderne du terme, bien que la théorie médicale n'en soit jamais absente.

Physiology is constrained and informed by anatomical understanding. The Egyptian language included words for brain, various parts of the head and skeletal structure, the heart, the stomach or stomach area, testicles, uterus, bladder, and liver, as well as the externally visible organs.[49] The materials compiled in the Ebers text included parts of a treatise (on the etiological entity *wḫdw*) identifying the *mtw* (singular *mt*), the vessels which

---

[48] See Ritner, R.K. (1990). 'O. Gardiner 363: a spell against night terrors', *JARCE* 27, 25–41, esp. 33 ff.

[49] Walker, J. (1996). *Ancient Egyptian Anatomical Terminology*; for which see much of the following. For the vexed issue of whether the Egyptians carried out medically relevant dissection, see 4.4, pp. 198–201, and 6.2, pp. 253–254.

distributed vital or pathological liquids throughout the body, to the limbs and major organs.[50] The model of the *mtw* is highly schematic with noticeable bilateral symmetry. Its relationship to observation is difficult to establish, as *mt* seems to refer to any string-like cord or vessel.[51] (Before the work of the Alexandrian anatomists in the 3rd century Greek writers on medicine used *neura* similarly, to refer to long stringy parts of flesh such as blood vessels, ligaments, tendons, etc.).[52] The *mtw* all meet at the heart and again at the anus.[53] At Berlin 163, their number is totaled as 22, in agreement with the rest of the text; the parallel passage at Ebers 856b gives 12, but this is probably a scribal error for 22.[54] Ebers 854 makes the total 52.

The references to the *mtw* form an allusive explication of some part of a physiological theory. They are said to contain air, the breaths of life and death, blood, urine, water, and semen.[55] At times they also carry mucus, feces or other pathological entities, notably *stt* and *wḫdw*.[56] The heart is described, in more than one text, as 'speaking' through each *mt*. This was probably a reference to the pulse, a diagnostic aid and physiological interpretation not much employed by the Greeks until Herophilos' work in third century Alexandria.[57]

If the *mtw* are blocked, or overwhelmed by too much of any substance, or twisted up, illness results and the pulse is silenced. The four *mtw* leading to the liver are 'those which cause all illness to appear because of over-flooding with blood,' according to Ebers 854l.[58] Ebers 855g describes a condition in

---

50 Eb. 856, with a very close parallel in Berlin 163 = *GdM* 4/1, 7–10 (translation); 4/2 (notes), 30–33; 5 (text in hieroglyphs), 11–17. Cf. Eb. 854.

51 Usually thought to include, without any categorical distinctions between, veins, arteries, muscles, tendons, ligaments, possibly nerves and perhaps the windpipe. Bardinet, *Papyrus médicaux*, 63 ff. argues that muscles etc. cannot be included, but the argument is not particularly persuasive. Symmetry: cf. Bardinet ibid., 117.

52 Nor was there much standardization later: Lloyd, *Science, Folklore and Ideology*, 149–167 ('The development of Greek anatomical terminology').

53 At the heart: Eb. 856b, Berlin 163b. At the anus: Eb. 856h, Bln. 163h, also Eb. 854o. Text: Grapow, *GdM* 5: 4, 12–13, 17. *GdM* 4/1, 3, 7–8, 10; 4/2, 26, 31–32; 5, 12. Bardinet, *Papyrus médicaux*, 5, 115, 117. Walker, *Anatomical Terminology*, 240 ff. argues that what is referred to is not the visible anus (*rt*), but the internal rectum (*phwy*(*t*)).

54 Cf. this chapter, p. 103.

55 For the *mtw* overall, see *GdM* 7.1, 400–408. A recent English translation is Ritner, R.K. (2006). 'The cardiovascular system in ancient Egyptian thought', *JNES* 65.2, 99–109. Cf. Nunn, *Egyptian Medicine*, 44–49, 54–56, 60–63.

56 *štt*: probably 'slime, mucus', *GdM* 7.2, 812–814. For *wḫdw* see below, 114 ff.

57 Ebers 854a and Smith case 1 gloss A: *GdM* 4/2, 1, 172; 4/2, 24–25, 140; 5, 1, 299. For Herophilos see von Staden, *Herophilus*, 267–288.

58 *GdM* 4/1, 3; 5, 4. Cf. 856h = Bln. 163h: *GdM* 4/1, 10; 4/2, 32; 5, 17.

which the *mtw* of the heart (*ḥ3tj*) contain feces (*ḥs*), causing the heart (*jb*) to become distended.[59]

The regulation of temperature is a normal physiological process which became pathological when it went wrong: at Ebers 855d the twisting of the *mtw* seems to have prevented the passage of air through them. They became hot, a heat that was passed on to the heart. As Bardinet, *Papyrus médicaux* 96, comments, this implies that a normal function of the air in the *mtw* was to keep the interior of the body cool, while heat is a cause of illness.

Substances transported through the *mtw* included blood, feces (*ḥs*, above), air (*ṯ3w*),[60] the demonic *ʿ3ʿ* and *stt*, and *wḫdw*, a leading pathogenic concept in Egyptian medicine. Ebers 856a–h, which concerns the *mtw*, was based upon or directly copied a text described as:

> The book concerning the movements of *wḫdw* in all the limbs of a man, that was found among the writings which were under the feet of [the statue of the god] Anubis of Letopolis. It was brought to the king of upper and lower Egypt, Usuphais, the justified.[61]

The word is extremely common in the medical papyri, but, like the noun *ʿ3ʿ*, was a technical, specialized word unattested outside these works. In four instances the termination is feminine, *wḫdw.t*.[62] The word is probably related to the verb *wḫd*, 'to suffer'. Because of this, von Deines and Westendorf, *GdM* 1961, 207, translated it as 'Schmerzstoffe' and 'Schmerzstoff-Dämon' (pain substances, pain demon; a translation retained by Westendorf, *Handbuch*). This has not found general favor, and like most recent commentators I have left *wḫdw* untranslated.

The meaning of *wḫdw* is a leading exhibit in the debate over the relationship between Greek and Egyptian medicine of the pre-Ptolemaic era.

---

[59] *GdM* 5, 9; 4.1, 5. The relationship between *ḥ3tj* and *jb*, the two principal terms for the chest area and heart is unclear. See, *inter alia*, *GdM* 7.1, 40–42; Bardinet, *Papyrus médicaux*, 188 ff.; Nunn, *Egyptian Medicine*, 54; Walker, *Anatomical Terminology*, 147 ff. For *jb* as mind, Allen, J. (2000, rev. ed. 2010). *Middle Egyptian*, 79.

[60] Eb. 855e (*mtw* of the heart (*ḥ3tj*)), cf. Eb. 856b = Bln. 163b. Walker, *Anatomical Terminology*, 158–159 thinks air must here be a metaphor for blood.

[61] Eb 856a–h = Bln. 163a–h. *GdM* 5, 11–17; 4.1, 7–10; 4.2, 30–33. *Wḫdw*: *GdM* 7.1, 207–215; Bardinet, *Papyrus médicaux*, 113 ff.; Nunn, *Egyptian Medicine*, 61–62. The *wḫdw*-treatise incorporated into the Ebers, then, claimed to date back to a first dynasty king.

[62] Eb 131, 242, 246, 385 = *GdM* 4/1, 14, 259, 260, 44; 4/2 35, 198, 199, 53; 5, 24, 442, 445, 75; see also *GdM* 7.1, 215.

3.2.1. *Comparing Greek and Egyptian Concepts:* Wẖdw *and Residues*

Wẖdw was morbid, mobile—presumably through the *mtw*—and could affect a large number of organs, including the teeth and eyes. The appropriate therapeutic response to its presence was eradication. The invocation against *wẖdw* at Ebers 131 listed male and female *wẖdw* as disease entities to be driven from the body, along with the influences of gods and the dead (also divided into male and female).[63] In a by-now-standard interpretation, Robert Steuer argued that *wẖdw* was a kind of disease-causing excrement, the result of the decay of food left too long in the bowels, and subsequently taken up and transported by the *mtw* to spread putrefaction and disaster in the rest of the body. This analysis was developed by Steuer and Saunders in 1959, arguing that it was very similar to, and must therefore have been influential upon, the *perittôma* (residue) theories of certain Greek theorists.[64]

Their argument that *wẖdw* was an etiological principle rather than a particular disease, and their reconstruction of its principal components, have both been widely accepted. The most doubtful among other commentators is Bardinet, *Papyrus médicaux*, who points out that no extant passage is explicit about *wkhdw*'s relation to ingested food. According to Steuer and Saunders, *wẖdw* produced coagulation and destruction of the blood, which led in turn to widespread putrefaction throughout the body: again, no Egyptian text actually described such a process.[65] A disease theory in which pathogenic feces, or residues of digestion, spreads upwards through the body is most clearly stated by a gloss (on a missing passage) at Ebers 855g: 'As to the heart spreads itself out, it means that the *mtw* of the heart contain feces', but the word used for excrement is the standard *ḥs*, not the special term *wẖdw*. Of course, the text may at this point be elliptical, assuming that *ḥs* is about to transform into pathogenic *wẖdw*; or it may be simply using a synonym for this early stage of the disease.

Support for a link in Egyptian thought between digestion and disease comes from Herodotos who, reporting or perhaps deducing what he un-

---

63 Eb 131 (*GdM* 5, 24; 4.1, 14; 4.2, 35).

64 Steuer, R.O. (1948). *Aetiological principle of pyemia in ancient Egyptian Medicine*. Steuer, R.O. and J.B. de C.M. Saunders. (1959). *Ancient Egyptian and Cnidian Medicine*. Cf. Yoyotte, J. (1968). 'Une théorie étiologique des médecins égyptiens', *Kêmi* 18, 82–83.

65 Bardinet, *Papyrus médicaux*, 128 ff. Accepted by Westendorf, *Handbuch*, 341 n. 526; Ritner, R.K. (2000). 'Innovations and adaptations in ancient Egyptian medicine', *JNES* 59.2, 107–117; cf. Nunn, *Egyptian Medicine*, 61–62.

derstood to be the views of the (fifth century) Egyptians of his time, said that they believed ingested food to be the cause of all disease: νομίζοντες ἀπὸ τῶν τρεφόντων σιτίων πάσας τὰς νούσους τοῖσιν ἀνθρώποισιν γίνεσθαι. This belief, he added, was behind the Egyptian emphasis on purifying the bowels with purgatives and enemas.[66] Four hundred years later, Diodoros of Sicily provided a similar account, though with a different nuance: it is a superfluity of food that is the problem: 'For they say that the greater part of the food ingested is a superfluity, out of which diseases are engendered; and so the therapy just mentioned [purging] by eradicating the beginnings of diseases, would best procure health.'[67] These accounts are to some extent supported by the numerous examples of remedies emphasizing regular and proper digestion in the medical texts.[68] The extent to which we can use Herodotos and Diodoros as reliable guides to Egyptian medicine of the fifth century, first century, or first two millennia BC is, however, limited.

In Greek literature, use of purgatives marked Egyptians off from Greek medicine and also physically differentiated their bodies from the Greek norm; a framework of emphasis that similarly guided ethnographic reports of its conceptual justifications. Such ethnographic accounts are presumptive of difference and liable to simplification. The differences between Egyptian medicine as presented in Greek accounts of it, and of the picture of Egyptian medicine that emerges from reading Egyptian texts, demonstrates this clearly. It is reasonable to conclude, for instance, based on both Greek accounts and internal Egyptian evidence, that problems with the digestion and expulsion of food were indeed a significant feature of Egyptian pathological theory, and were related to many of their treatments. But Greek accounts of Egyptian medicine also leave much out, such as the frequent use of invocations and topical applications, and the important Egyptian concept of demonic or divine invasion of the flesh.

---

66 Herodotos 2.77. Morgan, G. (1991). 'Nourishing foods: Herodotus 2.77', *Mnemosyne* 44.3/4, 415–417, argued that τρέφω here meant 'solidifying' rather than nourishing, with constipation as the symptom.

67 1.82: φασὶ γὰρ πάσης τροφῆς ἀναδοθείσης τὸ πλέον εἶναι περιττόν, ἀφ' οὗ γεννᾶσθαι τὰς νόσους ὥστε τὴν προειρημένην θεραπείαν ἀναιροῦσαν τὰς ἀρχὰς τῆς νόσου μάλιστ' ἂν παρασκευάσαι τὴν ὑγίειαν.

68 Remedies to expel worms, *wḥdw* at e.g. Eb. 50–61, 90–103. Enemas: e.g. Bln. 164. See 4.2.2.1, pp. 159–163.

3.2.2. *The Knidos Connection*

Given this rhetoric of difference, it is perhaps not surprising that none of the Greek accounts of Egyptian medicine draw any parallels with contemporary Greek medicine. But according to Steur and Saunders, Greek theories of disease-causing food 'residues' (*perittômata*) had been heavily influenced by an Egyptian idea of pathogenic fecal matter (*wḫdw*) that spread throughout the body and disrupted the normal motions of blood and air. At the time they were writing, doxographical theory held that residue theory was one of the identifying characteristics of a particular group of Greek physicians, the so-called Knidian 'school'; a rival to the 'school of Kos' associated with Hippokrates.

The author of *Regimen in acute diseases* was sharply critical of a now lost work, 'Knidian Sentences' (Κνίδιαι γνῶμαι); apparently the work of authors from the island of Knidos. It seems to have put forward a model of medicine that involved classifying variant symptomatologies as different diseases, offered a small number of remedies—primarily purges, whey, and milk—and attached, in its critic's view, too little importance to the kind of prognostic account of a disease's course known from other medical texts of the classical period.[69] *Regimen in acute diseases* itself evidently represented another kind of view, one that was—according to much nineteenth and twentieth century scholarship—closely associated with Hippokrates of Kos and the 'school' of Kos.[70] This historical model was partially dependent on the analysis of various Hippocratic texts as being more or less closely linked to Hippokrates himself.

Several claims for Egyptian medical influence on classical period medicine, including the link between *wḫdw* and *perittôma*, have been argued partly on the basis that the parallels appear only in texts and views associated with the Knidian physicians, and not in those linked to Hippokrates and Kos. Hence the suggestion that Egyptian medical concepts influenced physicians of the Knidian school, but were rejected or ignored by rival thinkers of the school of Kos.

Jouanna, although generally cautious, has argued for the Knidian origins of several Hippocratic texts whose nosological approach, he thinks,

---

[69] 1–3 (2. 224–226 Littré).

[70] The Greek word is *hairesis*, but the word was for any medical grouping until the later third century BCE: see von Staden, *Herophilus*. The concept 'medical school' does not belong to the classical period, and the modern term "'school' of Kos" is in itself anachronistic.

owes something to Egyptian prognostics. Mansfeld views the Knidian therapeutics described (in hostile terms) by *Regimen in acute diseases* as having much in common with Egyptian purgative therapies.[71] As for residue theories, these are described in the Anonymus Londinensis, a second-century CE papyrus that has preserved part of a medical doxography from the later years of the fourth century BCE. This is probably the work attributed by later authors to Menon, a member of the Lykeion at around that time; it certainly displays Aristotelian terminology and concepts.[72] The so-called Menoneia arranged the views of twenty thinkers on medicine from the fifth and fourth centuries into two categories: those who held that diseases came from the residues of nutriment, and those who argued that disease was due to bodily elements. One theorist of the former group was Euryphon of Knidos, assumed to be naturally a member of any Knidian school:

> Euryphon of Knidos thinks diseases are produced in the following manner; he says that when the belly does not discharge ingested nourishment, residues are generated, which, when they have risen to the area of the head, bring about diseases; however when the belly is slender and untouched, digestion happens appropriately; whenever this is not so, the result is as described.[73]

Thus, in much relatively modern scholarship, the Knidians were identified as proponents of 'residue theories', with Euryphon involved in its origination as a Greek medical concept.[74] Hippokrates of Kos was the leading member of the humoral theories that eventually supplanted earlier Knidian concepts.

---

[71] Jouanna, J. (2004). 'Médecine égyptienne et médecine grecque' in Jouanna, J. and J. Léclant, *La médecine grecque antique*, 6; Mansfeld, J. 'Theoretical and empirical attitudes in early Greek scientific medicine' in Grmek, M.D. (1980). *Hippocratica*, 371–390.

[72] There is a new Teubner edition by Manetti, D. (2011). *Anonymus Londiniensis. De Medicina*, replacing Jones, W.H.S. (1947). *The medical writings of Anonymus Londinensis*. See also Manetti, D. '"Aristotle" and the role of doxography in the Anonymus Londiniensis (*PBRLibr*. inv. 137),' in Eijk, Ph.J. van der. (1999). *Ancient Histories of Medicine*, 95–141; Nutton, *Ancient Medicine*, 72–86 esp. 72–74. IV 26–28 (Manetti p. 8): οἱ μ(ὲν) γ(ὰρ) εἶπον γί(νεσ)θ(αι) νόσους παρὰ τὰ περισσώματα τὰ γινόμενα ἀπὸ τῆς τροφῆς, οἱ δὲ παρὰ τὰ στοχεῖα. 'For while some have said that diseases arise because of the residues from nutriment, others hold that they are due to the elements.'

[73] IV 31–40. My translation, text from Manetti: Εὐ̣ρυφῶ̣ν γ(άρ) τοι ὁ Κνίδιος οἴεται τὰς νόσους ἀποτελεῖσ̣[θ]α̣ι̣ τρόπωι τοιούτωι· ὅταν ἡ κοιλία, φ(ησίν), τὴν ληφθεῖσαν τροφὴν μὴ ἐκπονήσ̣η̣ ἀπογεννᾶται περισσώματα, ἃ δὴ ἀνενεχθέντα ὡς τοὺς κ̣(ατὰ) τ̣ὴν κεφαλὴν τόπους ἀποτελεῖ τὰ[ς νόσ]ους̣· ὅταν μ(έν)τοι γε λεπτὴ καὶ καθα̣ρ[ὰ] ὑπ(άρχῃ) ἡ κοιλία, δεόντως γίνεται ἡ πέψις· Galen attributes *Knidian Sentences* to Euryphon (*In Hipp. Epid.* VI *comment*. I, *CMG* 5.10.2.2, page 54.2–4 Wenkebach), but does not specify his source.

[74] In spite of the fact that Dexippos of Kos was the author of a residues theory: *Anon. Lond.* 12.8–14.

Over the last forty years, the notion that medical schools of thought existed at all in the classical period has been sharply attacked. So has the idea that we can identify any text in the Hippocratic corpus with Hippokrates himself, or that we know what Hippokrates' views were. The idea of the Koan and Knidian schools is now rejected by most modern scholars, though a modified version is still in play on the Continent.[75] This complicates and multiplies any story of Egyptian theoretical influence upon Greek medicine, because the division between Knidos and Kos and—critically—the association of residue theories primarily with the latter, strengthened the notion of indirect influence or even direct transmission from Egyptian medicine. If this subset did exist within Greek medicine, and if certain ideas did appear only within this subset and not in other Greek medical traditions, that would be evidence for a single point of origin (or transmission) of a theory that spread throughout that group in a relatively organized manner.

Just such a point of origin, and clear evidence for the take-up of Egyptian concepts in Greek language medicine, has been seen in another passage of the Menoneia. The manuscript text is at this point very lacunose and breaks down almost completely immediately afterwards. In his 1947 edition, W.H.S. Jones produced an interpretation that makes sense and does not contradict what Greek remains, but his reconstruction and translation is inevitably highly speculative:

> Ninyas of Egypt says, uniquely, that some conditions are congenital, but some have another origin, and the congenital originate within the body. He says that diseases that are formed from another cause do so in the following way; in that whenever nourishment that has been taken has not been distributed by the body, and instead remains inside, our heat generates residues out of it.[76]

The name Ninyas is attested twice—this being one of them—in Greco-Roman literature. Its other occurrence is the name attributed to a legendary

---

[75] See esp. Lloyd, G.E.R. (1991). *Methods and Problems in Greek Science*, 192–223. Smith, Wesley D. (1976). *The Hippocratic Tradition*. Nutton, *Ancient Medicine*, 74. For the alternative viewpoint, Jouanna, J. (1999). *Hippocrates*.

[76] Anonymus, as the lines IX 37–44 appear in the edition by Manetti:

ὁ δὲ Αἰγύπτιος Νινύ[ας
συγγενικὰ γί(νεσ)θαι πάθη . [
καὶ τὰ μὲν συγγενικὰ [
εἶναι. ὑπὸ δὲ ἄλ(λης) αἰ(τίας) . [
τὰς νόσους τρόπωι ṭ[οιούτωι
ἡ τροφὴ ληφθεῖσα μὴ [
ἀλλ' ἐμμείνῃ ἡ θερμό[της] πλεί[ω] χ̣[ρόνον
ἐξ αὐτῆς ἀπογεννᾶι [

Assyrian king, and derives from the toponym Nineveh. It was not an Egyptian name, though could of course belong to members of an Assyrian family resident in Egypt.

The Menoneia's referencing of an individual whose family or person came from Egypt, and who bore a non-Greek name, is good evidence that individuals of Egyptian origin or descent could adapt to Greek language and work as Greek physicians. But Ninyas the Egyptian has been taken as conclusive proof of the *wḫdw* concept's introduction into Greek medicine. As Vivian Nutton put it for *Brill's New Pauly*: 'N(inya)s' theory, which certainly has parallels in ancient E(gyptian) medical texts ... constitutes the most explicit acceptance of non-Greek medical ideas by Greek physicians.'[77] Steuer and Saunders were nearly as positive: Ninyas' Egyptian identity was 'doubtless more than a coincidence.'[78]

As Steuer and Saunders also pointed out, Ninyas' explicit views and his own language are concealed behind the doxographer's Aristotelian terminology and interpretation.[79] His theory is one of several that involved or relied upon a notion of pathogenic food residues within the body. An Egyptian origin cannot be taken as a demonstration that his views were Egyptian rather than Greek, when many Greeks held very similar theories; nor does the author of the Menoneia indicate that he was unusual in any respect. If we do assume that being 'of Egypt' included a knowledge of and respect for Egyptian medicine, Ninyas could be considered to have held a theory of residues explicitly and knowingly compatible with, and derived from, both Greek and Egyptian etiology; and so might any other number of residue theorists. It is also perfectly possible he came from an immigrant family which had Hellenized to a greater or lesser extent, and was unfamiliar with much of Egyptian medicine.

The Ninyas affair raises the question of what kind of contacts would be required for any 'influence'—a notoriously vague term—that Egyptian disease theory might have had on Greek ideas. Egyptian plants, and, more importantly, manufactured Egyptian compounds, were by the early classical period already part of the Greek pharmaceutical and perfumery

---

[77] 'Ninyas [2]', *BNP* 9.770. For the Assyrian Ninyas, see Frahm, E. 'Ninyas [1]', *BNP* 9.679; Diodoros 2.20f.

[78] Steuer & Saunders, *Egyptian & Cnidian*, 26. Cf. Yoyotte, 'Une theorie', 81: 'sans doute significative'.

[79] Περίττωμα is an Aristotelian medical term: τὸ τῆς τροφῆς ὑπόλειμμα: *GA* 724b26, cf. Diokles of Karystos fr. 182 ed. van der Eijk, Ph. (2000). *Diocles of Carystus* 1 (both reports rather than verbatim fragments). Περιττώματα included feces, phlegm and bile: Aristotle *History of Animals* 511b9.

repertoire, attesting to contacts between traders, Egyptians workers resident in Greece, and possibly to the acquisition or exchange of medically relevant information. The transmission of physiological-pathological theory is a somewhat different case. A basic concept of putrefying feces spreading throughout the body might have been casually, even repeatedly transmitted and become widely diffused within Greek culture generally. Aristophanes' joke about Egyptian purgatives (below, p. 161) relies on such an ethnocultural stereotype. A detailed, anatomically-based, conception of *mtw*, *wḫdw*, and related norms of physiological function would have required professionalized contacts and possibly textual transmission.[80] This is possible, but we have no definite examples.

Without independent evidence for the transmission of medical theory, the diffusion of particular theoretical concepts, or a doxographic story for the spread of *perittôma* theory, the argument for Egyptian influence depends on the strength of the parallels themselves. These are weak.

The writer of the Menoneian doxography interpreted the theories of physicians through the terms and categories of Aristotelian biology. *Perittôma* is unattested in the Hippocratic corpus; it may well have been a word favored by the doxographer rather than one utilized by the theorists he summarized, and the concept lying behind it might also have been less clearly defined or more variable.[81] The identification of the pathogenic substance as excrement, and its connection to bodily putrefaction is less clearly marked in Anonymus Londinensis than it is in the Egyptian texts. Problems with kinds of food and inadequacies of digestion are far from limited to residue pathologies in Greek medicine, as food and drink are important factors in the production and regulation of bodily humors, some variant on which is an equally common physio-pathological theory in the classical period and rapidly emerged as the dominant model.[82] As such, not only were purgatives and hemogogues important, but diet was the therapeutic preoccupation of Hellenic medicine (combined with prescriptions regarding exercise, bathing, etc.) and was very closely linked to the proper digestion of foods. The widely held Greek view that blood was derived from digested food is not mentioned in Egyptian texts. In both cultures early anatomy was far from standardized, and the best evidence on the *mtw* and their meeting places

---

80 Steuer & Saunders, *Egyptian and Cnidian*, 54–55; in more detail Yoyotte, 'Une theorie', 83.

81 Above, this chapter n. 79.

82 Not counting Erasistrateans, Empiricists, probably some Methodists, and unknowns.

does not find a match, in extant Greek works, for the number and arrangement of the body's vessels.

There are similar weaknesses in other arguments for the Egyptian origin of various elements of Greek medicine during the pre-Hellenistic period. In 1939, Erik Iversen observed the similarity between a gynecological prognosis test in a classical Greek text, and that of Carlsberg papyrus VIII, 4. The papyrus dates to around 1200, but its content is earlier.[83] In both tests, a strong-smelling foodstuff is placed in the woman's vagina for a night. If the smell can be detected on her breath the next day, she will conceive; if not, she will not. The foodstuff is an onion in the Egyptian text and a clove of garlic in the Greek example. The parallels are certainly striking, but an independent development is possible in both cases.[84] Greek gynecology of the time provided an explanatory model for the test on its own terms: menses might also emerge in the form of nosebleeds, and fertility, like health in both sexes, was associated with a lack of blockages.[85] The milk of a woman who has borne a male child is a medical ingredient in both pharmaceutical traditions. The parallel is again suggestive of Egyptian influence on Greek therapy, but exactly the same prescription is attested in China.[86]

3.2.3. *Comparing Other Disease Theories*

Other parallels can be observed between many features of Greek and Egyptian pathology theories. In both disease is frequently explained or perceived as an excess, deficiency, alteration or inappropriate location of naturally occurring internal substances. These range in the Greek texts from air

---

83 *On barren women* (= *Diseases of Women* 3) 214 (8.416 Littré); *P. Carlsberg* 8.4 = *Kahun Medical Papyrus* 28. Iversen, E. (1939) *Papyrus Carlsberg No. VIII, with Remarks on the Egyptian Origin of some Popular Birth Prognoses*; but see Totelin, L. (2009). *Hippocratic Recipes*, 181–183 (including other supposed parallels).

84 Cf. von Staden, *Herophilus*, who notes that the Herophileans of Hellenistic Alexandria, who had developed a much more anatomically accurate theory of gynecology, excluded this form of prognosis.

85 Classical views of female biology: Hanson, A.E. 'The medical writers' woman', in Halperin, D. et al. (1990). *Before Sexuality*, 309–338.

86 *Diseases of Women*, in particular 2.158.13 (8.336.7–9 and 36.7–15 Littré). 'Milk of a human male child', e.g. Ebers 109 and 17 other references in the medical papyri: see Dawson, W. (1932). 'A strange drug', *Aegyptus* 12, 12–15. Totelin, *Recipes*, 179, with n. 232, argues against this being an example of Greek borrowing from Egyptian medicine, for which view see Ritner, 'Innovations', 116 and Laskaris, J. 'Error, loss and change in the generation of therapies', in Eijk, Ph.J. van der. (2005). *Hippocrates in Context*, 177–186.

(*pneuma*), blood, and a multiplicity of possible humors, not to mention the residues of the Anonymus Londinensis. In the wrong places or amounts they interfere with the workings of the healthy body, viewed as the movement of such substances through hollow channels around the body, and also affect the intangibles associated with health, such as temperature.

In the Greek world the most obvious example of this kind of system is the numerous variations on some kind of humoral theory, but the Menoneia shows that residues were also a common approach, during at least the classical period of the fourth-fifth centuries BCE. Even the ideas of the Alexandrian physician Erasistratos, a rare example of a strictly mechanistic explanation based upon the behavior of fluids under pressure, similarly conceived of the body in terms of appropriate and inappropriate amounts, positions, and movements of, in this case, blood and *pneuma*. There was thus considerable common conceptual ground in the two cultures' notions of health and illness, and a limited degree of similarity in their theories of physiology and disease, but this is a notional and partial correspondence between meta-features of medicine in two ancient cultures.

The argument that one particular theory depends on a that of a different culture requires at a minimum demonstrating that this sort of theory is unusual, and therefore that even a broad similarity is likely to be due to more than chance. But notions of balance/imbalance and hot/cold, in particular, seem to be relatively widespread ideas. Chrisman, 'Transcultural care', groups modern world beliefs about illness into four groups: the germ theory of modern biomedicine, equilibrium or harmony systems, illness caused by the human agency of sorcery or witchcraft, and illness due to gods or spirits. The link between illness and being out of harmony or balance is common not only to Greek medical thinking, at least by the days of Alkmaion of Kroton, and classical Chinese medicine, but also occurs in many Native American medical belief systems; a balance between hot and cold is important in Hispanic folk medicine.[87] There are quite a few correspondences, in fact, between isolated passages or single concepts in the Egyptian medical papyri and the fragments or ideas of individual Greek physicians. For example, Ebers 854l attributes illness to a flooding of the vessels (to the liver) with blood.[88] Erasistratos argued that all disease was

[87] Chrisman, N.J. 'Transcultural care', in Zschoche, D. (1986). *Mosby's Comprehensive Review of Critical Care*, 65–66; and for another system based on the concept of balance within the body see Lambert, M. (1995). 'Ancient Greek and traditional Zulu medicine: a question of balance', *AClass* 38, 71–87. Cf. Laskaris, *The Art*, 2 n. 5.

[88] Eb. 854l (*GdM* 4/1,5; 4/2, 28; 5, 9).

caused by too much blood (*plêthora*) in the body's venous system, causing it to flood or disrupt the other passages of the body, including the arterial network. This is not, however, inexplicable in terms of Erasistratos' radical anatomical-physiological theory—which does not have a close Egyptian parallel—and his intellectual contemporaries and antecedents within the Greek tradition.

Greeks and Egyptians both viewed air, breath and blood as among the substances carried within the channels of the body: given the universality of respiration and circulation, this is again not a surprising coincidence. As noted above, one account of disease in the Ebers implies that air was believed to cool the blood in healthy persons. Aristotle thought something similar.[89] Dissection eliminated, rewrote and to a limited degree standardized many anatomical terms and related physiological concepts of Greek physicians of the third century and later, but until then both Greeks and Egyptians were empirically limited to what went into the body, what came out, and what of its structures were visible externally or through trauma, mummification, and animal butchery.

Though the ingredients and procedures of treatment often appear similar, this can be explained equally well as a consequence of the limited medical resources of the ancient world, as by direct influence. It is also important not to extend the types of contact, usage and adaptation readily available through trade in substances, or the few large features of a medical culture readily if stereotypically observed by the visitor, to the transference of professionalized concepts and precise diagnostic criteria between different languages, cultures, and systems of technical knowledge. Evidence for pre-Ptolemaic Greek physicians having any kind of detailed acquaintance with Egyptian texts and/or ideas is doubtful, though not disproven. We have no good grounds for supposing more than the minimum suggested by Egyptian drug ingredients and the stereotypical view of Egyptian medicine as largely purgative, as in Aristophanes (below, p. 161). Herodotos' investigations do not suggest that he thought contemporary medical writers already had a good grasp on Egyptian practices (or that there was much to grasp). We also have no evidence for Greek ideas or writings influencing Egyptian medical theory, but given the paucity of our evidence from the overlapping

[89] Bardinet, *Papyrus médicaux*, 83–84, translates Ebers 854 as saying that the heart is mobile under certain kinds of pathological stress (other editions translate the passage as a reference to the motion, i.e. beat, of the heart). In Greek medical thought of the classical era the uterus is similarly not securely fixed to a single place, although in healthy women it does not wander.

time period of about 650–300 BCE, as well as the ideological anonymity and universalism of Egyptian medical texts, that is not very surprising.

3.2.4. *A Difference in Approach? Rational Greeks and Irrational Egyptians*

As we have just seen, for some external observers, specific parts of Greek and Egyptian medical theory have appeared potentially both compatible and adaptable. On the other hand, other modern authors seem to regard Egyptian and Greek medicine as incompatible in their approach, or certainly as clearly distinct. The following quotations from James Longrigg and Mario Vegetti are typical of this view:[90]

> In ancient Egypt and Mesopotamia, then, the views of the physician on the causes of disease and the operation of remedies were so linked with belief in supernatural forces that a rational understanding of the organs and functions of the body or one of the operation of the remedies applied to it was impossible.

> ... it is astonishing to see the amply documented gap between traditional Egyptian medicine—with its static and timeless repetitiousness and its unrelenting blend of clinical experience with magical practice—and Hellenistic medicine. The latter may have developed in the Alexandrian circle, but there clearly was no intellectual or social contact with the Egyptian tradition.

Egyptian medicine involves 'magic', and consequently, for many authors, is 'irrational'; it is unchanging; it involves what Longrigg calls 'the nauseating practice' of coprotherapy, which is 'much in evidence';[91] it is 'obsessed' with purgatives and digestion.[92]

Some of these characterizations—especially the purgative stereotype—derive from Greek reports and attitudes, but the explicit distinction between 'rational' Greek medicine—by which is meant (most of) the Hippo-

---

[90] Longrigg, *Greek Rational*, 1, 3–4; with Julie Laskaris' comments on these remarks, *The Art*, 26–28. Vegetti, M. 'Between Knowledge and Practice: Hellenistic medicine', in Grmek, M.D. (1998). *Western Medical Thought from Antiquity to the Middle Ages*, 84. For Alexandrian medicine see ch. 6.

[91] So does Greek medicine, if you are female. See von Staden, H. (1992). 'Women and Dirt', *Helios* 19.1–2, 7–30, with Hanson, A.E. 'Talking recipes in the gynecological texts of the Hippocratic Corpus', in Wyke, M. (1998). *Parchments of Gender*, 71–94 especially 87–92.

[92] For a vigorous attack on this kind of attitude, though one that risks a mirror-image of Egyptian superiority, see Ritner, R.K. 'Implicit models of cross-cultural interaction: a question of noses, soap, and prejudice', in Johnson, J.H. (1992). *Life in a Multi-Cultural Society*, 282–290.

cratic corpus texts, Hellenistic period fragments and Roman era works[93]—and 'magical', 'supernatural', 'irrational' Egyptian medicine, is a modern one. For a start, much of Greek medicine was not exclusive of ritual procedure, appeals to the gods, incantatory formulae, belief in god-sent diseases, divine cures, the malign effects of curses, wishes, and the angry dead, and the innate powers of plants, minerals, or even excrement. The Hippocratic and Hellenistic medical texts, even if we lump them all together as taking a broadly naturalistic approach, were not particularly representative of Greek approaches to medicine. In other words, much of Greek medical tradition and practice contains elements of magic to a degree similar to that of Egyptian medicine; moreover Egypt's medical works include physiological, anatomical and pathological concepts and deal with material stuffs and processes. In Greek texts, 'naturalistic' and god-caused explanations of illness and recovery are not necessarily opposed.[94] The purifiers treated 'the sacred disease' with dietary and similar restrictions; an approach similar to the regimen treatments of contemporary *iatroi* (physicians). The same drugs and preparations were widely used by all kinds of practitioners; indeed the *iatroi* seem to have relied on the plant-collectors and drug-sellers for at least their ingredients. In Ptolemaic Egypt, almost identical prescriptions were given by 'the god' and by physicians to two correspondents of Zenon.[95] 'Drugs', wrote the Alexandrian anatomist Herophilos, 'are the hands of the gods'.[96]

In any case, it is a mistake to say that Egyptian medicine—or any other part of Egyptian thought—involves something we call the supernatural. As there is no Egyptian term for such a concept, its usefulness for describing Egyptian ideas is limited, whether we think we are imposing an objective category, a modern category, or the category developed in some Greek authors, of *para physin*. *Para physin* is like most modern references to the 'supernatural', which is not a culturally validated term in academic discourse and therefore tends to be dismissive or pejorative. It designates not another category of beings beside 'nature' (*physis*), but things mistakenly thought to be part of nature.[97] The supernatural cannot exist without its

---

93 But not traditional Roman medicine.

94 The idealizing meta-analysis of a medical system promulgated through its writings is moreover often not the same as that system as practiced. For biomedicine's failures to live up to the ideal of scientific process, see Gordon, D. 'Tenacious assumptions in western medicine', in Gordon, D. and M. Lock. (1988). *Biomedicine Examined*, 19–56.

95 *P.Cair.Zen.* III 59426, TM 1066 and *PSI* 4.413 (third century), TM 2096. See also above, 2.3.2, pp. 71–72.

96 von Staden, *Herophilus*, 416–418 (T248–T249) and 400 ff.

97 See Lloyd, *Magic, Reason and Experience*, 49 ff.

exclusion from some prior definition of the natural, but there is no equivalent distinction in Egyptian thought. Whatever else disease demons may be, in Egyptian texts they have the same existence status as the rest of the Egyptian cosmos—they are in this sense perfectly natural objects.

Equally anachronistic is the use of the terms 'rational' and 'irrational' to characterize, respectively, the Greek invention of naturalism, and Egyptian explanations involving gods, the dead, and *ḥkꜣ*. Such an analysis presupposes our own awareness that the former approach eventually (but perhaps not inevitably) led to the empirically demonstrable successes of modern biomedicine and science. It then backdates this confirmation, applying it to a set of theories and procedures that are not, in fact, those of science as it is now practiced and understood.[98] There is nothing 'irrational' about 'magic' or 'religion' if they work as well as other theories and associated treatments within a consistent view of the world that was as empirically validated as any other.[99] There was no empirical evidence for an excess of a substance such as phlegm, rather than a god, being the cause of a disease; and certainly no trial—let alone a statistically valid one—showed that treatments based on the former were more effective than those of the latter.

The differences between Egyptian and intellectualized forms of Greek medicine were located chiefly in the justificatory explanation offered for therapeutic practices, and in what other elements were included or excluded—for example, whether an incantation accompanied the topical application of a drug, or—especially in the Hellenistic period—how surgery was used, and for what conditions. The Hippocratic-era *Oath* implies that only some practitioners practiced 'cutting for the stone', but surgery for internal conditions, absent entirely from surviving Egyptian material, was developed much further among Greek practitioners in the Hellenistic and Roman periods.[100] Such differences, however, are more often a matter of

---

[98] For the issue as to what, if anything, should count as science in the pre-modern world, see Lloyd, G.E.R. (2004). *Ancient Worlds, Modern Reflections*, 12–23, 'Science in ancient civilizations?', with references.

[99] Greek medical texts and other philosophical works often appeal to empiricism in the form of eye-witness evidence and common or possible observations; but not to a degree, or with a consistent methodology, comparable to modern science; its purpose was to support and persuade more often than discover. See Lloyd, *Magic, Reason and Experience*, 146 ff. An empirically-grounded program of research was formulated for biology by Aristotle (*Parts of Animals* I 5) and continued by the Alexandrian anatomists, but dissection was far from routine and actual experiment very rare, especially outside physics and ballistics: the medical experiment of Erasistratos reported in Anonymus Londiniensis XXXIII 43–51 is an exception.

[100] See Celsus *Medicine* book 7.

emphasis than incompatibility. Epistemological argument and theoretically explicit naturalism is characteristic of Greek intellectual enterprise, together with a strongly narrative framework of explanation and action, but even this strand of medicine contained divergent views on disease causation. Medical and philosophical texts often recast divinity as the operation of, or as inherent in, natural law and materials: nature was itself divine. The purifiers' methods relied implicitly on the common religious view that gods prefer, reject or are manifest in certain materials or actions: so that avoiding polluting goat products acts as a protection against god-sent disease.[101] The explicit exclusion of gods as relevant to the natural world was very much a minority move, made only by the Epicureans and a very few others.[102] God(s) as natural law and materials, gods—or the dead—working through material entities and processes, and the explanatory description of those laws and materials, are often compatible and sometimes closely aligned.

This elaboration of otherworld causation into predictable material states of the body is visible in both Egyptian medical texts and terminology and at least some Greek writers, notably Herodotos. Indeed, the Egyptian emphasis, at least in the diagnostic and prognostic passages of the medical texts, is sometimes less explicit about which kind of demons or dead people are responsible, than they are about what is happening in the body in terms of processes and substances, such as a blockage in the heart or a rise in temperature. It is apparently these that most affect the appropriate prognosis and therapy. That is, the 'any dead person, deity or enemy' of the therapeutic spells identifies a general kind of problem, but in a specific person's body the disease entity is itself more individualized and consequently requires more analysis and description, couched in terms of the disruption of healthy processes as well as of specific morbid substances.

3.3. *Egyptian and Greek Medicine: Contemporary Perceptions*

The question remains as to whether, and if so how, Greeks and Egyptians, especially those of the Hellenistic period, perceived elements of medicine as specific to their own culture, or superior to that of others.

---

[101] *The sacred disease* 2.

[102] For Epicurean views see e.g. Long, A.A. and D.N. Sedley. (1987). *The Hellenistic Philosophers*. A summary of types of ancient atheism can be found in Auffarth, C. 'Atheism', *BNP* 2.232–233. The insult *atheos* often means a rejection of more conventional views, but not the notion of divine power itself; cf. *asebeia*.

The Greek ethnographers certainly identified a specifically 'Egyptian medicine', as discussed above. Egyptian sources, most of which drastically predate Greek texts, do not mention any foreign system of medicine, but medical works—usually the private and informal handbooks of practitioners listing plants and recipes—were acquired by cult officials and their families for temple scriptoria and personal collections in the Greco-Roman period.[103] Pharmaceutical exchange can be documented.[104] The ideologically governed conventions of Egyptian technical-ritual genres, however, precluded any explicit acknowledgment of a non-Egyptian cosmic order or kind of knowledge, in contrast to the comparative, anthropological approach common in Greek literature.[105] This is related to the distinction between Egyptian and Greek medicine made in two ancient sources and widely repeated in modern accounts, between the supposed unchanging homogeneity of the former, and its explicit or implicit contrast with the notoriously changeable and varied world of Greek medicine. According to Aristotle, '... in Egypt it is permitted for physicians to change [their advice] after the fourth day, but if earlier, it is a risk for them'. Three centuries later, Diodoros was in receipt of similar information:[106]

> For the physicians draw their support from public funds and administer their treatment in accordance with a written law which was composed in ancient times by many famous physicians. If they follow the rules of this law as they read them in the sacred book and yet are unable to save their patient, they are absolved and go unpunished; but if they go contrary to the law's prescriptions in any respect, they must submit to a trial with death as the penalty, the lawgiver holding that but few physicians would ever show themselves wiser

[103] van Minnen, P. (1998). 'Boorish or bookish? Literature in Egyptian villages in the Fayum in the Greco-Roman period', *Journal of Juristic Papyrology* 28, 99–184. School copying of Hippocratic works is also demonstrated. The majority are Roman period, or cannot be precisely dated other than as Greco-Roman. For Roman period texts in particular, see Hanson, A.E. 'Greek medical papyri from the Fayum village of Tebtunis: Patient involvement in a local health-care system?' in van der Eijk, *Hippocrates in Context*, 387–402. See further 5.2.1, pp. 221–222.

[104] Totelin, *Hippocratic Recipes*, 153–156. See further 4.2.3, pp. 167–177. Pharmaceutical exchange may well be something of an iceberg, with most of the relevant material unexamined or unrecognized, in the study of ancient Greek and Egyptian medicine, since there have been few experts in both languages: Hanson, A.E., personal communication, 2011.

[105] Cf. Baines, 'Literacy and society', 592: 'What is also missing in Egypt is the abstract form of textual argument that arose in Greece ... In Egypt no such mid-level metalanguage appeared.' For incorporated material from foreign sources see Ritner, 'Innovations'.

[106] *Politics* 1286a13–14: καὶ ἐν Αἰγύπτῳ μετὰ τὴν τετρήμερον κινεῖν ἔξεστι τοῖς ἰατροῖς, ἐὰν δὲ πρότερον, ἐπὶ τῷ αὑτοῦ κινδύνῳ. Diodoros 1.82, trans. Oldfather. For comments on the extent of this practice, Nunn, *Egyptian Medicine*, 121. For its uses, Ritner, 'Innovations', 107 n. 1.

> than the mode of treatment which had been closely followed for a long period and had been originally prescribed by the ablest physicians.

Greek and Latin texts meanwhile commonly represent Greek medicine as polemical and inconsistent, resulting in a perception of unreliability and lack of authority. The author of *Regimen in acute diseases* observed:[107]

> Yet the art as a whole has a very bad name among laymen, so that there is thought to be no art of medicine at all. Accordingly, since among practitioners there will prove to be so much difference of opinion about acute diseases that the remedies which one physician gives in the belief that they are the best are considered by a second to be bad, laymen are likely to object to such that their art resembles divination.

Nature of man opened with a denunciation of monists; *The sacred disease* with an all-out assault on a common and widely accepted view of that condition.[108] References to the incorrect opinions and varying ability of predecessors and contemporaries were commonplace, especially in opening remarks.[109] Even in more technical fields, dealt with in books such as *Fractures*, practice was divergent: '... I know practitioners who have got credit for wisdom by setting people's arms in positions which ought rather to have given them a name for ignorance'.[110] Any reader of Celsus, Rufus, or Soranos, among others, is familiar with the later doxographic maze of medical allegiance and argument. Galen's creation of his own image is achieved largely through conflict with other doctors and schools. He aligns himself rhetorically with past authorities, notably Hippokrates and Plato, against present rivals, but his take on classical medicine is a heavily interpreted one. Tradition had authority, but it has to be the right tradition, and there was no single canon for Greek medical practice until Alexandria in late antiquity and the early Islamic period.[111]

In contrast to the variation of theory and approach offered by the Greek medical works is the apparently more unitary form of Egyptian healing texts. Egyptian works do not draw attention to divergence or reference

---

[107] Ch. 8 (2.240–242 Littré). Cf. *Law* 1 (4.638 Littré): 'Medicine is the most distinguished of all the arts, but through the ignorance of those who practice it, and of those who casually judge such practitioners, it is now of all the arts by far the least esteemed.'

[108] *Nature of Man* 1 (6.32 Littré); *The sacred disease* 1–5 (6.352–366 Littré).

[109] E.g. *Regimen* 1 (6. 466 Littré); *Regimen in acute diseases* 6 (2.238 Littré); *Ancient medicine* ch. 1, ch. 15 (1.570, 604 Littré).

[110] *Fractures* 1 (3.414 Littré), cf. *Joints* 1 (4.78 Littré).

[111] See Nutton, V. (1995). 'Medicine in late antiquity and the early Middle Ages', in Conrad, L.I. et al, *The Western Medical Tradition*, 71–87.

disagreement or, for that matter, individuals, although some medical texts are associated with a particular god (as their author). Their contents are presented as collective, authoritative knowledge without use of the first person. They state rather than persuade.[112]

Geoffrey Lloyd has argued that the agonistic context of small scale *polis* society produced Greek culture's dominant rhetoric of competitive disagreement. Among doctors this tendency was reinforced by competition among practitioners for patients and pupils, as well as for intellectual status.[113] Oral debates and readings took place alongside the circulation of written texts in which particular methodological, epistemological and medical standpoints were explicitly argued and alternatives criticized: the audiences included prospective pupils and other doctors, but also other intellectuals and all interested parties and onlookers, as part of a public, face-to-face and agonistic society. In Egypt, on the other hand, technical materials circulated internally among literate professionals, with temple scriptoria as the chief mode of horizontal and vertical transmission. They may even have been subject to restrictions of usage and availability.[114]

Thus part of the perceived difference in approach is actual, and was due to the different social context and function of medical works in classical Greek and Late Egyptian society. A large part of the distinction is nonetheless one of presentation rather than content, or even methodology. Egyptian medicine is less static, and Greek theorists less radical, than the explicit assertions of the latter would lead one to suppose.

The cultural stereotype of Egypt as unchanging, in other aspects than medicine, is common among Greek authors. It derived not only from Egypt's demonstrable antiquity, but also from Egyptian self-presentation.[115] Elite Egyptian institutional culture coded power as the written word itself and its associations with authority and agreement. The codification of medical knowledge in written form has therefore a different cultural value from

112 A structure common to both medical and mathematical works is a system of a sequence of cases introduced by the phrase, 'If you find …': Parkinson, R.B. (2002). *Poetry and Culture in Late Middle Kingdom Egypt*, 55.

113 Lloyd, G.E.R. (1991). *Methods and Problems in Greek Science*, 417–434 ('The invention of nature'). Dean-Jones, L. 'Literacy and the charlatan in ancient Greek medicine', in Yunis, H. (2003). *Written Texts and the Rise of Literate Culture in Ancient Greece*, 98–99, argued that written texts attracted medical apprentices from outside the family.

114 See Baines, J. (1990). 'Restricted knowledge, hierarchy and decorum: modern perceptions and ancient institutions', *JARCE* 27, 1–23, esp. 15 ff.

115 E.g. Herodotos 2.100.1, 2.142–143 on the length of Egyptian royal history, cf. Diodoros 1.69.9 and Manetho's Greek language presentation of dynastic chronology.

that of Greek medical texts. Variation is downplayed in written contexts, which instead display a rhetoric of a consistently valid and unitary knowledge among largely technical domains, including the cultic, medical, and astronomical.[116] Egyptian narratives were repeatedly re-edited, re-composed and, in the late Egyptian and Greco-Roman periods, translated and adapted into Greek.[117] Although Egyptian physicians must have learnt partly through training and experience, their knowledge and authority is portrayed as dependent on consultation of eternally true and canonical texts: the authority of the expert depends officially not on their ability to interpret past authorities, to make discoveries, or to apply written knowledge to individual cases, but in their ability to read and reproduce the power of the word. An official inscription from the pharaonic period describes one physician as 'reading the papyrus rolls daily'.[118] The tomb of Weshptah, the vizier of king Neferirkara (2475–2455 BCE), tells the story of its occupant's dramatic collapse. In response 'the king summoned lector priests and physicians and had them consult books of medicine and magic'.[119] The authority of such writings derived from divine authorship. A text incorporated into the Ebers papyrus was said to have been found under the feet of the statue of Anubis (Ebers 856; quoted above, p. 114).

The reports of Aristotle and Diodoros are a reflection of this ideological idealization of medicine. The status of Diodoros' written law (νόμος ἔγγραφος) for the physicians of Egypt is unclear, but as with references to prohibitions and penalties concerning famous 'magic' texts, it is the expressive declaration rather than a practically enforced set of procedures that matters.[120]

The Greek rhetoric of disagreement and rival truths, and the Egyptian depiction of an unchanging and single field of knowledge, created a mirage of medical practice that by emphasizing those aspects served to obscure others. The vigorously expressed differences of Greek medical writers

---

116 For a brief summary see Tait, J. 'The wisdom of Egypt: classical views' in Ucko, P. and T. Champion. (2003). *The Wisdom of Egypt*, 26 ff.

117 See Jasnow, R. (2002). 'Recent Trends and Advances in the Study of Late Period Egyptian Literature', *JARCE* 39, 207–216.

118 Jonckheere, F. (1958). *Les médecins de l'Égypte pharaonique*, no. 62.

119 Breasted, J.H. (1906). *Ancient Records of Egypt* 1.242–249 (no. 246).

120 For the dangers of knowledge in the wrong hands, and prohibitions against this occurrence, see the demotic story cycle of Setne Khaemwese: Lichtheim, *Literature*, 3.125–138. For the reliability of Diodoros' accounts of Egyptian history and *nomoi* see e.g. Africa, T.W. (1963). 'Herodotus and Diodorus on Egypt', *JNES* 22, 254–258; Murray, O. (1975). Review of A. Burton, *JHS* 95, 214–215.

distracts the reader from noticing that these are often variations on a theme, and that the number of themes is limited. Greek writers on medicine resisted any hypothesis of contagion and employed variants on humoral or residue theories of imbalance and blockage in bodily vessels, related to seasons, qualities and elements.[121] Anatomical knowledge underwent what should have been a paradigm shift in the early third century, thanks to the efforts of Herophilos and Erasistratos, but it did not transform medical theory and had a limited degree of penetration into medical practice outside the elite. Some five centuries later Galen was still having to make the case for the usefulness of dissection in medical practice. In the second century CE the philosopher Calvisius Taurus, visiting Aulus Gellius in Attica, was acquainted with the difference between veins and arteries, discovered in Alexandria some four to five centuries previously: the local physician was not.[122] The Stoic Khrysippos refused to recognize the anatomists' empirical proof that the hegemonikon was within the head; preferring on several grounds the traditional location of the heart.[123] Medical methodology, meanwhile, problematized both deduction and empirical investigation but could not solve the question of how they related; the late Hellenistic methodological sects locked many practitioners into a defensive and doxographical mode of justification, not investigation.[124]

Within the extant material on Egyptian medicine, at least some of the concepts at work—*wḫdw, ꜣḫj, mtw* etc.—appear reasonably consistent. However, the few works that survive do not always agree on anatomical and theoretical detail, while a multiplicity of treatments is routinely cited for a single illness.[125] The extant New Kingdom copies of the Ebers and Smith

---

121 The obvious exception is Erasistrateanism, and to a lesser degree Asklepiades' *poroi*: Vallance, J.T. (1990). *The Lost Theory of Asclepiades of Bithynia*. For miasmic seeds as a theory of contagion, see Nutton, V. (1983). 'The seeds of disease', *Medical History* 28, 1–34, repr. in ibid. (1988). *From Democedes to Harvey* ch. 11.

122 Aulus Gellius *Attic Nights* 18.10.

123 See e.g. Tieleman, T. (1996). *Galen and Chrysippus on the Soul*, 51, 233 ff., on the Stoics' arguments against the location of thought in the head, and on the validity of poetry as a form of knowledge.

124 For the origins of the methodological schools of the Hellenistic period see von Staden, *Herophilus* part II: 'The Herophileans'.

125 For the multiple additions of alternative remedies and terms under the rubric, 'Another', 'another book said', 'otherwise said', see *GdM* 7/2, 899–902; cf. Ritner, 'Innovations', 109–110. For catalogues in Greek medical literature see van der Eijk, Ph.J. 'Towards a rhetoric of ancient scientific discourse: some formal characteristics of Greek medical and philosophical texts (Hippocratic corpus, Aristotle)' in Bakker, E.J. (1997). *Grammer as Interpretation*, 95 ff. These include not only the Hippocratics (e.g. *Diseases of Women* 1.84 (8.127–186 Littré)) but

papyri glossed older terminology and diagnoses in more contemporary kind: either medical terminology or medical concepts or both had evidently changed in the meantime. As we have seen, Egyptian cult officials in the Ptolemaic and early Roman periods collected Greek medical texts or used them for pedagogical purposes, including a commentary or variation on the classical period work *Regimen*.[126] The major differences between Greek and Egyptian technical works on medicine remain the lack of methodological or epistemological controversy in Egyptian texts as opposed to Greek and Latin ones, and no sense at all of the self-consciously critical and eristic nature of Greek discourse. The genre had different functionalities within each society.

3.4. *In Greek Egypt*

The question then becomes: do we have any evidence for transmission of medical ideas or practices between Egyptians and Greeks within Ptolemaic Egypt? Greek soldiers were present in sizable numbers in Egypt from the sixth century BCE. Some settled there. Doctors or semi-specialist healers, like makers of equipment, camp-followers, and other trades must have accompanied these immigrants and formed part of the population of Memphis, Naukratis, and other settlements throughout the countryside. In the Ptolemaic period, such immigration and settlement reoccurred on a much larger scale. Larger towns acquired quarters of different cultural and ethnic characters, while in smaller villages and new foundations Greek immigrants and Egyptians lived in close proximity to people of different linguistic and cultural backgrounds; the predominance of males among early settlers necessitated intermarriage from a very early stage. For some dwellers in the countryside, in particular, access to physicians of a particular language and kind of medical training must have been restricted or difficult. The plants, foodstuffs and other ingredients of diet and drugs had to be either local or expensively imported. Diseases and poisonous animals were not always

---

also numerous Greek *receptaria* on papyrus (see, e.g. Andorlini, I. ed. *Greek Medical Papyri* II 5.). The similarity between this catalogue form in Greek and Egyptian medical literature was noted by Goltz, D. (1974). *Studien zur altorientalischen und griechischen Heilkunde; Therapie, Arzneibereitung, Rezeptstruktur*, 150–165, but see also G. Harig's review of Goltz. (1975). *Deutsche Literaturzeitung* 96, cols. 654–658.

[126] First described as P.Tebt. III 897, this papyrus was published in full as *P.Bingen* 1, MP3 539, TM 60195.

identical to those of Greece, the Aegean islands, or western Asia Minor, while the original immigrants must have brought new pathogens with them. A degree of adjustment and acquisition between both patients and the professionals faced with treating them seems likely and has some support, but its particulars are less easily assumed.

One important piece of evidence has already been discussed in the context of temple medicine, which is to say within the context of Egyptian professional medicine. Greek works on medicine have been found on the sites of Egyptian temples, where they were at least acquired and probably copied for temple scriptoria. They may also have been used by cult officials for treatment, as Egyptian medical texts written in hieroglyphs, hieratic and demotic were, but that remains speculative. It is also worth noting that Greek medical texts crop up in Ptolemaic Egypt as pedagogical materials, alongside Homer and Athenian tragedians, implying that such works were viewed as a legitimate part of Greek literary culture, but not necessarily in a way that excluded other systems of medicine in cases of actual illness (or its prevention).

The suggestion that Egyptian professionals, at least, were not only acquiring but reading and to some degree utilizing Greek works, is supported by the instances of drugs and ingredients in late demotic papyri that are used in Greek medicine but unattested in earlier Egyptian texts, and, in some cases, are from outside Egypt.[127] In itself, as I argued above in reference to Greek use of Egyptian materials, this type of cross-cultural borrowing does not necessarily mean anything more than Egyptian physicians investigating Greek trading stock.[128] A demotic text of the Roman period, however, employs technical words used with precision and corresponding closely to their usage in Greek medical texts.[129] Jacco Dieleman, discussing this papyrus, observes that:

---

[127] A second century CE papyrus from Krokodilopolis was thought by its editor to mention several substances from the Mediterranean region previously unattested in Egyptian medicine: Reymond, E.A.E. (1976). *A Medical Book from Crocodilopolis: P.Vindob.D.6257* (LDAB 55973, TM 55973). Many of these identifications are doubtful: Dieleman, *Priests, Tongues* (below, n. 129), 111 n. 23. See further nn. 129–130, this chapter, and also 4.2.3, p. 167, n. 107.

[128] See chapter 4, especially 4.2.3–5, pp. 167–183 for discussion of the use of drugs or ingredients from different medical systems.

[129] P. London-Leiden, first edited by Griffith, F.Ll. and H. Thompson. (1904). *The Demotic Magical Papyrus of London and Leiden.* (P. London 10070+P. Leiden I 383: together LDAB 55973, TM 55955). Dieleman, J. (2005). *Priests, Tongues, and Rites. The London-Leiden Magical Manuscripts and Translation in Egyptian Ritual (100–300 CE).*

> The medical terminology used in P. London-Leiden is, though, limited in number, in line with the terminology of the medical papyri of the pharaonic period, except for 7 Greek loanwords ... Since the use of Greek medical terms is restricted to a single spell each, every instance is an isolated one-time usage rather than a completely accepted loan word. The Greek terms are spelled in alphabetic Demotic signs, or in one case in cipher, and integrated into a running demotic sentence. The term *podakran*, written in Greek script serves as heading to a demotic prescription against gout.[130]

We can cautiously conclude that by the early Roman period, and possibly before, Egyptian technical literature incorporated novel nosological classifications and their accompanying Greek-language terminology. This indicates a continuum of approach with the pharaonic era adoption of Semitic disease entities (in the form of demons), which were likewise transliterated rather than translated. We can speculate that multiple routes of transmission included oral contacts between professionals, reinforced by the diagnostic expectations of patients with a Greek linguistic background, to a degree sufficient for some degree of textual penetration. There is a considerable difference between such classifications of a disease and the details of its nature or cause; and we cannot determine from the above whether the inclusion of *podakran* entailed, for instance, use of humoral theory, or whether it was recast in terms of more traditional Egyptian physiology. It does however demonstrate that Greek medicine was not discounted by or entirely irrelevant to Egyptian physicians: instead it was used to extend their knowledge, their capacity to act against disease, and probably their client base. Exposure on a large scale to Greek professionals and patients did not rewrite Egyptian medicine as that of Greek professional, post-classical medicine—humoral (usually), regimen-oriented, tending to mark itself off from divine modes of explanation and therapeutics—but allowed it to incorporate useful elements of diagnosis, treatment and possibly theory on their own terms. The accumulation of these additions was legitimized by being unmarked: like other innovations, such foreign novelties were written into Egyptian use and literature as part of its permanent record.

The relation of Greek physicians to Egyptian medicine was similar. In the second century CE Galen attributed a recipe to the temple of Hephaistos

130 Dieleman, *Priests, Tongues*, 117–118. For the medical Greek loanwords of P. London-Leiden see ibid. appendix 4.2, p. 312. This is unusual: Dieleman adds that the demotic medical papyrus edited by Reymond, *Medical Book* (LDAB 55973, TM 55973; above, n. 127) contains no medical terms from other languages. Reymond's example is wrong: see Dieleman, 118 n. 41.

(Ptah) at Memphis.[131] The claim, whether or not it was doxographically accurate, shows Greek incorporation of Egyptian knowledge, rendered authoritative not by silence, as in Egypt, but by singling out a remedy to a particular origin. The origin point was itself a claim to authority by virtue of its invocation of the Homeric trope of Egypt's reputation in drugs.[132] As we saw in section 3.2.3, other instances of Egyptian influence upon Greek theories are more difficult to establish, especially when discussing disease concepts rather than specifics of terminology or procedure. Independent developments can rarely be ruled out. This is also the case for the development of Herophilean pulse theory and diagnostics in Ptolemaic Alexandria, or for the use of dissection by the anatomists on the possible model of Egyptian embalming procedure.[133] Ninyas, in the classical era, wrote nothing not explainable in terms of Greek medicine and language of the time; the 'Egyptian physicians' of Roman period texts refer again to physicians present physically in Egypt but operating professionally in Greco-Roman cultural and medical contexts. This sort of thing might hint that a medical Hellenism or a bilingual orality was possible, as in the creation of Greco-Egyptian literature, the magical-religious synthesis and its philosophical relatives, or, more simply, the ability of numerous inhabitants of Ptolemaic Egypt to operate successfully in both Greek administrative and distinctively traditional contexts, at least of oral communication. On this model, at least some Greek and Egyptian theories were understood as compatible or equivalent alternatives, not as excluding markers of a unique validity. But Ninyas might also be an example of just such an exclusively Greek theorist: his name and geographical epithet merely fossilized indications of a largely discarded identity.[134]

A working theory of Greco-Egyptian medical interaction, in the arena of theoretical concepts as understood by professionals, is compatible with a separatist model of identity, but allows for significant points of contact

---

131 *The composition of drugs according to place* 9.5 (13.294 Kühn).

132 Préaux, C. (1956). 'Les prescriptions médicales des ostraca grecs de la Bibliothèque Bodléenne', *CdÉ* 31, 147–148, suggests that Greek adoption of Egyptian drugs was much rarer than the converse, pointing as an example to the absence of the common Egyptian ingredient beer in Greek prescriptions. On the other hand this may indicate adaptation rather than rejection, since beer was often used as a liquid base, and Greek moisteners were more likely to be honey, wine, oil or water.

133 See further 6.2–3, 251–258.

134 Cf. Hanson, A.E. 'Egyptians, Greeks, Romans, Arabs, and Ioudaioi in the first century A.D. tax archive from Philadelphia: P. Mich. inv. 880 recto and P. Princ. III 152, revised', in Johnson, *Life*,133–145.

between the systems as a whole (one is not 'more rational' than the other) and between specifics of recipes, practices and, potentially, theoretical concepts such as a relation between excrement, anatomy, and illness. Some theoretical systems were exclusive of others. Caelius Aurelianus says that [a] 'follower of Herophilos, thinks that indigestion and spoiled food are what must be examined' in looking for the cause of cardiac disorders.[135] This sounds, again, rather like *wḫdw* theory, but Herophilos' work on anatomy would have necessarily excluded the anatomy of pharaonic medical texts, which was closely linked to the pathology of *wḫdw*. In general concepts are more compatible, their elaboration into explicit, anatomically-detailed theory less so. The relationships between Greek and Egyptian-trained physicians are thus more likely to have been exclusory than those between Egyptian physicians and Greek patients, or vice versa; but they also offered opportunities for the adaptation, assimilation, and expansion of medical knowledge.

As in other societies in which more than one system of medicine is available, the stance of patients was probably multivalent and their preferences contingent upon the availability and local authority of practitioners, as well as upon the degree to which the patients were linguistically or otherwise embedded in one culture rather than the other (or both). Greek forms of medicine were more heterogenous, and Egyptian practice more flexible, than is often allowed: an individual's preferences for amulets, purgatives, or regimen were as much founded on their positioning within their own culture's choices as they were about a choice between cultures. In the next chapter, we shall investigate the evidence for the navigation of this territory by patients and practitioners in the form of responses to illness: diagnosis, prognosis, and treatment.

---

[135] Caelius Aurelianus *Acute Diseases* 2.39.225 (*CML* 6.1.1, 282.5ff.) = von Staden, *Herophilus*, T214.

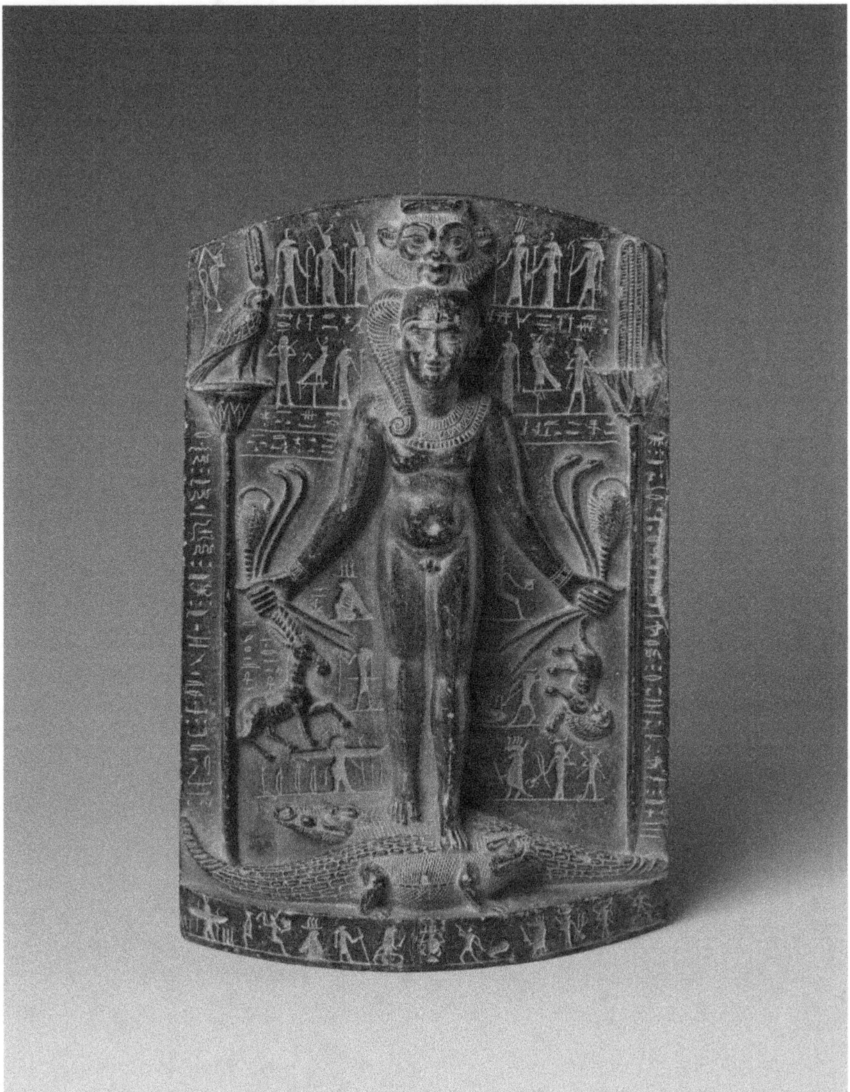

Figure 2. Cippus of Horus.

CHAPTER FOUR

RESPONSES TO ILLNESS

Responses to illness—diagnosis, prognosis, therapeutics—articulate the relationship of an individual or small group to broader explanatory models and values within a society or social sector.[1] One definition of a therapeutic procedure is the organized application of techniques with the aim of achieving a goal; that goal being an improvement in the state of a person who is ill or otherwise medically incapacitated. This can include palliative as well as curative care, and the improvement might be only temporary or relative. Aelius Aristides, for instance, was chronically ill with both long-standing and novel complaints, but still regularly perceived certain events as marking transitive improvements in an illness, in his work, or in his quality of life.[2] For an individual experiencing illness, therapeutic choices are one means by which personal and social identity is negotiated and displayed. The therapeutic process aims at reintegrating the patient within the norms of social and individual expectations, or to put it another way, at reestablishing their ability to cope with daily life.

Therapeutic decisions were principally made on the basis of diagnosis and its underlying theories, but a fatal prognosis could eliminate the patient's access to medical intervention altogether. The explicit recommendation that practitioners, in cases where the patient was not expected to recover, ought not to treat, was common to both Egyptian and Greek medicine.[3] This part of the medical encounter was therefore one in which the patient had limited power, but they had some room for maneuver by seeking out alternative practitioners and kinds of medicine. Therapeutic recommendations could be ignored or adapted, as the author of a classical period Greek text irritably noted;[4] surgery could be refused. Among

---

[1] In the work of the anthropologist Arthur Kleinman (n. 9), this kind of interaction is called a 'semantic illness network': an individual's involvement in a set of shared concepts, experiences or symbols.

[2] Behr, C.A. (1968). *Aelius Aristides and the Sacred Tales.*

[3] Smith case 6, 'An ailment for which nothing is done' (except palliative care): p. 75 in the translation by Allen, J. (2005). *The Art of Medicine in Ancient Egypt.* Cf. cases 7, 8, 13, 17, 24, 31, 33, 37, 44. Greek classical period: *Art* 8 (6.4–6 Littré), and see below, 4.1.2, pp. 149–150.

[4] *Art* 7,10–12: καὶ μὴν πολύ γε εὐλογώτερον τοῖσι κάμνουσιν ἀδυνατεῖν τὰ προστασσόμενα

practitioners, the process of diagnosis and therapy articulated their power and agency within and via social expectations of the healing role. Oral debate and written argument were both part of medical and intellectual culture in Greece as early as the fifth century,[5] but the personal reputation of doctors and other healers was largely achieved through the healing encounter. Diagnosis, prognosis, drug prescription and preparation, surgical skill, or expertise in ritual or regimen, formed part of an individual healer's modus operandi compared to that of his competitors. Successes and disasters could make or break a career, but effect was also achieved through a theater of healing. Among *iatroi*, that included displays of deduction that amounted to prophecy, use of technical jargon, crowd-pleasing treatments or elaborate bandaging, quoting poets, and even exoticism of dress (or the rejection of same).[6] In folk medicine, Theophrastos described dramatic displays by two drug-sellers, who demonstrated their power over *pharmaka* by swallowing large quantities of hemlock. In a separate incident, a shepherd's ability to ingest a whole bundle of roots undermined the reputation of a drug-seller, previously famous for being able to eat one or two without ill effect. The drama of the situation is underlined by the death of one of drug-sellers.[7]

The unifying ideological stance of Egyptian medical texts obscures any similarly competitive aspect within Egyptian medicine, but the performative, real-time nature of the encounter with the patient shows up even more strongly through their handbook format with its instructions for preparation and application: 'Next you shall say (diagnosis) ... Then you need to make him a potion (ingredients) ...; it is crushed and often drunk, so that he will be healthy.'[8]

ὑπουργεῖν, ἢ τοῖς ἰητροῖσι τὰ δέοντα ἐπιτάσσειν. 'It is a good deal more probable that the sick are unable to follow instructions, than that doctors do not order what is necessary.'

[5] Thomas, R. (2000). *Herodotus in Context*, esp. 249 ff. Lloyd, G.E.R. (1979). *Magic, Reason and Experience*, 96–98.

[6] On the importance of prognosis to reputation and medical skill see *Prognosis* 1; cf. *Fractures* 35, *Joints* 9 and 58, *Epidemics* 1, ch. 5; and below, 4.1.2, pp. 149–151. For other elements of physicians' self-presentations see especially *Decorum*, esp. ch. 2 and *Precepts*, esp. chs. 10, 12, both probably composed in the Hellenistic era.

[7] *Enquiry into Plants* 9.17.1–2; 9.16.8. Also below, 4.2.4, pp. 177–178, n. 156. (Theophrastos attributed this ability to survive to an individual's steadily increasing the amount ingested, thus increasing that person's tolerance; but in one case he also reported the use of an antidote for an overdose).

[8] Ebers 202. German translation *GdM* 4/1, 92: 'Dann sollst du dazu sagen (... diagnosis) .... Dann sollst du ihm ein Trankmittel machen: (... ingredients ...); werde durchgepreßt, werde getrunken oft, so daß er sofort gesund wird.'

The medical discourse of the practitioner might differ, in some cases sharply, from a particular illness as experienced by an individual patient, from the explanations of other kinds of practitioner, or from lay understandings of medical concepts. In 1980, Arthur Kleinman published an influential analysis of health care systems, in which he distinguished between medical sectors within any society: 'popular', 'folk' and 'professional'. The first consists of those with no particular interest or expertise in healing beyond the norm; the second of specialists in health care who have no official, professional standing; and the third of 'acknowledged' specialist professionals, often with official, organized or institutional status.

There are difficulties with the application of this division to antiquity, not least in defining the recognition of professionals *vis-a-vis* that of folk-sector healers. For the purposes of this chapter, the point is that whatever forms of recognition applied to practitioners of healing, the performative encounter between practitioner and patient was a form of negotiation within, or between, one or more of Kleinman's 'semantic illness networks'.[9] In the rest of this chapter, we shall explore elements of the patient-practitioner encounter one by one, beginning with diagnosis.

The overwhelming majority of the evidence for this encounter is textual material, in most cases derived from the upper-status end of Kleinman's 'professional' sector, that is from texts written and used primarily by Greek *iatroi* and Egyptian *swnw*, 'physicians'.[10] As we shall see, some practices, such as offering a diagnosis or the use of pharmaceuticals, were in more general use, with differentiation taking place primarily according to external criteria such as availability, expense, or the degree of expertise of local practitioners. Even among such common procedures, however, explanatory models varied—particularly between Egyptian models and those of Greek *iatroi*, or, within the Greek sector, between *iatroi* and other healers; details of usage varied frequently. Other procedures were more specifically tied to specializations among practitioners; some seem, for the beginning of the Hellenistic period at least, to have been unique to either Egyptian or Greek medical practice.

This raises several questions. In Ptolemaic Egypt, did patients or medical practitioners perceive there to be such a thing as 'Greek' or 'Egyptian'

[9] Kleinman, A. (1980). *Patients and Healers in the Context of Culture*. For his notion of semantic illness network, see n. 1. For more on distinguishing 'professional' and other categories of healer, see especially 5.1.1, pp. 206–212; 5.3.3, pp. 236–238.

[10] Other terms for physician, e.g. *wʿb*-official of Sakhmet and *sȝw*, appear to identify subsets of this category. See 5.1.1 and below, p. 145 n. 14.

medicine, with distinctive characteristics? To what degree did semantic illness networks, embedded in the culture and social structures of pre-Ptolemaic Egypt and Greece, translate? Were elements of medical practice defined, adopted, or resisted in terms of ethnocultural preferences? Is medicine an example of a separation of cultural systems within Ptolemaic Egypt,[11] or did patients make health care choices among an expanded range of alternatives and practitioners without regard to ethnocultural criteria?

4.1.1. *Diagnosis*

Even self-medication requires some framework, however limited, of medical knowledge, by which particular substances or procedures are associated with symptoms. Few adults call up their doctors to find out what to do in case of headache; they lie down or take a painkiller on their own. Recognizing a sting as that of a nettle, and applying a dock leaf, is still part of the lay folklore of British families.

In ancient Egypt, papyri like the Brooklyn snake papyrus carefully described the appearance of poisonous animals, the effects of their bites, and the therapeutic options, but much of this knowledge must also have been acquired through experience and observation; it was then communicated orally. Only when it was written down was its information available only to a single language group, and its bilingual origin, available in oral form to speakers of both Greek and Egyptian, was forgotten. Certainly everyone could recognize the scorpion genus, even if they could not instantly distinguish between less and more dangerous species.[12] Most cases of illness and injury in antiquity were self-diagnosed. In the lay sector of widely held beliefs and commonplace medical knowledge, diagnosis

---

[11] Claire Préaux argued specifically for separate medical systems: (1956). 'Les prescriptions médicales des ostraca grecs de la Bibliothèque Bodléennes', *CdÉ* 31, 148: 'Tout semble indiquer que les Grecs se sont installés dans le pays égyptien avec un bagage médical apporté de chez eux, et qui ne changera guère au cours des siècles, comme ils ont apporté avec eux leur droit, leur notariat et les auteurs qu'ils lisaient dans leurs écoles.' For the 'separation' model of Ptolemaic Egypt see 1.3.1, p. 30.

[12] The Brooklyn Museum Papyrus 47, 218.48 + 47, 218.85 differentiates carefully between different species of snakes and the effects of their bites. Ed. and trans. Sauneron, S. (1989). *Une traité égyptien d'ophiologie. Papyrus du Brooklyn Museum No. 47.218.48 and 85*, dating it to the early Ptolemaic era. A date in the 27th dynasty (525–404 BCE) might be more likely: Verhoeven, U. (2001). *Untersuchungen zur späthieratischen Buchscrift*, 306. See also chapter 1, p. 6.

was essentially implicit in the selection of treatment and based upon such basic associations as that between a scorpion bite and a stinging pain; treatment of other problems, such as nosebleeds, did not require a causal analysis at all (for purposes of treatment).

For most kinds of healer, in both Egypt and Greece, the classification of disease was a crucial part of their practice. In classical period Greece, texts describing symptoms and diseases offered a particular kind of medical discourse, that of the *iatroi*, from which other explanatory models were more or less excluded.[13] Egyptian medical works, which included diagnostic materials, specifically declared themselves to be for the use of specialist healers, and were available to literate individuals as a group.[14] Material evidence, such as statuettes that protected homes or vulnerable sleepers from attacks by disease-demons, indicate that the basic concepts of disease causation expressed in Egyptian medical texts were also at work within lay and folk conceptions of illness.[15] The specialized, authoritative domain of the expert was marked by the detailed symptomalogical accounts of disease classification to be found in several of the Egyptian medical texts. Diagnostic passages took the healer through the steps needed to identify the disease: 'If you see a man suffering from his stomach and he is vomiting much, ... his two eyes are bloodshot ....then you should say concerning it: it is a product of putrefaction of his mucus.'[16] An Egyptian work on traumatic conditions distinguished carefully between 'a wound in the head which has reached to the bone of his skull without gaping' (case 1) and 'a gaping wound in his [head], which has penetrated to the bone and violated [his skull]' (case 2).[17] Diagnosis of the immediate cause was often followed by a precise description of its effects upon the physiological system:

---

13 *The sacred disease* described the classificatory systems of purifiers, but this is a rare example. Below, p. 148 n. 30. Gordon, R. 'The healing event in Graeco-Roman folk medicine', in van der Eijk, P., H.F.J. Horstmanshoff and P.H. Schrijvers. (1995). *Ancient Medicine in its Socio-Cultural Context* 2.363, identifies five kinds of 'magical' healer in addition to the *iatroi*.

14 The medical texts of the Ebers and Smith papyri describe themselves as for the use of *swnw*, *w'b*-officials of Sakhmet, and *s3w*: Ebers 854a; Smith case 1, gloss A. Chester Beatty 6.6 declares itself a 'manual of a collection of remedies of the *swnw*. The Brooklyn medical papyrus describes the remedies used by the *ḫrp šrḳt*. A single individual might hold one, two or more of these and other medically relevant titles: see chapter 5.

15 Below, section 4.3.2, pp. 188–189.

16 Ebers 192, trans. Nunn, J. (1996). *Ancient Egyptian Medicine*, 88.

17 Edwin Smith papyrus case 1, 1–2, 2. Ed. and trans. Allen, *Art of Medicine*, 72–73.

> ... his heart, it comes in fear, his face pale, his heart, it knocks: if you examine him you will find his heart hot, his belly distended. [Then you will say:] this swelling is a blockage of animal flesh; he has eaten sharp roasted meat.[18]

Medical texts from the classical and Hellenistic periods of the Greek world reveal a diagnostic process equally dependent upon specialized close observation by experts.

> In pneumonia (περιπλευμονίη), the following happens: there is violent fever, and the patient's breathing is rapid and hot; he is distraught, weak and restless, and beneath his shoulder-blade he suffers pain that radiates toward his collar-bone and nipple; he has a heaviness in his chest, and he is deranged. In some patients there is no pain until they begin to cough; this pneumonia lasts longer and is severer than the one with pain from the beginning.[19]

The detailed case histories of *Epidemics* are well known. Although the reason for their collection is not made explicit, it was probably to clarify diagnosis and prognosis through observation and collocation, in particular through the association of symptoms with fever periodicities.[20]

In both medical systems, illness was categorized on the basis of the symptomatic group—fever/heat, phlegmatic disease, tumors—or took the analysis a stage further in identifying the underlying cause, whether this cause was identified as the maleficent dead or as an excess of blood (see chapter 3). But in spite of such efforts, diagnosis was not an exact science. Terminology was not standardized, except to some degree by common frameworks of use. Anatomical vocabulary, in particular, was used inconsistently.[21] In the extant Egyptian medical papyri there are many explanatory glosses by later copyists and editors. In the Hellenistic period, Alexandrian physicians produced medical glossaries and exegesis of earlier texts, for the sake of both clarity and as a weapon in theoretical and methodological disputation.[22]

---

[18] Ebers 207; German translation *GdM* 4/1, 94: '... sein Herz (ib), es gerät in Angst, sein Gesicht ist blaß, sein Herz, es klopft: wenn du ihn untersuchst und du findest sein Herz heiß, seinen Bauch aufgetrieben. [Dann sollst du dazu sagen]: das ist eine tiersitzende Anschwellung; er hat scharf gebratenes Fleisch gegessen.'

[19] *Diseases* 3.15 (Translation Potter 1988: Loeb *Hippocrates* VI). It continues on the subject of pneumonia symptoms.

[20] Potter, P. 'Epidemien I/III: Form und Absicht der zweiundvierzig Fallbeschreibungen' in Baader, G. and R. Winau. (1989). *Die Hippokratischen Epidemien*, 9–19; Lloyd, *Magic, Reason and Experience*, 154–155.

[21] For vague and varying terminology in classical period texts, see e.g. Craik, E. (1998). *Hippocrates: Places in Man*, 12–13. Development of anatomical terms: Lloyd, G.E.R. (1983). *Science, Folklore and Ideology*, 149–167.

[22] von Staden, H. 'Hairesis and heresy: the case of the "haireseis iatrikai"', in Meyer,

The level of diagnostic consensus between healers is today described as the interpractioner rate of agreement, for aspects of medical practice that vary between practitioners.[23] It depends partly on a shared theoretical framework and the precision of accepted diagnostic criteria; partly on the ease and experience with which it can be put into practice. Some conditions are simply hard to diagnose: meningitis in children is notoriously difficult to differentiate from less dangerous fevers. In antiquity, some differences in diagnosis, and consequently in therapy, were due to individuals or groups holding incompatible beliefs, for instance that epilepsy is caused by excess of phlegm, rather than by a god.[24] Even doctors with apparently the same nosological views could interpret symptoms very differently, especially when multiple diseases were explained by relatively few and ill-defined theoretical concepts (e.g. blockage, humor, balance, invading entity).[25]

Remarks in a number of Greek and Latin works also paint a vivid picture of physicians disagreeing vigorously at their patient's bedside, and it seems to have been quite usual, for those who could afford it, to consult more than one expert.[26] *Regimen in acute diseases*, *Joints*, *Fractures*, Soranos' *Gynecology* and the collected works of Galen all contain many references to incorrect opinions or treatments, contrasted with the author's own approach. The patient was thus left with the task of navigating the contradictory recommendations of his physicians.[27]

B.F. and E.P. Sanders. (1982). *Jewish and Christian Self-Definition in the Graeco-Roman World*, 76–100, 199–206.

[23] E.g. Davis, P. et al. (2000). 'The "supply hypothesis" and medical practice variation in primary care: testing economic and clinical models of inter-practitioner variation', *Social Science and Medicine* 50 (3), 407–418.

[24] These are not in fact necessarily incompatible as I have formulated them—the god could be responsible for, or present as, phlegmatic excess—but the author of *The sacred disease* explicitly excludes the latter.

[25] *Breaths* is an extreme example—all diseases are due to air. Theories involving more than one kind of humor allowed greater differentiation in disease causation, but still to a limited degree.

[26] For physicians having to compete with each other during consultations, and in other arenas of persuasion, e.g. *Joints* 1; *Decorum* 3. Disagreement in debate: see Craik, *Places in Man*, 9–10.

[27] Menander 659 Jaekel, πολλῶν ἰατρῶν εἴσοδός μ' ἀπώλεσεν, 'the visiting of multiple doctors destroyed me'; cf. Pliny *Natural History* 29.5.11, the funerary epigraph *turba se medicorum perisse*. Hadrian is said to have uttered a variant on this 'popular saying' (τὸ δημῶδες): ὅτι πολλοὶ ἰατροι βασιλέα ἀπώλεσαν, 'Many physicians killed the king': Cassius Dio *Roman History* 69.22.4.

In Egypt, ideological conventions framed medicine as objective, collective, and unchanging knowledge. In practice, however, amid competing claims to personal authority, individual variation in diagnosis and therapy must have occurred. The text of the Edwin Smith papyrus repeatedly uses a word meaning 'knowledge gained from practical experience' at the beginning of each of its 48 diagnostic categories, or cases.[28] Two glosses to the original text mention another treatise, 'The nature of wounds', in support and explication.[29] One or more additional author-copyists have added these and other glossing explanations; if we have no evidence for the assertion of difference in written medicine, there is certainly a role for individual assessment and the selective use of information. The multiplicity of drug recipes and incantations cited for the same conditions in the Egyptian texts also testifies to the generation of new alternatives and their acceptance within even the ideologically coherent written tradition.

Few of the precise nosological entities familiar to Greek physicians were readily identifiable with those of Egyptian medicine. The outstanding exceptions are in the category of trauma, together, to an extent, with other externally visible conditions such as cataracts or external deformities, mutilations, and growths. Many symptoms or groups of symptoms, including fever and pus, were commensurable in themselves, but the selection of what counted as a symptom, its evidentiary value, and in particular the extension of symptamologic criteria into a diagnostic classification were more specific to a particular professional culture and its explanatory models. The attribution of illness to divine or demonic presence, sometimes with particular symptoms associated with a particular god—as in the 'swellings of Khons' at Ebers 874—is well attested for both professional and folk sectors in pharaonic Egypt, and among Greek purifiers, but not among Greek physicians.[30]

---

28 Allen, *Art of Medicine*, 9: *ssзwj*.

29 Smith case 5 gloss 1; case 41 gloss 1.

30 See Borghouts, J.F. 'Divine intervention in ancient Egypt and its manifestation', in Demarée, R.J. and J. Janssen. (1982). *Gleanings from Deir el-Medina*, 1–70, esp. 29; Westendorf, W. (1999). *Handbuch der Altägyptischen Medizin*, 374. For Greek purifiers classifying madness by correlating gods with symptoms: *The sacred disease* 4. In Egyptian healing ritual, parts of the patient's body were identified with the corresponding body parts of gods, and his body as a whole with Horus, e.g. BM 10309 incantation 2, ed. and trans. Leitz, C. (1999). *Magical and Medical Papyri of the New Kingdom*, 22–28; P. Leiden I 348, spell 12: ed. Borghouts, J.F. (1971). *The Magical Texts of Papyrus Leiden I 348*.

4.1.2. *Prognosis*

Diagnosis was closely related to prognosis, which in turn impacted treatment. Prognosis was a major part of the interaction between physician and patient, as well as with any other individuals involved, such as family, friends and neighbors. Its most essential form is the assessment of mortality. The late fifth-century Greek treatise *Wounds in the head* put it this way:[31]

> When anyone is going to die from wounds in the head, and it is impossible to make him well or even save his life, the following are the signs from which one should make the diagnosis of approaching death and foretell what is going to happen.

The topic of wounds in the head was shared by the trauma text of the Smith papyrus, which employed three categories of prognosis—good, bad, and uncertain. These were expressed in terms of the physician's response: 'an ailment I shall treat', 'an ailment with which I shall fight', and 'an ailment I shall not treat'. The first two of these have parallels in other Egyptian medical works, but the refusal-to-treat category is unique to the Smith.[32] The healer uttered the diagnosis and prognosis aloud and, it seems, in the wording formulated in the text.

We lack the patient's point of view on such pronouncements. A fatal prognosis in antiquity was usually made at a late stage of an acute disease—unlike today, when modern testing can result in a death sentence years removed, or for patients who do not yet feel themselves to be ill—and was unlikely to have been a surprise. When a patient was delirious or unconscious, the accuracy of the prognosis—for the remaining course of the disease—served partly to impress the physician's skill upon the surviving members of the household.[33] When the patients were able to react, a favorable prognosis from a trusted authority must often have induced the placebo effect; its antithesis, the corresponding nocebo effect.[34] The author of *The Art* justified declining to treat in such cases as a simple recognition of his profession's limitations: 'to refuse to undertake to cure cases in which the disease has already won the mastery, knowing that everything is not

31 *Wounds in the head* 19.

32 The first formula is found in the Smith, Ebers, Hearst (once) and Berlin (twice); the second only in the Smith and the Ebers (twice).

33 *Prognostic* 1 (2.112.11–12 Littré) complains that physicians were often brought in at too late a stage; the last days of such cases are vividly depicted by the *Epidemics*' case histories.

34 The nocebo effect: summary of recent research by Pilcher, H. (2009). 'The science of voodoo; when mind attacks body', *New Scientist* 2708, 30–33.

possible in medicine.' The fact he had to justify the practice suggests, however, that not everyone was happy with physicians refusing treatment, an implication the author confirms: 'some find fault with the healing art because of those who are not willing to attempt treating patients overpowered by diseases.'[35] Other Greek works also make it clear that the practitioner's reputation was at stake. 'One should especially avoid such cases [those requiring reduction of the thigh or upper arm] if one has a respectable excuse, for the favorable chances are few and the risks [to the patient] many.'[36] The author of *Diseases of women* recommends that if one cannot avoid refusing to treat a particular condition, the doctor should 'treat it only after first announcing your prognosis', apparently in an effort to avoid high expectations on the part of the patient.[37] In some circumstances, evidently, practitioners did treat 'incurable' cases.[38]

Prognosis was an aid to the decision choices of the practitioner, Egyptian or Greek, as much as information for the patient. It also, and this was crucial, demonstrated his command over the subtle technicalities of medical observation, his mastery of a hidden world of demons and/or internal processes, and his ability to integrate these into an understanding of the future.[39] Greek prognoses were often detailed predictions of the course of the patient's illness; and in this respect a fatal prognosis demonstrated the practitioner's ability in lieu of a cure. *Prognostics* supplied the prognosticator's manifesto in its opening chapter:

> If he is able to tell his patients in advance when he visits them not only about their past and present symptoms, but also to tell them what is going to happen, as well as to fill in the details they have omitted, he will increase his reputation as a medical practitioner and people will have no qualms in putting themselves under his care.[40]

---

35 *Art* 3, 2; 8, 1–7 (6.4–6, 12–14 Littré; *CMG* 1, 1,10.21 ff.). For fatal or incurable prognoses in general, see von Staden, H. 'Incurability and hopelessness: the *Hippocratic Corpus*,' in Potter, P. et al. (1990). *La maladie et les maladies dans la collection hippocratique*, 75–112. Refusal to treat: 103 ff.

36 *Fractures* 36 (3.540.9–12 Littré); cf. *Prognostics* 1 (2.112.10 f. Littré): 'by realizing and announcing beforehand which patients were going to die, he would absolve himself from any blame.'

37 *Diseases of women* 1.71 (8.150.12–13 Littré).

38 E.g. *Joints* 11 (4.104.21 Littré) criticizes practitioners who 'do not even try' to cure patients with dislocated shoulders. On this see Wittern, R. (1979). 'Die Unterlassung ärztlicher Hilfeleistung in der griechischen Medizin der klassischen Zeit', *Münchener medizinische Wochenschrift* 121 no. 21, 731–734; cf. von Staden, 'Incurability', 107 ff.

39 Physicians were usually male. For women as medical practitioners, 5.1.2, pp. 214–216 and 5.1.3, pp. 218–219.

40 2.110 Littré, cf. 2.112; *Joints* 58 (4.252.14–17 Littré).

The physician's display of knowledge of the hidden and the future was a crucial and highly competitive feature of Greek medicine.[41] It also assimilated the medical practitioner to the figure of the prophet; a display of personal charisma that some practitioners carefully fostered. The classical period author of *Prorrhetic* 2 attacked the circulation of 'amazing' (θαυμασταί) predictions as improbable and not based upon clinical signs.[42] In the second century CE, Galen was careful to tell his readers that his rivals called him a seer (*mantis*), as did astonished clients and onlookers—at least until Galen explained how he did it all by deduction on the basis of medical theory.[43] This recurrent motif implied that Galen's unique ability to analyze the present was equivalent to the prophet's certain knowledge of the future, even as his disavowal reinforced his rationalist credentials. In a (possibly semi-fictionalized) case history Galen took care to conceal the details of his medical detective work from his patient's family, who are subsequently suitably astonished by an apparently telepathic diagnosis. The readers, however, are let in, like Watson by Holmes, on the attention to detail that made it possible.[44] At a time when the physiological effectiveness of most therapeutics ranged from dubious to harmful, prognosis was the expert's chance to shine.[45]

For the patient, a believable diagnosis-prognosis, subject to confirmation as the stages of the disease progressed, reinforced the authority of the healer and of any treatments he carried out. It enabled her to construct her illness in terms of the objective entity described by the physician and determined its temporal framework, even to some extent its outcome. It gave the disease a name and pinned down its properties.

---

41 *Epidemics* 1.11.9–10 (2.634.6–7 Littré); *Fractures* 35 (3.538.6 Littré), *Joints* 9, 58 (4.100.4, 4.252.14 f. Littré).

42 *Prorrhetic* book 2, chs 1–2; cf. *Regimen in acute diseases* 3 (2.242.3 ff. Littré).

43 Galen *Prognosis* 5 (*CMG* 5.8.1, p. 94): ὁ δ' ὡς ἐκ μαντικῆς αἱ προρρήσεις καὶ οὐκ ἐκ θεωρίας ἰατρικῆς γίνοιντο; cf. 7. 6 ff. (*CMG* 5.8.1, pp. 106–107); *Examinations by which the best physicians are recognized* 4.2 (*CMG Suppl. Or.* 4.63).

44 *Prognosis* 6.18–19 (*CMG* 5.8.1, pp. 100–104). Flemming, R. (2000). *Medicine and the Making of Roman Women*, 263–264, suggests this story was heavily or entirely fictionalized, based on a closely parallel case in the literary-historic tradition involving Erasistratos and the Seleucid royal family, a model to which Galen explicitly draws attention. For other versions of this tale, including its inclusion in stories of Hippocrates, see Pinault, J. Rubin. (1992). *Hippocratic Lives and Legends*, 60–77. I owe the comparison between Galen and Sherlock Holmes to Mattern, S. (2008). *Galen and the Rhetoric of Healing*, 79.

45 Except via psychological effects, such as the placebo.

4.2.1. *Therapies*

Therapeutic choices are dependent not only on a partially empirical base of local tradition including, for example, botanical knowledge, but also on the theoretical framework and diagnostic choices of the healer, which may diverge sharply both between and within the medical culture(s) of a particular society.

There was considerable overlap between broader characteristics of therapeutic practice in Greek and Egyptian medicine. Treatment usually involved the use of *materia medica*. Such substances were applied topically, ingested orally, or administered through fumigations, pessaries, and suppositories; they were often combined with oral or gestural formulas. In cases of injury practitioners additionally employed methods including manipulation, bandaging, surgery, and cautery. Preventative or prophylactic care formed a related and sometimes overlapping category characterized by the use of amulets, statuettes or similar artifacts, and *cippi* (see 4.3.3), as well as attention to diet.

Some aspects, however, were relatively specific to Greek or to Egyptian medical systems. Egyptian physicians employed substantive drugs within an accompanying oral and performative ritual that was itself embedded in a mythological-theoretical framework. (I discuss this in much more detail below, at 4.2.2).[46] '*Ḥkꜣ* ('magic') is strong in combination with a medicine,' according to the Ebers papyrus.[47] On the other hand, many Greek *iatroi* excluded personalized or external entities from disease theory and diagnosis, eliminating traditional therapies such as oral incantations or amulets on the same grounds; this was the dominant understanding of the Greco-Roman social elite (although possibly a minority view overall, and sus-

[46] For a summary, Westendorf, *Handbuch*, 524–528.

[47] Ebers 3. There is no good translation for *ḥkꜣ*, at least in anything less than a 3-sentence definition. Ritner, R.K. (1993). *The Mechanics of Ancient Egyptian Magical Practice*, 4–28 argued for the term 'magic' as useful for a category of Egyptian acts and actors (unlike 'religion') if anachronistic aspects and pejorative use are discarded; cf. Baines, J. 'Display of magic in Old Kingdom Egypt', in Szpakowska, K. (2006). *Through a Glass Darkly*, 1–3. Stephen Quirke prefers to reject 'magic', 'religion' and 'medicine', as 'not having been successfully defined for the Pharaonic context', e.g. (1997). *JEA* 83, 244; cf. (1992). *Ancient Egyptian Religion*, 113. I have generally preferred 'religious' terminology, because in modern society 'religion' implies social authority and widespread intellectual validity where magic does not, but the modern reading of 'religion' as distinct from the workings of a 'physical' world, or 'science,' is also anachronistic. I have used 'medicine' as largely synonymous with 'healing', since it implies something broader than therapeutics.

ceptible to considerable nuance on what was and was not included).[48] The excluded items are precisely the type of explanation and therapeutic response central to all we know about Egyptian medicine. The practice of naturalistic medicine was certainly not without its performative aspects, but these had very different justifications.

Secondly, dietetic rather than pharmacological prescriptions had become a crucial part of (higher status) Greek medicine before the Hellenistic period. Iain Lonie remarked that, as early as the classical era: 'If we exclude diet [and the gynecological texts], therapy in Hippocratic texts reduces to a few simple formulas for purges and emetics'.[49] (Such purges and emetics were however widely used in both cultures: pp. 157–163). Regimen could be curative, as the title given to the classical text *Regimen in acute diseases* implies, but also often preventative: *Regimen* and *Regimen in health*.[50] In contrast, long-term prescription of daily regimen, especially as a preventative measure, did not appear in Egyptian medicine. (Herodotos' claim that Egyptians purged themselves preventatively for 3 days a month is not supported by Egyptian sources; see 4.2.2.1, pp. 161–162). I shall argue below that this difference is a consequence of differing views on disease causation: for Egyptian healers, ill health was ultimately the result of attack from outside. Medicine was remedial and prevention defensive. For Greek physicians, at least those who subscribed to the naturalistic approach, illness was the result of a failure—innate or chosen—on the part of the patient. It could therefore be prevented by ensuring that the patient conformed to his environment; an act of agency and self-control closely related to Greek moral and political ideology.[51]

A third possible distinction was in attitudes to invasive surgical intervention for internal conditions. Egyptian texts testify to the excision of visible tumors and problems, and to intervention in cases of injury, but do

48 As Lloyd, *Science, Folklore and Ideology*, 129 notes, the authors of the 'Hippocratic' texts never mention amulets, either favorably or unfavorably. Since non-medical contemporaries do mention the use of amulets and associated beliefs, albeit often with skepticism, this exclusion seems programmatic: Theophrastos in Plutarch, *Life of Perikles* 38; Plato, *Charmides* 155e–156e; cf. Polybios *Histories*, 8.17. See further 4.3.2, pp. 187–188 with nn. 192–198.

49 Lonie, I.M. 'Literacy and the development of Hippocratic medicine' in Lasserre, F. and P. Mudry. (1983). *Formes de pensée dans la Collection Hippocratique*, 153.

50 Littré 6.466 ff. and 6.70–87. For an overview of Hippocratic-era dietetics: Craik, E. 'Hippocratic *diaita*', in Wilkins, J. et al. (1995). *Food in Antiquity*, 343–350.

51 The distinction is not absolute: Greco-Roman folk medicine, in particular, retained notions of externality and attack; while Egyptian texts also sometimes link behavior to disease, e.g. crimes that offend the gods, or overeating (4.2.2.1, p. 162).

not describe other forms of surgery. No certain surgical scars have been identified on over thirty thousand mummies examined in the last two centuries, suggesting that it was at best extremely rare.[52] This is also the case for classical period Greek medicine, with the partial exception of embryotomy and excision of bladder stone ('cutting for the stone') carried out by some practitioners but not others.[53] Surgical methods, however, including internal operations, developed rapidly among practitioners of Greek medicine during the Ptolemaic period, especially among elite physicians.[54] Similarly, many Greek physicians used phlebotomy regularly, but the practice is entirely absent from Egyptian medicine, and examples of cauterization are much more limited in the extant Egyptian literature than in the Greek. On the other hand, several of the central characteristics of Egyptian medicine—oral, performative, artifactual and pharmaceutical modes of affecting illness—informed healing methods in other sectors of Greco-Roman society; and Egyptian drugs expanded the pharmacological repertoire of Greek physicians. Commensurable aspects of Egyptian and Greek practice, moreover, might well have reinforced tendencies and trends in both, e.g. the use of enemas, purgatives, and possibly dissection.

In particular, quantification and a degree of polypharmacy are characteristics of much Egyptian medicine previous to the Ptolemaic period; perhaps Egyptian influence was responsible for their appearance in Hellenistic and later Greco-Roman pharmaceutics. Similar questions arise for the Herophileans' introduction of the pulse as a diagnostic tool, an understanding attested in Egyptian texts but absent from earlier Greek medicine.

4.2.2. *Conceptualizing Drugs*

'*Pharmaka* [drugs] are the hands of the gods', said the third-century BCE Alexandrian physician Herophilos.[55] He probably meant the common natu-

---

[52] Rowling, J.T. (1989). 'The rise and decline of surgery in dynastic Egypt,' *Antiquity* 63 (239), 316. Below, 4.4., pp. 118–120.

[53] *Oath* lines 22–24 (4.630 Littré): οὐ τεμέω δὲ οὐδὲ μὴν λιθιῶντας, ἐκχωρήσω δὲ ἐργάτῃσιν ἀνδράσι πρήξιος τῆσδε ('I will not cut, even for the stone, but I will leave such procedures to the men who carry out that craft'), implying that other physicians did operate on bladder stone. Cf. the third- or second-century BCE text *Physician* 14 (9.220 Littré).

[54] 4.4, pp. 193–196. Since the majority of surviving texts comprise diagnostic-pharmaceutical handbooks or collections of oral formulas, it is possible that surgery and related therapies in Egyptian medicine are invisible rather than absent.

[55] Four sources attribute this remark to Herophilos: T248a, b, c (with Wellmann's emendation) and T249 in von Staden, H. (1989). *Herophilus: the art of medicine in early Alexandria.*

ralistic identification of divinity with the workings of nature, though a more traditional assertion of direct creation by gods is also possible. The sentiment expressed, in any case, seems commensurate with a near-contemporary Egyptian observation: 'He [god] created remedies to end illness, wine to end affliction.'[56] (The second half of this remark also has many parallels in Greek culture). Egyptian gods created remedies: 'Another remedy which Isis made for Ra, to expunge the pain in his head.'[57] In Greece, Hermes tells Odysseus how to obtain and use the root moly in his defense against Kirke.[58]

Many societies, including those of ancient Egypt and Greece, assess the medicinal or affective qualities of plants, animals and minerals though analogical reasoning. The squirting cucumber was employed in classical Greek medicine as a purgative, an emmenagogue and to induce birth; the latter two at least probably on the basis of the forceful ejaculation of its seeds, and perhaps empirically confirmed by its actual laxative effects.[59] In case nine of the Edwin Smith papyrus, the wound has 'fractured the shell of his skull.' The prescription includes a powder made from ostrich eggshell. When the bandage is taken off, on the third day, the 'shell' will have healed, and now has the same constitution as an ostrich egg(shell).[60] The frangibility, curvature and protective function of shell and skull are aligned, so the shell's properties of strength and wholeness can be transmitted to the skull bones as well.

Some Greek theorists extended this kind of approach into the theory of similars by similars. The property that is supposedly shared between the patient or illness on the one hand, and the plant or other substance used to treat it, need not be as obvious as the case of the squirting cucumber. Indeed, it often requires the eye of the expert, which is convenient for the

---

[56] *Papyrus Insinger* 32.12, translated by Lichtheim, M. (1983). *Late Egyptian Wisdom Literature*, 230.

[57] Ebers 247 = Hearst 75, cf. Ebers 242–246: remedies made by gods (Re, Shu, Tefnut, Geb, Nut) for themselves or each other. Gods were also responsible for the properties of drug ingredients: the tears of Re turned into honey-producing bees: Derchain, Ph. (1965). *Le Papyrus Salt 825, II, 5–7*, 137.

[58] *Odyssey* 10.304–306.

[59] King, H. (1998). *Hippocrates' Women*, 153. In other cultures, plants that produce flowers, fruits or seeds noticeably or in quantity are associated with enhanced fertility. See Etkin, N. 'Ethnopharmacology', in Johnson, T.M. and C.F. Sargent. (1990). *Medical Anthropology: Contemporary Theory and Method*, 152–153, for these and other types of cross-cultural associations between efficacy and plant property.

[60] Translation by Allen, *Art of Medicine*; cf. the slightly variant version of Westendorf, *Handbuch*, 720–721. Ostriches lay the largest eggs of any living species: the shells are thick but contain small pits, possibly reinforcing the similarity to a human skull.

expert. The alternative system of treatment by opposites, allopathy, could be equally subtle in its reasoning, and disagreement over the properties (drying, moistening, binding, loosening etc.) of conditions, foods, and drugs was a common cause of inter-physician disputes.[61] The lengthy classical work *Regimen* offered an extremely detailed analysis of the specific properties of food substances, varying by preparation: 'Wheat is strongly nourishing, more so than barley, but both it and its gruel are less laxative. Bread made of it without separating the bran dries and passes through, but purged of the bran it nourishes more, but is less laxative. Of the various breads themselves ...' (42).

That kind of analysis derived from and reinforced a Greek concept of health, developed in the classical period, as being qualitatively in balance with the rest of the substantive universe. A small number of elemental materials could be 'chemically' understood in terms of their qualities—usually hot, cold, wet and dry. Larger scale structures, such as bodily structures and humors, were explained by the relative proportions of such properties. More complicated versions of this model extended or varied the numbers of humors and properties—the fourth century theorist Praxagoras of Kos argued for eleven humors of relative saltiness, sweetness and so on, as well as hotness and coldness.[62] The human body (including the mind) reflected the qualities of its local environment, transmuted into biological properties through breathing in the winds, drinking the water, and eating foods that had been nourished by the earth. If these were such as to maintain a balance between bodily elements and their qualitative properties, health resulted; if not, the body became imbalanced, dysfunctional, and ill. Different species of plants, foodstuffs and other substances, and different regional varieties, had varying qualitative effects upon individuals because of their own constituent qualities. These kinds of explanations downplayed the visual or functional analogies that were probably originally responsible for the existence of particular ingredients within the pharmaceutical repertoire. Instead they redescribed empirical experience and folk tradition within a naturalistic model that excluded most amulets or spoken remedies, although Galen was able to explain his observations of one amulet's effectiveness in terms of the vapors emanating from the plant remains it included.[63]

---

[61] Aristotle *Nicomachean Ethics* 2.3.1104b18: 'medicines work naturally by means of oppositions'. Cf. [Hipp.] *Aphorisms* 2.22, 5.19; *Breaths* 1.

[62] Frs. 50–52, 54–60: Steckerl, F. (1958). *The Fragments of Praxagoras of Cos and his School.*

[63] *The temperaments and properties of simples* 6.10 (11.859.12–860.8 Kühn), cf. 10.19 (12.207

Other substances used for their repulsive or dramatic qualities—narcotics, cathartics, odiferous plants like garlic—were incorporated into the 'chemical imbalance' model, although different physicians drew the naturalistic line in different places. Within the theoretical framework of many Greek *iatroi*, although a person is to some extent at the mercy of their local environment or inherent variations in constitution, they can continually readjust their internal condition through diet, exercise, bathing and other forms of *diaita*, 'regimen'. More elaborate regimens were effectively restricted to those with disposable time and income, but basic dietary formulas could have been widely followed. Acute illness was primarily treated with the more drastic realignments of *pharmaka*, from milder diuretics to emetics and powerful laxatives; as well as cautery and phlebotomy.[64] In the earlier fourth century, Plato offered a man-on-the-street summary of the kind of therapeutics on offer: 'When a carpenter ... is sick, he expects his physician to give him a drug in order to vomit the disease out, or get rid of it by purging downward, or using cautery or the knife.'[65]

Cathartics—laxatives, emetics, and (for women) emmenogogues—were easily justified in terms of the imbalance model, but they were also continuous with the socio-religious concept of purification. The same words were used for both: *katharsis*, *katharmos*.[66] As a medical belief, this survives in modern society under the name of detoxification, not to mention colonic irrigation. Evidently it has enough emotional force to withstand a certain lack of scientific rigor, and in antiquity, of course, there was no actual scientific explanation with which it could be compared. Cathartic drugs, along with their procedural cousin phlebotomy, were a consistent and significant part of Greek medicine for as long as we have records of it. Herophilos' widely reported aphorism on hellebore equated it to a brave general:

Kühn) on Galen's test of the medicinal properties of green jasper for the health of the stomach. Galen found the stone effective in itself, rather than the healing design prescribed in the astrological-medical tradition.

64 For this approach e.g. *Places in Man*, *Aphorisms*.

65 *Republic* 3.15, 406d–e. The 'carpenter' and his ilk rejects the 'kind of doctor' who prescribes (lengthy) dietetics. Cf. *Aphorisms* 7.87: 'What diseases are not cured by *pharmaka*, iron (i.e. surgical instruments) cures; whichever diseases iron does not cure, fire (cautery) cures; whatever fire does not cure, should be considered incurable.'

66 The classic work on purity and pollution in ancient Greece remains Parker, R.A. (1983 repr. 1990). *Miasma*. Recent experimental research indicates that physical activities such as cleaning hands can reduce feelings of guilt and immorality: Chen Bo-Zong and K. Liljenquist. (2006). 'Washing away your sins: threatened morality and physical cleansing', *Science* 313 (5792) 1451–1452.

'... for when it has aroused all inside, it itself marches out in the vanguard.'[67] Purging through emetics and laxatives was the principal purpose of drug use. *Aphorisms* includes multiple references to purging, as do the gynecological works, from which survive the great majority of recipes known for that period.[68] Emetics and enemas were widely prescribed by the author of *Regimen*: emetics in the winter, to push out phlegm above the diaphragm; enemas in summer, to draw down bile from the groin and reduce colic.[69] *Pharmaka* were often qualified by the adjective ἐλατήριος/ον, 'purgative'. For a patient with quartan fever, one treatise prescribes, in succession: a purge of the head, an upwards purge, a purge downwards and finally, if these do not work, a cleansing with warm water in addition to a *pharmakon*.[70] Pneumonia became incurable if the patient was not purged at the right moment.[71] Traumatic medicine also involved this method of rebalancing the body: purging is good for those with wounds of the head, the belly, joints, and wounds at risk of gangrene or that need stitching with sutures.[72]

The principal Egyptian model of illness, as we saw in chapter 3, emphasized external cause and personified it as a hostile entity, whether the invasion was prospective or already successful.[73] (The evidence of wisdom texts, however, as we shall see in 4.2.2.1, pp. 162–163, links at least some digestive complaints to gluttony and its avoidance to virtuous moderation: a value set entirely compatible with Greco-Roman culture). Within this physical-causative framework, the health-causing powers of foods and

---

[67] E.g. Pliny *Natural History* 25.23.57–58 = von Staden, *Herophilus*, T255. Hellebore was the exemplar of the purge and thus of drugs in general. It seems sometimes to have been known simply as *to pharmakon*: *Epidemics* 5.2 with Smith, W.D. (1994) ad loc. (Loeb *Hippocrates* VII, 153). Girard, M.C. 'L'hellébore: panacée ou placébo?', in Potter, *La maladie*, 393–405.

[68] *Aphorisms* e.g. 2.8–10, 29, 35–36 (cf. 1.23), 37; 4.2, 3–14, 18–20, 41; 6. 47. Ṭotelin, *Hippocratic Recipes*, 111 note 1: 81.63% of the 1551 recipes in the Hippocratic corpus are from the gynecological treatises.

[69] *Regimen in health* 5. See Scarborough, J. 'Theoretical assumptions in Hippocratic pharmacology', in Lassere & Mudry, *Formes*, 307–325.

[70] *Affections* 18 (6.226.4–228.5 Littré), cf. *Diseases* 2.42–43 (7.58.22–60.24 Littré).

[71] *Regimen in acute diseases* 11 (1.464.5–6 Littré); cf. (mistakes in purgation) *Diseases* 4.47 (7.576.1–5 Littré); *Drugs* 41 ed. Schöne, H. (1924). 'Hippokrates περὶ φαρμάκων', *Rh. Mus.* 73, 434–438.

[72] *Wounds* 2 (6.404 Littré).

[73] Traces of a similar concept of disease agency, which probably remained relatively common in Greek lay and non-elite disease conceptualization, can be seen in verb choices of classical period medical texts. von Staden, 'Incurability', 101 with n. 55: the incurable disease is an entity or agent 'living with' and 'dying with' its victim; which it also 'kills', 'puts to death', 'destroys', etc.; also as 'not exiting' the body (e.g *Internal Affections* 36 (7.280.16 Littré)); 'the disease exits if treated' is a formulaic phrase.

other substances in prescriptions were due to the involvement of the gods and the resonances of their creative actions, which produced, *inter alia*, life, power, fertility, violence, skill with words, heat, and order. This was a different kind of chemistry—one that in modern terms is less like the periodic table and more like the metaphor of personal chemistry between individuals.[74] Drugs were understood through their 'symbolic' associations, which in Egyptian terms were actual, not symbolic. Disease was defeated largely by the expulsion of its embodied causes, which also put a stop to their deleterious effects upon the body. Powers of regeneration and fertility were often also evoked to maximize restoration and growth for what had been damaged; and defensive powers utilized before evil could occur.

4.2.2.1. *An Obsession with Purgation? Egyptian Medicine in the Greek Imagination*

Expelling or attracting disease entities and products from the body was the explanatory model responsible for the prominence of purgative drugs, enemas and many suppositories in Egyptian medical texts. Ebers 132–164 contains thirty-three recipes for treatment of the rectal area, which included gastrointestinal complaints in general; the Chester Beatty VI papyrus also contains a section (of 26 remedies) on the topic.[75] Some Egyptian physicians used the title 'shepherd of the rectum.'[76] Because of the difficulty in identifying ingredients, it is difficult to establish how many of these were purgative drugs;[77] a number were milder enemas or suppositories, several of which are described as 'cooling' or 'refreshing' the rectal region.

---

[74] The modern world offers both: recent works on depression include psychotherapist Peter Kramer's *Prozac Nation* (rev.ed. 1997) and Andrew Solomon's 2001 personal memoir, *The Noonday Demon*.

[75] Westendorf, *Handbuch*, 212 for a closer analysis. Nunn, *Egyptian Medicine*, 158 estimated that a quarter of remedies within the Ebers text were for gastrointestinal and rectal problems.

[76] *Pḥwy, pḥwyt* have both usually been translated 'anus' but Walker, J. (1996). *Studies in Ancient Egyptian Anatomical Terminology*, 221–245 extends the meaning to the internal passage; i.e. the rectal or pelvic area (associated in women with childbirth). The Greek translation was *iatroklystes*, 'enema doctor': see 5.1.1, p. 206 with n. 6. 'Shepherd of the rectum/anus', which tends to startle the modern reader, sounds a lot less odd if translated into familiar terms as rectal specialist, gastroenterologist, or colorectal surgeon. The word translated as 'shepherd' or 'herdsman' (*nery*) does not occur together with any other medical specialists; it may be relevant that this practitioner is not titularly identified as a *swnw* (physician).

[77] Grapow, H. *GdM* 3, 28ff.

None of this is particularly surprising, especially in view of the fact that the anatomy and pathology of the heart, stomach, and chest were all closely connected with what we would regard as the digestive system: the rectal specialist's handbook of Chester Beatty VI included references to the bladder, heart, chest cavity and rib area.[78] For Egyptian anatomy-physiology, the lower body is to a large extent a unity: a spell in the London papyrus mentions what Westendorf translates as the viscera of the abdomen and anus. Leitz offers a somewhat different reading of the same text, as meaning 'entrails of the abdomen and of the belly', with a meaning in which blood is blocked within the womb by entrails that seal its opening.[79]

One case identified 'rectal' problems with death of *mtw* (probably here meaning arterial vessels) in the legs: an effect of progressive arterial disease.[80] In Egyptian anatomy, the rectum was a meeting-point for the *mtw* of the whole body, which, according to Ebers 854o, were affected when the rectum was engorged with feces. Drugs delivered by suppository or enema were thus the equivalent of slow-release drugs administered by mouth.[81]

From a diagnostic or explanatory standpoint, feces, vomit, urine and menstrual blood are the only indications of internal activities and pathogens for observers in non-technological societies. Moreover, indigestion, constipation and diarrhea are common illnesses at all times; in antiquity the last in particular often signified death, especially among children. In Egypt, specialists existed for such commonly referenced problems, as did eye specialists for the also frequent eye conditions.[82] If Greek medicine is used as a comparison, then as we have just seen, we find an equivalent therapeutic emphasis on purging through laxatives or emetics, or more subtly diuretics; the use of enemas for these purposes;[83] and a nosological and prognostical

78 Westendorf, *Handbuch*, 212. Cf. Walker, *Anatomical Terminology*, 235, who remarks that CB VI is more a handbook for chest complaints than a treatise on conditions of the rectal area.

79 London Medical papyrus (BM EA 10059) 33 (10, 7): *mẖ.tw n pḥwj.t ẖ.t.* German translation by Westendorf, *Handbuch*, 205: 'Eingeweiden des Afters und des Bauches'. Leitz, *Magical and Medical Papyri*, 71, with n. 192.

80 Ebers 856h = Berlin 163.

81 Enemas do deliver substances into the bloodstream, though in lesser amounts than via oral ingestion.

82 Eyes, teeth, belly and enema-specialists are mentioned in earlier literature; Herodotos 2.84 describes specialists in the eye, teeth, head, belly and 'invisible diseases', the last a loaded Greek medical term: see Thomas, *Herodotus*, 41. Westendorf, *Handbuch*, 473ff. and this volume, 5.1.1, p. 208 with n. 14.

83 For the use of enemas (κλύσμα, κλυσμός) in classical period remedies, usually for female problems of the womb: Totelin, *Recipes*, 52 (cf. also for fomentations, fumigations, infusions, suppositories et cetera).

fascination with bodily excreta. Rectal specialists are absent from Greek records, but so are eye-doctors, dentists, surgeons and gynecologists;[84] not because Greek doctors did not work in these areas but because they did not present themselves as specialists in any single area or technique of medicine (preferring differentiations on the grounds of ability, methodology, or occasionally exclusion, as in the *Oath*'s catalogue of forsworn activities).

It is then particularly interesting that several Greek writers singled out purging as the defining characteristic of Egyptian as opposed to Greek medicine, given that purging was central to their own health behaviors as well. As in other comparisons of Greek and Egyptian medicine, they framed this disjunction in terms of Greek superiority.[85] Aristophanes invoked purgative medicine as an easily recognized, but evidently derisible, stereotype: 'These are the fair-maidened currents of the Nile, who in lieu of heavenly distilment floods the flats of bright Egypt, for a people much given to laxatives' (*melanosurmaiai*).[86] Herodotos had previously identified purgation as an identifying ethnographic characteristic not just of Egyptian medicine, but of Egyptian society as a whole (or at least those 'who live in the cultivated parts of the country'): 'Every month for three successive days they purge themselves, with emetics and enemas, in the belief that all diseases come from the food a man eats.'[87] The report is in two parts: a factual assertion of regular purging, and a rationale for it: all diseases come from food. Diodoros' recapitulation makes this specifically a preventative measure: 'consequently the treatment just mentioned, by removing the beginnings of disease, would be most likely to produce health.'[88]

---

[84] There are of course Greek medical treatises on specific subjects, including diseases of women and dentition, but these are not necessarily linked to clear categories of specialists.

[85] Cf. Demokedes' curing Darios' ankle injury where Egyptian physicians failed: Herodotos 3.129.1 ff. Below, 4.4, pp. 192–193.

[86] *Women at the Thesmophoria*, ll. 855–857, trans. Henderson, also quoted p. 41; other English renditions of this passage are less explicit about its laxative implications. *Melanosurmaios* has a double meaning of black robes and fond of purges, and Aristophanes is punning on the famously black silt left behind by the Nile.

[87] *Histories* 2.77. συρμαίζουσι τρεῖς ἡμέρας ἐπεξῆς μηνὸς ἑκάστου, ἐμέτοισι θηρώμενοι τὴν ὑγιείην καὶ κλύσμασι, νομίζοντες ἀπὸ τῶν τρεφόντων σιτίων πάσας τὰς νούσους τοῖσι ἀνθρώποισι γίνεσθαι.

[88] *Library* 1.82: Τὰς δὲ νόσους προκαταλαμβανόμενοι θεραπεύουσι τὰ σώματα κλυσμοῖς καὶ νηστείαις καὶ έμέτοις, ένίοτε μὲν καθ' ἑκάστην ἡμέραν, ἐνίοτε δὲ τρεῖς ἢ τέτταρας ἡμέρας διαλείποντες. φασὶ γὰρ πάσης τροφῆς ἀναδουείσης τὸ πλέον εἶναι περιττόν, ἀφ' οὗ γεννᾶσθαι τὰς νόσους·ὥστε τὴν προειρημένην θεραπείαν ἀναιροῦσαν τὰς ἀρχας τῆς νόσου μάλιστ̓ ἂν παρασκευάσαι τὴν ὑγίειαν.

Given our uncertainty as to Herodotos' sources for his account of Egypt, including some remaining doubt as to whether he was actually there, we should be wary of taking his assertion as a factual statement of widespread Egyptian practice. Nowhere in our extant Egyptian sources are there any direct instructions for regular prophylactic purging, let alone for three days every month.[89] It is moreover unclear from the Greek whether the disease theory was Herodotos' own assertion or derived from some other source, and if so whether it was this person's own understanding or a formal principle of medical theory.

The demotic wisdom text of Papyrus Insinger (and associated fragments), which may date to the Ptolemaic period or the 4th century, and in which self-restraint is the leading virtue, is clear on the link between gluttony and illness. It may also draw a more general link between food and disease. The relevant instructions are 6.11 and 6.12: 'Illness befalls a man because the food harms him', and, 'He who sates himself with too much bread becomes ill and suffers'.[90]

The link between stomach complaints and eating—especially eating more than usual, or eating unfamiliar foods—does not require much in the way of disease theory. A key theme of P. Insinger and other wisdom texts is the difficulty of managing transitions between hunger and plenty, and of moderation in dealing with the latter. The formulations above might indicate either a theory along Herodotean lines, that (excessive) food becomes a nosological entity that causes most kinds of illness, or it might refer only to the commonplace symptamological categories of indigestion, constipation, and diarrhea, induced by eating too much. P. Insinger 6.18 implies not that purgatives prevent illness, but that gluttony causes loss of bowel control: 'His (the moderate man's) belly does not relieve itself in the street because of the food in it.' Arguably this notion could be extended into a view that evacuation always relieved illness, at least that of a certain type, but it is a

[89] For Herodotos and his sources see 1.4.1, pp. 39–40. Perhaps the three-day figure for purgation was derived from the commonly prescribed period of four days for all treatments in Egyptian medicine: cf. Lloyd, A.B. (1976). *Herodotus Book II,1–98*, 331. Herodotos makes these remarks just after commenting on the number and antiquity of written records in Egypt, which implies a temple context for his information. Assuming that his claim has something specific behind it, the three days of purging might have been part of a ritual performed by cult officials.

[90] Trans. Lichtheim, *Late Egyptian*, 202. Cf. 6.15, 6.16, and 6.13 on too much wine. For P. Insinger in general: ibid. 107 ff. For additional bibliography see Jasnow, R. 'Insinger Papyrus', in Redford, D.B. (2001). *The Oxford Encyclopedia of Ancient Egypt*, 2.167–169.

long way from a declaration that Egyptian medicine consisted essentially of purging morbid amounts of food. Such a theory is not explicit in the medical texts. (The view that Egyptian *wḫdw* was such a pathogenic food residue has been widely accepted, but is itself based largely on the remarks of Herodotos and Diodoros, and is therefore, as I argued in 3.2.1, pp. 115–116, unproven).

The absence could be due to drug compendia having survived in much greater quantity than theoretical explanations, but in what does survive of Egyptian theories, disease is persistently explained as a divine or demonic attack on the body. That concept is quite lacking from Herodotos' and Diodoros' accounts. The theoretical basis for the importance of the pelvic and rectal areas in Egyptian nosology and therapeutics probably had more to do with the Egyptian anatomical-physiological model of the body, than with morbid amounts of food.

Herodotos and Diodoros, then, understood Egyptian practices in terms of contemporary Greek medical preoccupations, which included the notion of food as the cause of all disease. A Greek observational framework necessarily construed Egyptian medicine largely through what the latter did not involve: phlebotomy, dietetics, humoral or pneumatic or similar theories, extensive cautery, and regular use of surgery. This left digestion-related treatments as the dominant feature, from a Greek viewpoint of Egyptian medicine. As a result, they emphasized Egyptian uses for purgation, constructing it as an exaggerated version of Greek *perittôma* theories and preventative dietetics. Other theoretical, physiological and therapeutic aspects of medicine attested in Egyptian sources went unrecorded.

Medicine in the fifth century was evidently a fertile arena for Greek cultural chauvinism. The absence of any clearly Egyptian theory, procedure, or indeed physician in Greco-Roman medical culture of the Ptolemaic and Roman eras suggests that the identification of Greek medicine as not just different but superior was largely retained by subsequent generations of those who identified themselves as Greeks. Choices within medicine can function as a means of displaying economic (e.g. ability to pay for the best specialists) or intellectual superiority (e.g. a modern preference for biomedicine over alternatives), and the exercise of such choices also helps to construct such a hierarchical framework. The fact that Greeks sometimes explicitly constructed medicine in ethnographic terms allowed Hellenizers and Greeks to display superiority through the exercise of medical preference.

4.2.2.2. *Contexts of Repulsion: The Meanings of Feces for Demons, Doctors and Historians*

Crocodile dung, virgin's urine, human milk, and remedies against human bites tend to strike modern readers as outlandish or peculiar; as a result they attract a disproportionate share of attention in modern literature. We are particularly little used to remedies involving animal products. Substances derived from humans and other animals—placenta, blood, fat, bile, internal organs, meat, milk—were widely used in both Greek and Egyptian medicine, although they are more common in extant Egyptian texts. Animal products were relatively high-value rarities (with the arguable exception of urine and excrement, and within that category hippopotamus dung was less easily obtained than that of goat or cat). A late wisdom text, The Instruction of Ankhsheshonqy, composed in the Ptolemaic period or shortly after, included the advice, 'Gather dung, gather dirt, but do not make a profession out of scavenging'.[91]

In particular, modern authors single out the medicinal use of animal or human feces. In classical period Greek medicine the excrement of fowls, cows, goats, donkeys and mules was applied externally, often through fumigations, but also internally. Such recipes were numerous, but, uniquely, their use was restricted to female complaints.[92]

Coprotic ingredients were also a significant part of Egyptian therapeutics. Sixty-seven remedies in papyri of the pharaonic period included feces from nineteen different animals, including humans. The majority were for external use in the form of topical unguents and eye ointments, suppositories, and fumigations.[93] Crocodile feces, dissolved in sour milk, formed a contraceptive pessary.[94] Three recipes prescribed feces to be taken orally.[95]

---

[91] 17.24. Translated Lichtheim, *Late Egyptian*, 82.

[92] Excrement appears in only the gynecological texts of the Hippocratic corpus: von Staden, H. (1992). 'Women and dirt', *Helios* 19, 7–30. See also Hanson, A.E. 'Talking recipes in the gynecological texts of the Hippocratic Corpus' in Wyke, M. (1988). *Parchments of Gender*, 71–94 especially 87–92, who argues that such ingredients were derived from pre-existing remedies using a 'magical' conceptual paradigm of purity and repulsion, and reconceptualized by the Hippocratics and their successors in a way that eventually allowed for excrement as a treatment for men as well as women, as is already the case in the Hellenistic period.

[93] 67+4 parallel passages: *GdM* 6, s.v. *ḥs*, pp. 358–363. The majority (55) are from the Ebers. The species are human (4 occurrences), donkey, sheep, fly, lion, cat, dove or pigeon, crocodile, ostrich, goat, pelican, lizard, pig, gazelle, dog, hippopotamus, goose, cattle, and panther.

[94] Kahun 21, Ebers 326, Ebers 782.

[95] Donkey dung (Hearst 208); bird droppings (Eb 326); feces of a fly on the wall (Ebers 782).

Their use has attracted more comment on the nature of Egyptian medicine as a whole than have the similar prescriptions within the Greek tradition. The comment of Herman de Meulenaere is fairly typical: 'Chose très remarquée, la Dreckapotheke y occupe une place importante'.[96] Stronger remarks often appear prompted by concerns about hygiene.[97]

It is not entirely a modern bias. Greco-Roman writers also described remedies or procedures that they found improbable, bizarre, or disgusting, and these often involved similar things. Galen's rejection of the ingestion of feces, sweat, urine, or menstrual blood, as prescribed by Xenokrates of Aphrodisias in the first century CE, or by the first-century BCE Alexandrian physician Apollonios Mys, were vigorously phrased and not only emphasized his own disgust, but seemed to be trying to create it in the reader:

> But drinking sweat and urine and a women's menstrual blood is outrageous and disgusting, and so are feces, no less than these. Xenokrates describes what cures feces can effect when they are smeared all over the parts at the mouth and throat and then swallowed down into the belly ...[98]

In fact, Galen himself viewed many kinds of excrement as having a medically useful 'most powerful expulsive force', prescribing them repeatedly in his work on drug simples.[99] In this he was in line with much of mainstream intellectual Greco-Roman medicine, which, far from throwing out *Dreckapotheke*, extended their use from their gynecological base into prescriptions for both sexes from the beginning of the Hellenistic period. In Egypt, the local ingredient of crocodile dung was among the animal products utilized by Herophilos in the mid-third century.[100] Thanks to Galen's rhetoric, we know that Apollonios Mys, in the early years of Roman Egypt,

---

96 de Meulenaere, H. 'Arzt', *LÄ* 1.458.

97 Nunn, *Egyptian Medicine*, 183: 'The frequent appearance of the excrement of various animals [in remedies for burns] is disconcerting.' Bodily substances, including feces and urine, are routinely used in the local pharmacopoeias of many societies, see e.g. for 18th century Brazil, Edler, F.C. 'Medical knowledge and professional power: from the Luso-Brazilian context to imperial Brazil', in Bala, P. (2009). *Biomedicine As A Contested Site*, 54.

98 Galen, *The temperaments and powers of simple drugs* 10.1 (12.249.1–6 Kühn). Xenokrates reported successful uses for human blood, brain, liver, muscle meat, bone ash in medicines: ibid (12.248.8–17 Kühn).

99 Expulsive power: *The temperaments and powers of simple drugs* 10.2.18; cf. 10.1, 10.2.15, 18–30 (12. 290–291; 12.245 ff. Kühn); *The composition of drugs according to place* 3.1 (12.247, 284–288, 290–309; 12.633 Kühn). The apparent variation in Galen's views seems to be due partly to the relative seriousness of the condition: disgusting remedies should be employed only when absolutely necessary.

100 *Medical books* 7.48 (*CMG* 8.2, 303 Olivieri) = von Staden, *Herophilus*, T260 (pp. 423–426). Below, 4.2.3, p. 175 and n. 148.

listed camel urine as a cure for dandruff and hot donkey urine for a sore throat. These appeared in his work *Common Remedies*, so it seems that animal feces and urine were single-ingredient, relatively accessible substances with reasonably general appeal, utilized by some prestigious physicians.[101] The first century CE pharmacopoeia of Dioskourides listed forty-three applications for animal dung; Celsus' *Medicine* includes them within book 5, and Pliny reproduced many excrement and other disgust-based therapies from a variety of sources.[102]

The use of such substances was not alien to Greek medicine, insignificant in extent, or reserved for the superstitious, ignorant or disgust-proof. It was part of mainstream pharmacology. The degree and kind of appropriate use of excrement, urine, and blood, however, was also part of a discourse of appropriateness and epistemological justification within Greek naturalistic, intellectualized medicine. It is within this discourse that Galen imported the social norm of disgust at bodily fluids into the medical arena, in which their power to disgust was otherwise either neutralized through professionalization, or reconfigured as usefully 'expulsive.' The categorization of feces (*ḥs*) in non-medical Egyptian texts, as being eaten only by the unjustified dead, was, for that matter, also a comment on the awfulness of excrement.[103] The dead were a principal cause of disease, so fecal suppositories, pessaries and anal-vaginal fumigations seem to have been rationalized as lures for ghosts or demons acting within the body.[104] Honey was anathema to such spirits, as their polarities were entirely reversed. At the same time foul or bitter-smelling and tasting plants, including garlic, also worked against diseases.

> I have made for him [child] an amulet against you [demon] of evil-smelling herbs, of garlic which is harmful to you and of honey which is sweet for men, but horrible to ghosts.[105]

---

[101] Urine was used in classical-period Greek recipes and in Egyptian medicine, often with connotations of fertility or sexuality. Egyptian conception test: Ghalioungui, P. et al. (1963). 'On an ancient Egyptian method of diagnosing pregnancy and determining foetal sex', *Medical Historian* 7, 241–246. Greek fertility tests: *Barren women* 2.214–216 (8.424–428 Littré). Cf. the story of king Pharos' test for a pure woman: Herodotos 2.111; Diodoros 1.59.1; also extant (unpublished) in demotic: see Ryholt, K. (1998). 'A parallel to the Inaros story of P. Krall', *JEA* 84, 151. Its use as an eye ointment is more distinctively Egyptian: Ramesseum III A, 19–20.

[102] Dioskourides *Medical Materials* 2.80.

[103] 'As you [child of 1–3 years] grew and your excrement disgusted [your mother] …'. The Instruction of Any (ca. 1550–1295), in Lichtheim, M. (1976). *Ancient Egyptian Literature*, 2.141.

[104] Coffin Text 6, 29 5 j: 'Your tribute is feces'; cf P. Hearst 7, 6, in which demons are lured by feces to their doom.

[105] This spell is discussed by Nielsen, E.R. (1993). 'Honey in medicine', *Atti del Sesto*

The deliberate use of animal and human substances, including those socially accepted as repulsive and in other contexts polluting, was, then, common to both Greek and Egyptian medicine of the Hellenistic period, as to many other societies. It is the Hippocratic corpus' restriction of feces to gynecology that requires explanation. The extension of coprotherapy to either gender, exemplified by Herophilos' adoption of crocodile dung as a remedy, was arguably stimulated, or at least reinforced, by local Egyptian pharmacological norms.[106]

4.2.3. *The Ptolemaic Pharmacy*

Most of the medical recipes of Egypt known to us come from texts composed and copied at relatively early periods in its history, before the end of the New Kingdom. Agriculture and pharmaceutical traditions evolved considerably over later pharaonic history and especially during the Ptolemaic period, when settlers and imports introduced new crops, varieties or drug preferences on a significant scale. Demotic texts from the second and third centuries of Roman rule demonstrate that the pharmaceutical repertoire of Egyptian medicine had by then greatly expanded. An unillustrated herbal from Krokodilopolis, copied in the second century CE, included over 65 plant and mineral substances previously unattested in medical contexts.[107] On the verso of another Roman period papyrus, written in demotic with elements of hieratic and Greek, are recipes with still more ingredients previously unattested in Egyptian language medical works.[108] Imported goods

Congresso internazionale di Egittologia 2.419. For its original publication see ibid. 419 note 9. For the inverted world of the dead, in which honey is repulsive and excrement attractive: Borghouts, J.F. 'Magie', *LÄ* 3, 1137–1151: 1145.

106 In French Indo-China in the early 20th century, the Vietnamese reaction to the imposition of French biomedical concepts, vaccines and drugs was complex. Hormone extracts were among the most popular new remedies, possibly because animal derivatives were already familiar in Sino-Vietnamese medicine: Monnais, L. 'Rejected or elected? Processes of therapeutic selection and colonial medicines in French Vietnam', in Bala, *Biomedicine*, 123.

107 P.Vindob.D.6257 (LDAB 55973, TM 55973) in Vienna, ed. and trans. Reymond, E.A.E. (1976). *A Medical Book from Crocodilopolis: P.Vindob.D.6257*. See also Dieleman 2005 (n. 108 below), 111–112; Ritner, 'Innovations', 113 and n. 39. Reymond's original identifications (*Medical Book*, 244–292) are often problematic: Devauchelle, D. and M. Pezin. (1978). 'Un papyrus medical démotique', *CdÉ* 53, 57–66 and reviews by Smith, M. (1978). *BiOr* 35 53–57; Brunsch, W. (1980). *WZKM* 72, 155–160; Johnson, J.H. (1982). *JNES* 41 (301–303). See further 3.4, pp. 135–136 and nn. 127, 130.

108 P. London-Leiden, first edited by Griffith, F.Ll. and H. Thompson. (1904). *The Demotic*

represented a source of medicinal materials largely independent of internal agriculture, if also largely restricted to use by the elite.

It is often very difficult to assign the original cultivation of a new crop in Egypt to a particular period, let alone to identify the point of their assimilation into indigenous medical tradition. In some cases archeological remains or unambiguous depictions demonstrate the presence in Egypt of a particular plant, but its Egyptian name (or names) remains unknown, so that even experts in this field are unable to say whether such an item was included in the medical texts, whose specialized botanical and biological vocabulary contains many words of dubious or unknown meaning.

The opium poppy, *Papaver somniferum*, (μήκων) is a good example of this kind of situation. Use of its opiate qualities requires internal ingestion of a substance taken from the liquid within the poppy's head; this is extracted by incising the unripe seed pod, as described by Theophrastos for fourth century Greece (*Enquiry into Plants* 9.8.2). The liquid contains an alkaloid form of morphine. Other components of the plant, including the seeds themselves, the flower and the leaves, do not contain opium in any quantity.

Several species of poppy, known generically as μήκων (Latin *papaver*) were common in Greece. Theophrastos mentions the corn or field poppy (L. *Papaver rhoeas*) and the yellow-flowering horned poppy of coastal areas alongside the opium poppy, which itself came in 'white' and 'black' varieties, after the color of their seeds.[109] Poppies and their seeds were regularly used in Greek medicine, often as purgatives or combined with other cathartics, such as hellebore, but opium poppy seeds were also used as a food or spice and, when crushed, made a useful oil.[110] The narcotic and pain-killing effects of the opium poppy's milky sap are also well attested in classical and later Greek literature. The corpus of classical period medical texts includes several references to poppy (μήκων), poppy juice (ὀπός), meco-

---

Magical Papyrus of London and Leiden. (P. London 10070 + P. Leiden I 383: together LDAB 55973, TM 55955). See also Dieleman, J. (2005). *Priests, Tongues, and Rites. The London-Leiden Magical Manuscripts and Translation in Egyptian Ritual (100–300 CE)*. 3rd century CE, with content probably not earlier than the first or second century CE. Cf. 3.4, pp. 135–136, n. 129.

[109] Theophrastos *Enquiry into Plants* 9.12.3–5. The 'garden poppy' of *Iliad* 8.306 is probably *P.somniferum*: Herzhoff, B. 'Poppy', *BNP* 11, 615–616. Dalby, A. (2003). *Food in the Ancient World from A to Z*, 268 views 'black poppy' as the corn poppy *P.rhoeas* and the ancient μήκων ἡ ῥοιάς as a hybrid.

[110] Theophrastos *Enquiry into Plants* 9.12.4 and 1.244 f. For opium seeds as a food, Andrews, A.C. (1952). 'The opium poppy as a food and spice in the classical period', *Agricultural History* 26.4, 152–155.

nium (another word for the crude sap), and opium or opion (τὸ ὄπιον).[111] In prescriptions later ascribed to the fourth century physician Diokles of Karystos, the use of the word *opion* was sometimes rather casual: it is prescribed for toothache and for pain, but in the latter case is roasted, suggesting the seeds rather than opium proper.[112] Opium was an ingredient in several Herophilean remedies, and Dioskourides mentions the view of Andreas, Ptolemy IV's court physician, that opium caused blindness.[113]

The opium poppy was originally probably native to Anatolia; and cultivated in the region by about 2000, spreading to the eastern Mediterranean sometime between about 1500 and 500.[114] Evidence for the date of its introduction into Egypt specifically, as a cultivated or wild-growing plant, or for Egyptian trade in its products, is controversial. The hypothesis of R.S. Merrillees, that opium was imported into Egypt from Cyprus in the 1500s in Cypriot juglets of the base ring I type, was based upon a resemblance between this kind of juglet and an inverted poppy seed pod. In addition, Merrillees argued that the decoration on some of these juglets is reminiscent of the incisions of poppy heads made during extraction of the juice.[115]

There is however no definitive evidence for opium's use in Egypt at this time, or at any time before the Ptolemaic. In the early 20th century, chemical analysis of a juglet from the tomb of Kha (d. ca. 1405) found evidence of opium, but a more recent examination of six possible candidates for this container could not replicate the finding.[116] A Cypriote juglet dating from 1600–1450 does contain morphine alkaloid, but as its provenance and

111 *Diseases of women* 2.117 (8.252.18, 21–22 Littré).

112 Opium: 148a, 1 (toothache); 147, 4 (against pain, roasted), cf. 92, 17 (fumigation for peripneumonia). Poppy: 196, 7; juice of poppy: 131, 120, 5, 111a, 29, 128, 10 (against gastrointestinal problems; purges). Fragments ed. van der Eijk, Ph. (2000). *Diocles of Carystus* 1.

113 Opium in Herophilos' recipes: von Staden, *Herophilus*, T257, T258, T259. Pliny says that Erasistratos condemned it as fatal and another third-century Alexandrian physician, Andreas, as damaging to eyesight unless adulterated: *Natural History* 20.76.200 (on poppy in general 20.76.198–20.82.215). Cf. Dioskourides *Medical Materials* 4.64.6.

114 For an overview, Merlin, M.D. (1984). *On the Trail of the Ancient Opium Poppy*; Scarborough, J. (1995). 'The opium poppy in Hellenistic and Roman medicine', in Porter, R. and M. Teich, *Drugs and Narcotics in History*, 4–23; and in brief, Germer, R. (1985). *Flora des pharaonischen Ägypten*, 45.

115 Merrillees, R.S. (1962). 'Opium trade in the Bronze Age Levant', *Antiquity* 36, 287–292.

116 Bisset, N.G. et al. (1996). 'Was opium known in 18th Dynasty Ancient Egypt? An examination of materials from the tomb of the chief royal architect Kha', *Ägypten und Levante* 6, 199–201; cf. in the same volume, Koschel, K. 'Opium alkaloids in a Cypriote base ring I vessel (bilbil) of the Middle Bronze Age from Egypt', 159–166.

history are unknown, later contamination cannot be ruled out.[117] Renate Germer has argued that the shape of the base ring I juglets can be explained in terms of their aesthetic descent from older Cypriot ceramics based on the gourd, rather than as a derivation from the poppy seed pod.[118]

The demotic medical text on the second century CE papyrus from Krokodilopolis includes *mḳn*, a demotic transliteration of the Greek *mêkôn*, 'poppy.'[119] It is unattested in other demotic and Coptic texts, and no other Egyptian name for any kind of poppy is known from the pharaonic period. The Ebers papyrus, from c. 1500, offers a remedy for crying children, of which one of the two principal ingredients is '*spnn* of *spn*'; this is the only occurrence of the word *spn* in Egyptian literature. It has been identified as opium on the basis of the condition it was supposed to remedy, but the identification is obviously extremely uncertain.[120]

A Greek loan-word such as *mḳn* is surprising if the poppy was used in earlier Egyptian medicine, but makes more sense if its products were introduced into local pharmaceutical practice during the Ptolemaic and early Roman era. Evidence from papyri of Greco-Roman Egypt makes it clear that this species of poppy (in both 'white' and 'black' varieties) was cultivated during the late third century on Greek-run estates in the north Fayum.[121] The product of this short-lived agricultural enterprise, however, was not opium, except perhaps incidentally, but oil made from poppy seeds. Since opium, as Dorothy Crawford points out, never occurs in any Ptolemaic lists of imports or goods transferred from one region to another, she draws the conclusion that the opium poppy was cultivated in village allotments for individual, or locally sold, medicinal and narcotic use, in addition to the wild plants that tend to grow on the edge of arable fields. A brief glimpse of this kind of activity is provided by a papyrus of CE 37, which mentions a

117 Bisset, N.G. et al. (1996). 'The presence of opium in a 3.500 year old Cypriote base-ring juglet.' *Ägypten und Levante* 6, 203–204. The jug is in the Martin von Wagner museum of the University of Würzburg (inventory no. A 39).

118 Germer, R. (1981). 'Einige Bemerkungen zum angeblichen Opiumexport von Zypern nach Ägypten', *Studien zur altägyptischen Kultur* 9, 125–129.

119 Reymond, *Medical Book*, no. 77, p. 264.

120 Ebers 782 (*GdM* 4/1, 292). The identification is not accepted by the authors of *GdM* 6, 489–490 or by Germer, *Flora*, 45. *Spnn* reoccurs on its own at Smith case 41 (*GdM* 4/1, 194–196): it might mean seeds, but *GdM* 6, 490 translate 'fruit'. Nunn, *Egyptian Medicine*, 153–156 reviews the literature on both words, and points out that even if *spnn* does mean seeds, poppy seeds contain virtually no opium.

121 For the following see Crawford, D.J. 'The opium poppy: a study in Ptolemaic agriculture' in Finley, M.I. (1973). *Problèmes de la terre en Grèce ancienne*, 223–251.

sale not just of poppies, but specifically of opium: ἀπὸ τιμ(ῆς) ὀπίου, while some brief medical recipes in Greek from the late third century BCE include mention of poppies, though other specifics are lacking.[122] The evidence, however, attests principally to Greek medicinal use of the opium poppy, with eventual Egyptian incorporation into demotic prescriptions at some point before the second century CE. It may have been primarily a wild plant, like its close relative the corn poppy.[123]

The most readily available and commonly used *materia medica* were local foodstuffs, supplemented by other plants. Many of these were common to pre-Hellenistic Egypt and Greece; barley and emmer wheat (*olyra*, *zeia*), the principal products of Egyptian agriculture, were routinely used in Greek prescriptions of the fifth and fourth centuries. So were vegetables and wild plants like leeks, radishes, onions and garlic; the latter two were also common in Egyptian medicinal recipes. European root vegetables such as turnips and parsnips are not attested. Cucumbers from India probably reached the Mediterranean world around the sixth century, but are almost impossible to distinguish, on the basis of depiction or description, from melons of the time, which had the same shape and were less sweet than they are today. The ripe melon was labelled part of a bad diet at *Epidemics* 5.71, but the wild melon or squirting cucumber was used as a purge.[124]

True figs and honey provided familiar sweeteners for food and medicine, to which Greek settlers could add locally grown dates, 'figs' of the country's ubiquitous sycamore, and the large sweet fruits of the 'doun palm', unknown outside Egypt.[125] The sycamore fig made its way into the Greek pharmacology of the Hellenistic and Roman period.[126] Those Greeks who could not afford imported olive oil from Palestine and Greece had to change to local sesame and safflower oils. D.B. Sandy, in a detailed study of oils in Ptolemaic Egypt, argues that oils preferred by the Greeks were in fact in short supply. 'Thus, as *P.Rev.* shows, the Ptolemaic government catered to the residents of

---

122 Opium sale: *P.Ryl.* II 141.21–22, TM 12927. Ptolemaic recipes: *SB* 8.9860 text a22 and text c9, MP3 2391.6, LDAB 6922.

123 *Papaver rhoeas*, depicted several times in pharaonic and Greco-Roman art: Germer, *Flora*, 44.

124 Hence its name τό ἐλατήριον, 'the purge'; also ὁ ἄγριος σίκυος. *Epidemics* 5.71 with Jouanna ad loc.; Theophrastos *Enquiry into Plants* 9.4.1–2; Dioskourides *Medical Materials* 4.150. Above 4.2.2, p. 155.

125 Dalby, *Food*, 113, 123. The date tree grew in Greece, but would not fruit.

126 Dioskourides *Medical Materials* 1.127, 5.33; Pliny *Natural History* 13.56.8, 23.134.

Alexandria by allowing foreign oil to be marketed there.'[127] Castor oil, bitter to the taste, was used in Egypt for lighting and in medicine as a purgative.[128] Dill, coriander, juniper berries, and cumin were common in Egyptian prescriptions; black cumin and garden-cress were almost certainly also used medicinally.[129]

The staple cereals were planted in the majority of annually irrigated fields, for taxes and home consumption. Late period Egypt was beginning to shift from growing emmer to growing wheat; new strains introduced by Greek settlers might have rapidly become popular among Egyptians, in a country where at least 30 different kinds of cakes and bread were already known. Villagers supplemented this basic diet with vegetables and fruits grown in the hand-irrigated village gardens and orchards. Common undomesticated plants were gathered from the banks of canals or the edges of fields. Other items—delicacies, preferred but rare varieties, industrial crops like the vital oils—were cultivated only in some locations, and traded between regions, or imported from abroad. Sheep, and especially cattle, were pastured mainly in the delta; wine was sold by village or regional specialty; preferred varieties of garlic appear to have been grown only in specialist areas.[130] The pomegranate, probably the carob, and perhaps the apple, were grown in small amounts in Egypt, but imports supplied much of the demand for these luxuries.[131] Peaches and citrons entered Greek gastronomy in the Hellenistic period. Two varieties of arum, used for medicine by the Greeks and possibly also the Egyptians, were imported into pharaonic Egypt from Asia Minor or the Greek islands.[132]

---

127 Sandy, D.B. (1989). *The Production and Use of Vegetable Oils in Ptolemaic Egypt*, 29. (Outside Alexandria, protection of internal markets meant that imported oils were unprofitable). For oils in Egypt, see Brewer, D.J. et al. (1994). *Domestic Plants and Animals. The Egyptian Origins*, 41 ff.; in the Greek world: Dalby, *Food*, 297, 289. Sandy, *Oils*, 31 argues that demotic *nḥḥ*, usually translated 'sesame oil' is in fact a generic term for all oils (except castor oil); evidence for the cultivation of sesame seed oil is found only after the beginning of the Ptolemaic era.

128 Castor oil is not used in classical period Greek prescriptions. Authors from Herodotos to Dioskourides (see the list at Sandy, *Oils*, 39–40) mention the Egyptians' use of it for lighting and often its inedibility, but do not know of its medicinal uses (see Ebers 251).

129 Germer, R. 'Ancient Egyptian Pharmaceutical Plants and the Eastern Mediterranean', in Jacob, I. and W. Jacob. (1993). *The Healing Past*, 71–72.

130 Ptolemaic period food-growing: Thompson, D.J. (1984). 'Agriculture', *CAH* 7.1^{2}, 363–370.

131 Pomegranate, employed against worms in Egyptian medicine, came chiefly from Palestine. Apple (*mêlon*) is again easily confused with other sweet round fruits, including pomegranates and citrons.

132 Germer, 'Ancient Egyptian', 78–79: *Dracunculus vulgaris Schott* and *Arum italicum Mill*, depicted in Karnak's 'botanical chamber'.

The arrival of large numbers of Greeks had a predictable impact on Egyptian viticulture. Vines had been a well-established minor crop in pharaonic Egypt but their products were chiefly drunk by the wealthy; the increase in wine production under the Ptolemies resulted in it outpacing beer by the first century.[133] Greeks normally drank wine, usually watered, and it was also a crucial part of medical regimen and a common oral or topical ingredient in remedies.[134] Native varieties were traded under the names of their village or region; according to Strabo wine from Egypt was notably sweet.[135] Individuals probably planted preferred crops or species in their own gardens or land as well, and there was a large import market for seeds, delicacies and preferred strains of wine, honey or oil. One of Zenon's correspondents was told by his physicians to obtain wine from Khios or Lesbos, indicating that these were considered better for health than local varieties, either on grounds of quality (indicated by expense as well as taste) or because of the properties of the soil.[136] Wine from Khios, exported to Ptolemaic Egypt in large quantities, was very expensive. Lesbian wine had also become popular by the fourth century. Further medicinal wines, as recommended by the physician Apollodoros to one of the Ptolemies, were also Greek: Naspercenite, Oretic, Oeneate, Ambraciot, Leukadian and Peparethon.[137]

---

133 Athenaios *Sophists at the Dinner Table* 1.34b: Egyptians who cannot afford wine drink beer. Wine overtakes beer: Thompson, D.J. 'Food for Ptolemaic temple workers' in Wilkins, J. et al. (1995). *Food in Antiquity*, 316–325. For the reasons why: van Minnen, P. 'Dietary Hellenization or ecological transformation?', in Andorlini, I. (2001). *Atti del XXII Congresso Internazionale di Papirologia, Firenze 1998*, 1265–1280. He opts for the latter. Cf. above 1.5, p. 42.

134 Wine was a common base for drug recipes: Totelin, *Recipes*, 111. The classical era *Wounds* 1 (6.400 Littré) says wine is the preferred treatment for wounds and ulcers; cf. 17 and *Use of liquids* 5 (6.128–130 Littré). Dioskourides' section on medicinal wines (book 5) shows they were used primarily as digestive remedies and diuretics; as well as emetics, antidotes to poisoning and occasionally as topical skin remedies. In phlebotomy, the area was often first swabbed with wine: *Epidemics* 5.6.3 (5.206 Littré). For the use of (antiseptic) wine or vinegar in treating wounds, including soaking bandages, see Salazar, C. (2000). *The Treatment of War Wounds in Graeco-Roman Antiquity* and von Staden, *Herophilus*, 14–15 (contrasted with Egyptian use of meat, fats and honey, as in the majority of Smith cases).

135 Egyptian wine varieties: Herodotos 2.60, Strabo 17.1.14, Athenaios *Sophists at the Dinner Table* 1.33d–f.

136 *PSI* IV 413, TM 2096 (third century), cf. 2.3.2, p. 72 with n. 104. Galen and Dioskourides also describe these wines as medicinal: Galen *Antidotes*, 14.162 Kühn (wine from Khios); Dioskourides 5.6 (wine from Lesbos).

137 Pliny *Natural History* 14.9.

The relatively well-off, a group in which Greeks were well-represented, ate most kinds of meat on a fairly frequent basis, but fish supplemented by wildfowl were the commonest source of animal protein.[138] Greek names for the extreme variety of the plentiful Nile fish were sometimes borrowed from Egyptian; others were extensions of older Greek words.[139] Shellfish such as Venus clams were to be found in the sea near Alexandria.[140] Domestic animals were not greatly different from those of Greece: goat, sheep, pig, goose, donkey (for milk as well as draught work) and pigeon, although some pastured animals were largely restricted to the delta area. Cattle were traditionally an uneconomic species used primarily by the elite of Egypt, but a surprising number of recipes in the pharaonic medical corpus involve parts of this animal, implying a clientele who could afford expensive remedies.[141] Similarly, most Greek pre-Hellenistic recipes were vegetal, but quite a few also specified cattle milk, urine, flesh, bile, marrow and liver.

The reputation of Egypt for both the power of its ingredients and the expertise of its inhabitants in producing *pharmaka* was a standard trope of Greek discourse for centuries.[142] Pre-Ptolemaic Greek medicine had included several medical ingredients unique to Egypt, which were now more readily available to Greek immigrant families or physicians: 'Αγύπτιος κρόκος (probably not crocus, but safflower), 'Αγύπτιος βάλανος (acorn), 'Αγύπτιος κύαμος (the pink lotus, named the 'Egyptian bean' because of the shape of its seeds), and 'Αγύπτιος ἄκανθα.[143] Plants imported from Egypt had been used not only for medicine but also for religious ritual, cookery, and the perfume industry; in the last case not only the ingredients but the technicalities of the industry were closely associated with a specifically Egyptian

[138] Thompson, D.J. (1995). 'Food for Ptolemaic temple workers', in Wilkins, J. *Food in Antiquity*: in the second century low-status inhabitants of the Sarapieon complex could afford fowl and on occasion, very expensive beef. For fish in Greek culture, see Davidson, J.N. (1997). *Courtesans and Fishcakes*.

[139] Dalby 2003, 231–232. For a list of Nile fish, see e.g Athenaios (a native of Naukratis), 7.311 f.–312b.

[140] *Natural History* 32.147. Pliny discussed almost 150 varieties of wine and grape in total.

[141] For a summary of cattle products in pharaonic recipes see *GdM* 6, 607; for an overview of wild and domestic animal products in pharaonic medicine: Nunn, *Egyptian Medicine*, 148–151.

[142] *Odyssey* 4.220–232; Aristophanes *Peace* 1253; Aelius Aristides *Oration* 36, 124. Theophrastos *Enquiry into Plants* 15.1, citing the *Odyssey* passage.

[143] Totelin, *Recipes*, 153–155. The pink lotus' bean-like seeds: Theophrastos *Enquiry into Plants* 4.8.7.

expertise.[144] Dioskourides' first century CE pharmacopoeia, which drew on recipes and ingredients from the eastern Mediterranean, included some sixteen recipes for medicinal perfumes, including one for the compound incense κῦφι. This was very much an Egyptian product: the Greek term is derived from the Egyptian *kʿpt*, meaning 'to be smoked', and Dioskourides describes it as being manufactured in Egypt by temple officials; recipes are recorded on temple walls at Edfu and Philae. Ebers 852 records its use as a medicinal fumigation: the ingredients listed are very similar to those given by Dioskourides.[145] The uses recorded by the latter—in antidotes and against asthma—appear, however, to be independent of Egyptian tradition.

The works of Dioskourides and Pliny confirm that Greek medicine used many more Egyptian materials in the early Roman era than it had in the fifth and fourth centuries BCE. A large number of such local substances appeared for the first time in the drug recipes of Greek physicians from the Herophilean sect in Hellenistic Alexandria. Some of these were used by Herophilos himself, as early as the mid-third century.[146] It remains unclear whether this interest of physicians like Herophilos was mediated through Egyptian physicians and based on indigenous beliefs about treatments, or whether it simply reflected a locally available resource. The remark attributed to him, that 'there is nothing which cannot be accomplished by plants, but the powers of most plants are unknown,' suggests both an interest in new plant-materials and acquiring information about them.[147]

Herophilos' work *Eyes* included the remedy: 'For those who cannot see in the daytime, twice daily rub on an ointment [of] gum, the manure of a land-crocodile, vitriolic copper, and the bile of a hyena made smooth with honey, and give the patient goat-liver to eat on an empty stomach.' Aëtios of Amida, who preserved this fragment, commented that, 'my guess is that one should rather do this to people who cannot see at night.'[148] Greek medicine of this and later periods distinguished between day- and

[144] Four kinds of Egyptian oils and perfumes appear in Hippocratic texts; several comic fragments indicate that Egyptian perfumers were established in Athens at the time: Totelin, *Recipes*, 153. Pliny *Natural History* 13.32–50 also mentions Egyptian perfume manufacturers and the tight control exercised over recipes for high-priced perfumes.

[145] Dioskourides 1.25; Ebers 852. Philae and Edfu: Manniche, L. (1989). *An Ancient Egyptian Herbal*, 57–58.

[146] von Staden, *Herophilus*, 17–19.

[147] von Staden, *Herophilus*, T255.

[148] *Books on Medicine* 7.48 (*CMG* 8.2, 303 Olivieri) = von Staden, *Herophilus*, T260 with notes (pp. 423–426).

night-blindness; the latter is also mentioned by Aristotle in the fourth century. 'Darkness by day' is a frequent lament of Egyptian writings, although it may be often metaphorical and does not occur in the large sections of the medical texts that concern eye problems. The concentration of unusual ingredients does not necessarily indicate a non-Greek derivation for the recipe: it might reflect the condition's resistance to treatment, prompting the use of locally available exotics. In addition, Herophilos and other Greek physicians could have been influenced by the fact that a certain substance was used in Egyptian treatments, particularly if the substance itself was also novel, without necessarily taking on board the accompanying Egyptian theoretical framework. Differences between traditional Greek and Egyptian ingredients were between species rather than genus: although hyena bile, for instance, was not a product of Greece, other forms of bile, along with animal excrement, blood and urine, were independently employed in both traditions; awareness of their use was probably reinforcing rather than transformative.[149] Minerals were employed in both traditions, though more frequently in Egyptian medicine.[150]

Drug recipes and other medical texts circulating on Greek-language papyri and ostraka, from the Roman and occasionally the Ptolemaic era, share much of their material with classical period theoretical works and recipe collections, from which they may have derived.[151] There is little evidence

---

[149] The listing of 'milk of a woman who has borne a child' in both the Berlin medical papyrus Berlin (194), and some 700 years later in *Barren women* 214 (8.414.18–19 Littré; the variant text of Kühn, p. 123 is closer to the Egyptian) might be an Egyptian ingredient incorporated into early Greek pharmaceutics via foreign born midwives or wet-nurses: Laskaris, J. 'Error, loss and change in the generation of therapies' in van der Eijk, Ph. (2005). *Hippocrates in Context*, 173–189. It is however used for different purposes, except in birth prognoses, a group in which other Egyptian-Greek parallels are well known: Iversen, E. (1939). *Papyrus Carlsberg No. VIII, with Remarks on the Egyptian Origin of some Popular Birth Prognoses*. See, however, Totelin, *Recipes*, 179 with n. 232 on the existence of an ancient Chinese parallel for kourotrophic milk. Independent development is difficult to rule out.

[150] Nunn 1996, 145 (table 7.3) lists 28 such substances: 20 as securely known, 6 as tentatively identified, and 2 as unknown. One of these, *jmrw*, a word which appears only in the Smith papyrus, where in 8 cases a patient is bandaged with it, is translated 'alum' by Allen, *Art of Medicine* (cases 32, 35, 36, 38, 43, 15, 37, 30: see *GdM* 6, 33–34).

[151] About 10 Greek papyri from the Ptolemaic period carry medical recipes, some very fragmentary: see Marganne, M.-H. (1981). *Inventaire analytique des papyrus grecs de médecine*. Among the earliest are *P.Ryl.* III 531, TM 60196 (250–150 BCE) and *P.Hibeh* II 191, TM 65740 (299–200 BCE), discussed by Andorlini, I. 'Riflessi e applicazioni della terapia ippocratica nella testimonianza dei papiri', in Garofalo, I. et al. (1999). *Aspetti della terapia nel Corpus Hippocraticum*, 431–446. Prescriptions from ostraka, (mainly from the 2nd century CE and later): Préaux, 'Prescriptions', 135–148.

here of the kind of sizable utilization of Egyptian pharmaceutics seen in the narrower Herophilean tradition, but on occasion a more readily available ingredient seems to have been substituted for a hard to get original. *P.Rylands* 531 is very similar to the recipes of *Diseases of women book* 2, but prescribes otter's kidneys instead of castoreum.[152]

This must have been a relatively common problem in relation to wildlife, which differed more, between Egypt and Greece, than domestic animals. Parts of European hares, beavers, and deer had to have been either substituted for or imported. On the other hand, turtle liver or perineum, found in two classical Greek remedies as well as in Egyptian medicine, could have been obtained by the hunters, herdsmen or fishermen that frequented the wilder places of Egypt.[153]

4.2.4. *Obtaining Drugs*

In Greece, rarer ingredients could be bought from drug-sellers (*pharmakopôleis*). The root-cutters (*rhizotomoi*) were specialists in the collection of wild plants; not only in identifying them, but in knowing the correct rituals and methods for removing and preparing their medicinal parts. Thrasyas of Mantinea, whom Theophrastos described as a maker of new *pharmaka*, and his pupil Alexias, probably came from this kind of background.[154] There was clearly a widely accepted role for such specialists in traditional drug use (beyond any general knowledge of common medications for common problems), which was not the same as that supplied by *iatroi*. Some of these practitioners, at least in later centuries, were literate, with a field of knowledge that largely overlapped with that of *iatroi*.[155]

It remains unknown how often buyers from *rhizotomoi* or drug-sellers asked for their assistance in diagnosis or therapeutics. From Theophrastos' descriptions of *rhizotomoi* procedures, their operating understanding of

---

152 Otter's kidneys: *P.Ryl.* III 531 recto col. 4. Castoreum: *Diseases of women* 2.200. See Hanson, A.E. 'Talking recipes', 79–81; Andorlini, 'Riflessi e applicazioni', 440–445.

153 Turtle liver: *Diseases of women* 1.78. Perineum: 1.75 (8.174.7–9, 166.2–7 Littré). The 'one who is hidden' at the bottom of murky pools in Egyptian texts is probably the turtle: Wilson, P. (2003). *Sacred Signs*, 116–117. Turtle and tortoise shell in the medical works: *GdM* 6, 146 (gall), 195 (shell), see also 508; and in recipes on ostraka: Jonckheere, J.F. (1954). 'Prescriptions médicales sur ostraca hiératiques', *CdÉ* 29, 46–61: 55.

154 *Enquiry into Plants* 9.16.8.

155 Notably Krateuas, the famous second century expert on plants and drugs at the court of Mithridates of Bithynia, who was called *rhizotomos* by Dioskourides (proem 1, 1.1.12 f. Wellmann), cf. 6.2, p. 251; Diokles of Karystos wrote a *Rhizotomikon*.

pharmaka and therapeutics involved gods; and their authority included a degree of personal power over *pharmaka*. The drug-sellers were in the habit of demonstrating their control of powerful *pharmaka* by ingesting large amounts of hemlock.[156] Like the purifiers and other 'charlatans' cited in *The sacred disease*, they were alternatives to the *iatroi*, whose medical cabinet looked similar, but who used different explanations.

We have no direct evidence from Egypt for a specialized profession there of plant-collectors, such as the Greek *rhizotomoi*, but a Greek language illustrated herbal of second century CE Egypt uses the verb φύεται, 'grows', telling root-cutters or similar individuals where the plants in question could be found.[157] Many undomesticated plants were gathered from the banks of canals or the edges of fields; and hunters or herdsmen were in a position, like Greek shepherds, to acquire both wilder plants and many animal products. Ebers 294 implied that the professional healer personally collected some of the ingredients for his recipes.[158]

> ... A herb—*sn-wtt* is its name—growing on its belly like the *ḳ3dt*. It produces a flower like the water-lily. If one finds its leaves like white wood, then one should fetch it and rub it on the pelvis.

That this fragment is not unique in its approach, but derived from a technical genre of botanical-medical writings, is suggested by a much later parallel. A collection of papyrus fragments contains a text written in late hieratic, but as the fragments were detached owing to reuse as cartonnage, a late third century practice, the text must have been copied in the Ptolemaic period at the earliest.[159] According to Stephen Quirke, these fragments include 'a series of entries preceded by the rubric "survey (*m33*) of all plants of field ..." ... [which] specifies the properties of plants with reference in part to ailment.' Further support for a long tradition of descriptive botany in Egyptian technical literature comes from Ebers 251. This section of text lists only remedies that involve the castor oil plant (*dgm*). It begins: 'The knowledge of what one makes from the castor oil plant, according to what is found in the

---

156 *Enquiry into Plants* 9.17.2.

157 Hanson, A.E. 'Text and context for the illustrated herbal from Tebtunis', in Andorlini, *Atti del XXII Congresso*, 588. It is the earliest survivor of an illustrated herbal. This text might have belonged to the Greco-Egyptian family of cult officials at Sobek's temple: ibid., 604. See also 5.2.1, p. 222 and 4.2.3, pp. 167–168, nn. 107–108.

158 = Hearst 35 (*GdM* 4/1, 140). Cf. Nunn, *Egyptian Medicine*, 138–139. Translation from Nunn.

159 British Museum EA 10547 (unpublished); discussed briefly by Stephen Quirke. (1997). *JEA* 83, 243–245.

writings of old, for the benefit of mankind'.[160] Clearly not only the botanical information, but also the organizing framework, were derived from an earlier work. The long-term survival of this botanical genre is attested by a section of the Late period Brooklyn papyrus, a collection of anti-snake prescriptions, as this also has a section organized by plant—in this case the onion (41–42).

The kind of work from which these excerpts and fragments were taken has survived in a demotic text of the mid-2nd century CE, albeit in broken and corrupted form. The fragments of this work show that each section—marked by a short space in the line—concerned a single plant, listed in numerical order. The information consists of the plant's number, name, notable visual features or usual habitat, and one or two prescriptions involving its use.[161] Texts like these, circulated among professionals and copied between temple as well as private libraries, would have been easily adapted for compendiums like those of the extant papyri, in which the implicit practical knowledge of the professional replaced a more explicit botany, and into which items from foreign traditions or personal experience were easily incorporated.[162]

The texts are clearly intended for a readership of literate and professional experts in medicine, who diagnosed, prognosed, and treated on the basis of the instructions and definitions to be found in these handbooks. That they could sometimes find their way into private, personal archives is demonstrated by the provenance of Chester Beatty XIII, which came from the family of the 'scribe' Qenherkhopeshef, but literacy is in itself the basic qualification for medical professionalism in Egypt. Recipes also occur on ostraka, often, again, in the catalogue format: remedy title, recipe, 'another' (recipe for the same problem).[163] Neither the handbooks nor the more ad hoc collections of recipes can have circulated beyond these very restricted circles in this literary form, but the recipes themselves could have been much

[160] German translation *GdM* 4/1, 307: 'Die Kenntnis von dem, was man macht aus der Rizinuspflanze, als etwas, da gefunden ist in Schriften alter Zeit, als etwas für die Menschen Nützliches.'

[161] Tait, J. (1991). *Carlsberg Papyri 1*, 47–91. Another demotic text from the 3rd century CE, though fragmentary and largely illegible, might also have been organized by category or be concerned only with one subject; it contains 2 references to fish and 3 to the penis. See the comments of Tait, J. (1977). *Papyri from Tebtunis in Egyptian and in Greek* (*P.Tebt.Tait*), 67, no. 19.

[162] For an overview of pharaonic botany see also Dieleman, *Priests, Tongues*, 195–198.

[163] Jonckheere, 'Prescriptions', *CdÉ* 29, 46–61; Bardinet, *Papyrus médicaux*, 479.

more widely disseminated through oral transmission. The sheer number of remedies available for the same diagnosis indicates a steady incorporation of innovation, variation and adaptation into Egyptian pharmacology.

However communicated, empirical constraints and variation in the experiential use of medical recipes produced a considerable degree of adaptation, alteration and personalization among professionals, folk healers, and self-medicating users. These fed back into the written tradition, in which the emphasis on the demonstrated efficacy, in practice, of a particular remedy is a notable feature: 'Very effective, worked a million times', an interesting basis for authority in a medical culture that normally attributes virtue to written knowledge above all else.[164]

Having obtained the required ingredients, the Egyptian healer proceeded to make up the drug. Available evidence for healing suggests that prescriptions were often or usually formulated by the physician, following, approximating, or adapting written instructions.[165] A royal decree to the high priest of Amun from the office of Ramesses IX is a forceful complaint about the inadequacy of the galena mineral supplied by the Theban estates to the king's Delta residence:[166]

> ... you sent through him 15 deben of galena. When it was given to the physicians of the office of Pharaoh's physicians to be processed, it was discovered to be such weak galena that there was nothing in it suitable for the eye-paint of Pharaoh's use.

The Egyptian medical papyri offered a large number of compound remedies for different diseases, often including the specifics of preparation and application. As in Greek medicine, material substances could be applied topically, taken orally, and administered via fumigations or suppositories. The end results were the personal tools of individual physicians. The Metropolitan Museum of Art in New York contains a jar labelled 'special ointment' that belonged to the chief physician Harkhebi.[167]

---

[164] Similar claims in the Greek medical corpus before the early 2nd century CE are rare. *Diseases of women* 1.78 is a possibly unique example: 'You will not find anything better.'

[165] The same process of adaptation to circumstance applied to Greco-Roman pharmacology, and accounts for the catalogue-style listing of recipes for the same condition characteristic of pharmacological texts. Classical period prescriptions regularly offer a choice of ingredients. Pompey, prescribed out-of-season thrushes, recovered after finding an alternative ingredient: Plutarch *Life of Pompey* 2.6.

[166] Wente, E. (1990). *Letters from Ancient Egypt*, no. 35, cf. no. 36.

[167] Allen, *Art of Medicine*, 65, no. 56.

In Greek medicine, although a choice of ingredients was often given, complicated drugs compounded from a number of ingredients were relatively rare until the later Hellenistic period. In the classical era, Thrasyas' newly invented poison seems to have been a rare novelty item, although physicians were familar with manufactured Egyptian perfumes. Sufferers in Egypt could have bought these and perhaps other drugs from Egyptian unguent-makers, healers, or other specialists; just as they might also have bought amulets, statuettes, or ritual performance. More basic remedies, and the overlapping area of basic regimen, did not require this level of assistance: the doctors' recommendations for wine and honey to Zenon's correspondent (2.3.2, p. 72: *PSI* IV 413, cf. *P.Cair.Zen.* 59426 and above p. 173) were easily put into practice.

4.2.5. *Quantification and Polypharmacy*

Some degree of information sharing must have taken place in regard to initially unfamiliar drugs, though subsequently adapted by individual physicians to particular needs and experience. An indication of more significant interplay—a relatively complex and informed reaction on the part of Greek physicians—could be the Alexandrians' use of precise quantities for ingredients in medical recipes. An example taken at random from the fragments of Herophilos, for a plaster, specified: 'Mix 2 drachmas verdigris, 4 dr. frankincense powder, 12 dr. calf-fat, 3 dr. all heal juice, 80 dr. wax, 20 dr. pine-resin, and an adequate amount of vinegar.'[168]

This seems to have been a novel development in Greek medicine, which had previously rarely quantified anything except fever periodicities.[169] Egyptian prescriptions, however, sometimes gave the exact amount of ingredients, or, more often, specified the proportions of ingredients within a recipe.[170] Any such interplay was probably not so much a precise transference as an awareness of possibility: obviously the measures employed did not translate directly. A strict adherence to written quantities is, in any case, as unlikely as a rigid reliance upon one set of materials; as we have

---

168 12.843 Kühn = von Staden, *Herophilus*, 257. von Staden remarks (p. 19) that Hellenistic Herophileans and Empiricists, 'for the most part … become meticulous in their specification of measures.'

169 Ingredient amounts are only rarely supplied in recipes from classical medical works. Totelin, *Recipes*, 54–55.

170 E.g. Ebers 190: ingredients given as 1/32, 1/16, 1/8, to be cooked together and drunk on four days.

seen, substitution and variation was common in both Greek and Egyptian medicines. The common use of the term 'recipe' for an ancient prescription reflects a genre more akin to our cookbooks than our pharmacy manuals. G.E.R. Lloyd's suggestion that the Egyptian texts' emphasis on quantification was rhetorical rather than actual could also be applied to the Greek recipes.[171]

It is also quite possible that the quantification (rhetorical or actual) of Hellenistic pharmacology was driven by internal developments. The literary exegesis of medical texts and, around the second century, the establishment of an authoritative Hippocratic corpus, focused attention on textual transmission rather than oral or experiential learning within elite Greek medicine.[172] Another factor that might have played a role was the rise of the mathematically precise mechanics of the Hellenistic period. Herophilos' formula for the speed at which a wound heals according to its shape, his water-clock for pulse-taking, and his precise dosage system might be explained as much by such mathematization of medicine as by Egyptian influence.[173]

Polypharmacy is a similar issue. Egyptian medicine of all periods routinely featured compound drugs. The majority did not exceed five ingredients, comparable to classical practice, but others involved tens of substances: Ebers 663 runs to 37 items.[174] This contrasts sharply with Greek pharmaceutical recipes of classical period medicine, in which 4–5 ingredients, plus a vehicle such as wine or water, had been the norm. Six ingredients were very unusual.[175] In Ptolemaic Alexandria, on the other hand, the third-century recipes recorded in the fragments of Herophilos frequently involved

---

[171] Lloyd, G.E.R. unpublished, cited by von Staden, *Herophilus*, 19 n. 67; attacked by Ritner, 'Innovations', 116 n. 57. For examples of exaggerated or rhetorical quantification in Greek intellectual activity see Lloyd, G.E.R. (1987). *The Revolutions of Wisdom*, 215–284, e.g. on numerical periodicities in Hippocratic texts: '... spurious quantification and ad hoc numerological elaboration' (257).

[172] von Staden, 'Hairesis and heresy', 76–100 and 199–206.

[173] The impact of mechanical pneumatic systems on his contemporary Erasistratos went further: see Vegetti, M. 'L'épistémologie d'Érasistrate et la technologie hellénistique', in van der Eijk et al, *Ancient Medicine*, 2.461–472.

[174] Significant socioeconomic differentiation is also very probable within the Egyptian pharmacology. Not only the number of ingredients, but also the presence of more luxurious items such as wine, lapis lazuli, many animal products, and (probably) honey indicate a strong bias toward a clientele of the elite and sub-elites for the users and owners of the written texts, which may not have been representative of medicine among the rest of the population.

[175] Totelin, *Recipes*, 53.

over ten ingredients. The Herophileans, especially Herophilos himself, Andreas of Karystos, and Mantias, all made major contributions to the extension of pharmacological knowledge and the development of drugs compounded from multiple ingredients: polypharmacy.

The presence within the classical pharmaceutical corpus of relatively expensive ingredients indicates that the Greek pharmacopeia was already a socially differentiated one. Expensive exotica, the more the better, exemplified the remedies and preventatives available to the socioeconomic elite. The rationalization of such recipes, as the addition of qualitative elements, was well established among physicians and other intellectuals. Available materials expanded rapidly as a result of the military and economic reach of Alexander's expeditions and the establishment of the Hellenistic kingdoms.

In this environment, the polypharmacy of much Egyptian medicine seems to have reinforced the Greek trend towards increasing elaboration in its remedies and, among medical professionals, the co-optation of folk medical knowledge into an enormous and complex field of technical expertise and theoretical-therapeutic schemata, of the kind that eventually produced works like Galen's *Drugs according to place*.[176] Egyptian 'influence', so far as it went, was largely a matter of the reinforcing of existing tendencies and perhaps a kind of conceptual expansion, matching the geographic and botanical expansion of information and trade, rather than a matter of the incorporation of entirely novel techniques.

4.3.1. *Non-Material Therapies*

That the written pharmaceutical recipes of both Egypt and Greece were not intended to be sufficient for the practice of medicine is clear from the vital information that they often leave out. Dosage was almost entirely lacking in classical era Greek medical texts, some of which instead emphasized the need to tailor the type or quantity of drug to the patient's constitution and circumstances.[177] Similarly, although Egyptian remedies usually specified

---

[176] Compiling drug prescriptions by the place affected (κατὰ τόπους), an organizational scheme with approximate Egyptian precedents, seems to have been an innovation of Mantias, a Herophilean of the Ptolemaic period.

[177] Although quantification became commonplace in the Hellenistic period, the Herophileans' exactness in written prescriptions did not become the norm: Dioskourides' remarks on dosage are usually limited to dangerous substances. Riddle, J.M. (1985). *Dioscorides on Pharmacy and Medicine*, 67–69.

the proportions of ingredients as fractions of the whole, they rarely supplied the total dosage of either the ingredients or the compound; instead this must have been an oral and empirical component of even the most text-dependent medical expertise.[178]

A large part of the doctor's actual encounter with the patient is thus not included in a medical text, whether theoretical or prescriptive. In the questions surrounding dosage, we can at least see what is missing. Other aspects, taken as read in antiquity, may not even occur to us. The addition of oral formulas to the application of material drugs was an aspect of much Egyptian medicine and employed by many groups of Greek practitioners. In the Greek language the word *pharmakon* means 'spell' as well as 'drug' or 'poison': its basic meaning seems to be that of 'persuasive or effective item acting at a distance.'[179] Theophrastos also reported extensive use of ritual action and incantations by root-cutters, the professional purveyors of plant-derived *pharmaka*, when obtaining and preparing plant materials.[180] Although many Greek physicians of the classical and Hellenistic periods abandoned this form of treatment as ineffective and unjustified in a naturalistic cosmos, other practitioners and many laypeople continued to employ spells, amulets, and curse tablets.

'Through whom do amulet and spell become remedies?' inquired an Egyptian wisdom text of the Hellenistic era.[181] A distinction has traditionally been drawn between Egyptian medical works that deal with illness but have a high quotient of incantations, and those in which the latter rarely appear. In many of the medical and pharmaceutical texts, spells are included occasionally rather than routinely.[182] A large number of curative, prophylactic and other incantations are known from other sources; the diagnosis of many conditions, moreover, as caused by demons, ghosts or gods suggests that the therapeutic response similarly invoked the inhabitants of the otherworld.

---

[178] Nunn, *Egyptian Medicine*, 142, suggests that the reference volume was standardized.

[179] References to the multiple meanings of *pharmakon* are collected by Scarborough, 'Theoretical assumptions', 308 n. 7. The 'spell' meaning is attested as early as the *Odyssey*, 4.220, but this conceptual separation of oral formula from drug/poison is anachronistic.

[180] *Enquiry into Plants* book 9; for a summary see Lloyd, *Science, Folklore and Ideology*, 119 ff. Root-cutters: above 4.2.4, pp. 177–178.

[181] *Papyrus Insinger* 31.22. Translated by Lichtheim, *Late Egyptian*, 230.

[182] Westendorf, *Handbuch*, 529–532 gives the percentage of 'spells' in the medical texts. Excluding the short or fragmentary texts, this varies sharply, from around the 2% mark in the Smith and Ebers, to 60+% for the recto of the Chester Beatty VI and the London medical papyrus. The Brooklyn anti-venom text is at 10%.

Such oral or performative components of the healing action, although only rarely included in the genre of written medical instruction, were probably routinely practiced by the physician and consisted largely of variations on relatively generic spells. For example, the text of the Hearst papyrus includes five oral formulas suitable for application to the general-purpose ingredients fat, beer and honey, to be included in remedies for 'whatever you like.'[183]

Most scholars, however, still seem to be convinced that the treatment of injuries lacked oral or ritual action. The Smith papyrus on trauma contains only one such formula (case 9) among its 45 cases of externally visible injury. In contrast, the 12 remedies of the papyrus' verso, most of which are in the same handwriting as the recto, contain eight incantations against internal illness, suggesting that the crucial difference was in the subject matter. Modern writers have argued that because the proximate cause of fractures, dislocations and wounds is generally very clear, the gods are required as neither explanation nor recourse.[184]

In other cultures, however, traumatic medicine is not differentiated from internal medicine by the exclusion of divine assistance or of ritual modes. At *Odyssey* 19.455–458, the sons of Autolykos sing a blood-stopping spell over the hero's wound: 'The sons of Autolykos, working over Odysseus, skillfully binding up his open wound ... chanted (ἐπαοιδῇ) an old spell that stanched the blood'.[185] Roman medicine treated dislocations with incantation combined with an analogical procedure.[186]

In Egypt the workings of *ḥkɜ*, the non-material force that we inadequately translate as 'magic', were not restricted to causally cryptic categories of event; indeed Egyptians thought that the causes of even internal disease were often quite apparent. Nor was *ḥkɜ* an appropriate response only to the

---

183 *Papyrus Hearst* nos. 212–216 inclusive (*GdM* 4/2, 310–311, 5.534–536); Westendorf, *Handbuch*, 36.

184 Breasted, J.H. (1930). *The Edwin Smith Surgical Papyrus*, 11: 'the obvious result of observable physical causes, having no connection with the malignant demons of disease.' Cf. Nunn, *Egyptian Medicine*, 96; Allen, *Art of Medicine*, 10.

185 τὸν μὲν ἄρ' Αὐτολύκου παῖδες φίλοι ἀμφεπένοντο,/ ὠτειλὴν δ' 'Οδυσῆος ἀμύμονος ἀντιθέοιο / δῆσαν ἐπισταμένως, ἐπαοιδῇ, δ' αἷμα κελαινὸν / ἔσχεθον, αἶψα δ' ἵκοντο φίλου πρὸς δώματα πατρός. Translation: Fagles 1996. For parallels in other societies, Renehan, R. (1992). 'The staunching of Odysseus' blood', *AJP* 113 (1), 1–4. Treatment of wounds in the *Iliad*, however, involved only extraction of the missile, washing with water, sucking the wound, and the application of soothing drugs.

186 Cato *Agriculture* 160. Cf. Nijhuis, K. 'Greek doctors and Roman patients: a medical anthropological approach', in van der Eijk et al, *Ancient Medicine*, 1.49–67.

actions of demons or the dead, because *ḥkɜ* was present in all kinds of circumstances, including those of being lucky or unlucky. Hence the didactic Middle Kingdom text, 'Instructions for [king] Merikare', composed between c. 2100 and 1550, says that the gods gave *ḥkɜ* to men in order to 'forestall the untoward'. John Baines notes that this implied that 'its benefits [i.e. those of magic, *ḥkɜ*]—as against the ability to enact specific performances—were freely available.'[187] The emphasis is here on the preventative use of magic, but *ḥkɜ* could also be used for reduction of already apparent harm, such as a wound. The text of Papyrus Leiden I 348 (1290–1220), which offered a comprehensive defense against hostile entities' effects on the body, includes spells against burns, as do several spells in the medical papyri.[188]

A large amount of evidence attests to the use of non-material remedies for scorpion and serpent bites, in spite of the fact that these are, like physical injury, not mysterious events. If you overturn the wrong rock without sufficient care you get stung, or as the papyrus Insinger put it: 'The snake one treads on ejects a strong poison'. But they also clearly enact the malevolence of fate, through the agency of Seth or Apophis: 'One cannot remove the poison of the crocodile, the snake, and the evil one.'[189] Spells and amulets that prevent or cure these events are some of the commonest and best-known: the Brooklyn text against snakebite contains several incantations for use with remedies, as well as the more general recommendation of paragraph 27: 'If one should exorcise the wound, he will survive; since (the snake) is driven out by the magic.'[190]

It could be argued that toxic creatures are a special case of misfortune because they clearly have agency. They are self-motivated and unpredictable in a way that a falling rock, for example, is not. Workplace injuries and other accidents might therefore be viewed in a different causal category to that of snakebite, because these events are not maliciously inclined. In Egypt, however, disorder is itself a malicious entity, or at least a metaphysical force vulnerable to the countervailing metaphysics of order (i.e. *ḥkɜ* as described by the Instruction of Merikare). And even if we allow there to have

---

[187] Lichtheim, *Literature*, 1.106, with bibliography of publications, 98. Translation: Baines. J. (1990). 'Restricted knowledge', 15 with note 91; cf. Baines, 'Display of magic', 20.

[188] See Borghouts, *Papyrus Leiden*, 13; *GdM* 5, 372–375.

[189] P. Insinger 27, 14; P. Insinger 29, 15. Lichtheim, *Late Egyptian*, 224, 227.

[190] French translation: 'Si l' on exorcise le blessé, il survivra; car (la vipère) est exorcisée par la magie.'

been a subtle distinction between scorpion bite and falling rocks, most war wounds were caused by the malicious agency of enemy fighters. Egyptian thought experienced no difficulty rendering these as agents of evil.[191]

Prayer and other non-material remedies, then, might have accompanied most uses of substantive treatment in Egypt, and a large proportion of treatment among Hellenistic period Greeks, with the exception of that carried out by many *iatroi*.

4.3.2. *Prevention and Protection*

One form of response to illness is the response to the possibility of illness; that is, preventative measures. These were generally long-term and low-risk; the obverse of high-impact drugs or surgical interventions, and they could also be used to manage chronic illness or to actively maintain health, a concept not quite the same as defending against disease. Greek dietetics was an example of the former. Other preventative measures, common to Egyptian and Greek society, were the use of incantation and prayer, avoidance of dangerous situations, animals and places, and artifact-based defenses. Among the latter were wearable amulets.

Greek and Hellenized intellectual culture tended to be critical of amulets and their explanatory basis, representing amulet usage as a matter of traditional, common, and ill-educated belief, and (therefore) as particularly popular among women.[192] The amulet given to Sokrates against headache (to be combined with an incantation) was from the barbarian region of Thrace.[193] According to Theophrastos, via Plutarch, the dying Pericles wore an amulet against illness round his neck, given to him by the women of his household.[194] Soranos, writing in the later first century CE, said amulets were of no use, but also that they often improved the mood of (female) patients.[195] Galen approved plant-based or mineral amulets after personally testing examples, and regarded the explanation as naturalistic.[196] It is clear that amulets remained a common tradition among lower-status social

---

[191] For the identification of enemy armies with the forces of evil, see 1.3.2, pp. 32–37.

[192] Theophrastos *Enquiry into Plants* 9.19.2–3: most of what is said about them is the work of men 'who wish to magnify their own arts'.

[193] Plato *Charmides* 155e–156e: cf. 4.2.1, p. 153 n. 48.

[194] Plutarch *Life of Pericles* 35, 39: cf. 4.2.1, p. 153 n. 48.

[195] *Gynecology* 3.(10).42; cf. 1.(19).63 (amulets do not work) = *CMG* IV 121.29–31; 47.16–20.

[196] *The temperaments and properties of simples* 6.10 (11.859.12–860.8 Kühn) and 10.19 (12.207 Kühn). Cf. 4.2.2, p. 156 and n. 63.

groups and were by no means excluded from the health-seeking behavior of many upper class individuals. Some physicians accepted them as a traditional part of medical practice in less qualified terms than Soranos. The classical period texts include several medications to be fastened on (ἐπιδέω, τὸ ἐπιδετόν, περιάπτω, τὸ περιαπτόν);[197] Rufus of Ephesos, some four or five centuries later, included a recipe for an amulet (engraved with lion, moon and star) among *physika*, 'natural things.'[198]

In Egypt, amulets and statuettes constitute the main evidence for non-elite attitudes to religion, magic, threats and healing. Amulets were a sub-set of artifactual protection, in which power against disease and similar threats was focused through, or instantiated in, a material object. The amuletic form was potentially a highly personalized form of defense; while the fact that amulets could be worn continually and transported everywhere made them very reliable for ongoing protection of the individual. The wisdom text of papyrus Insinger, in a section on not undervaluing small things, advised: 'Do not slight a small amulet when it is time to seek it.'[199]

For the protection of the household, its family and goods, however, other kinds of artifacts were required. In Egyptian medical theory, as we have seen, diseases were often understood as invading entities which entered the body at night, through a demonic version of sex, carried out upon the sleeper. Nocturnal visits by (dangerous) animals were also to be feared. Written evidence from the New Kingdom onwards attests to a relatively standardized use of the rearing cobra uraeus, through artifacts and associated oral ritual, in guarding bedrooms and houses.[200] These artifacts have not usually survived, but clay cobras found in the houses from Akhenaten's fourteenth century city of Amarna probably defended their sleeping occupants against poison from night-time threats.[201] The survival of related amuletic and literary forms are good evidence that such items continued in use. 'He is wakeful at night against the reptiles of the dark,' according to the Hellenistic era P. Insinger.[202]

---

197 Totelin, *Recipes*, 65 ('five' such tied-on medications; although she lists only three on pp. 123–124).

198 Rufus fr. 90 (403–404 Daremberg and Ruelle).

199 P. Insinger 24, 4. Translated by Lichtheim, *Late Egyptian*, 222.

200 For this genre see Ritner, R.K. (1990). 'O. Gardiner 363: a spell against night-terrors', *JARCE* 27, 25–41.

201 Szpowaska, K. 'Demons in the dark: nightmares and other nocturnal enemies of ancient Egypt', in Kousoulis, P. (2011). *Ancient Egyptian Demonology*. Cf. Szpowaska. (2003). 'Playing with fire: initial observations on the religious use of clay cobras from Amarna', *JARCE* 40, 113–122.

202 P. Insinger 31.10. Translated by Lichtheim, *Late Egyptian*, 229.

The very young were particularly vulnerable to disease. Apotropaic ivory tusks (often known as 'wands') seem to have been used to mark out zones of protection around an infant's sleeping place, and probably the scene of childbirth (although these are only attested for the later Middle Kingdom). The surviving examples are carved with the images of suitable gods and mythic templates: the journey of the sun god (with the infant identified as the newly born sun), the protective hippopotamus goddesses Taweret or Ipet, or, especially from the Late period, the apotropaic dwarf god Bes.[203] The incantations of Papyrus Berlin 3027, copied around 1550 but composed earlier, are all for the protection of the mother and infant: one further specifies the shape and composition of the amulet with which it was to be used.[204]

Amulets and statuettes of this kind attest to the conventional, widespread status of the conceptions of disease causation that were to be found in the medical papyri used by practitioners within Egyptian medical discourse. They indicate a degree of commonality of approach to and explanation for illness throughout the social strata; between professional practitioners and folk remedies; and between those with access to literary authority and those dependent upon oral tradition and consultation. In the Hellenistic and Roman periods, as we saw for temple medicine, Greeks and Hellenizers frequently accessed religious power through Egyptian or syncretized forms. A number of Greeks, probably the majority, also conceptualized disease in terms of divinities and daimons. Local defensive forms against disease causation were utilized by many Greek or Greco-Egyptian inhabitants of Egypt alongside Hellenistic amulets, and they appealed to local gods, cults and oracles. The *PGM* and *PDM* have material counterparts in the evolution of amuletic forms, such as late Hellenistic gems used for the protection and management of the womb. These have both Greek and Egyptian antecedents, but on these amulets the gods depicted are always clearly Egyptian: most often Khnum, the Osirian triad, and Bes.[205] The anti-menorrhage 'Tantalus' genre of gems are more syncretic.[206]

---

203 Evidence and literature summarized and discussed, with further references, by Szpakowska, K. (2008). *Daily Life in Ancient Egypt: Recreating Lahun*, 26–30; cf. Allen, *Art of Medicine*, 10–11 with cat. nos. 19–22.

204 Westendorf, *Handbuch*, 72; *GdM* 4/1, 293; Parkinson, R.B. (1991). *Voices from Ancient Egypt*, 129–130.

205 Ritner, R.K. (1984). 'A uterine amulet in the oriental institute collection', *JNES* 43 (3), 209–221, with bibliography. For syncretic religious artifacts of the Ptolemaic era, Rottrof, S. 'The Greeks and the Other', in Coleman, J.E. and C.A. Walz. (1997). *Greeks and Barbarians*, 221–235.

206 Barb, A.A. (1952). 'Bois du sang, Tantale', *Syria* 29, 271–278; for Tantalos amulets see also Bonner, C. (1950). *Studies in Magical Amulets, chiefly Graeco-Egyptian.*

4.3.3. *Horus-on-the-Crocodiles*

In the Late and Ptolemaic periods, a particular kind of defensive-curative artifact became numerous. Monuments—often on a large scale but also including statuettes and even wearable items—carried depictions of 'Horus-on-the-crocodiles', which show Horus, in human shape, standing on crocodiles (hence the name) while restraining snakes and scorpions in both hands.[207] The scene was the culmination of the mythic cycle of the young Horus, showing not only his triumphant survival of the deadly marsh animals of his hidden childhood, but also his consequent victory over usurpation and disorder, also signified by these Sethian creatures. The image was often accompanied by a text relating and invoking elements from the myth. The most famous *cippus* is the spectacular Metternich stele, dating to ca. 360–343, now in the Metropolitan Museum of Art in New York.[208] It was originally the donation of a wealthy individual to the temple of Mnevis at Heliopolis (there is a dedicatory inscription on the back of the stele), but seems to have been moved to Alexandria at the beginning of the Ptolemaic era. The lengthy text is the story of how Thoth and Isis cured Horus-the-child of a poisonous bite in the marshes: a medical template against toxicity in particular and disease in general. The *cippus*, however, removed the need for a practitioner to read or to have memorized the incantation: its instantiation in this inscribed form devolved the power of the depicted word from the external expert to the sufferers themselves. Water (or any other liquid) that was poured over the stone acquired the power of the words and symbols on it. The water or other substance could then be drunk, or topically applied, as a kind of solid-state spell, for the purpose of either protection or cure, depending on the precise text used.[209] Some *cippi*, although not the Metternich, include a basin for the collection of this water.

There were also much smaller *cippi* and even *cippi* amulets.[210] The latter were worn on the body, and smaller stelae could have been erected in domestic contexts. The larger stelae found in sanctuaries were more potent,

---

[207] The imagery of a male infant holding or strangling snakes may have reminded ancient Greeks, as well as modern-day classicists, of Herakles' defeat of hostile serpents in his cradle. I owe this point to Ann Ellis Hanson.

[208] See the recent publication in the Metropolitan's exhibition catalogue by Allen, *Art of Medicine*, no. 52, pp. 49–63.

[209] The text makes a difference: Allen, *Art of Medicine*, 64.

[210] See e.g. Allen, *Art of Medicine*, 63–64, nos. 53 (a small Ptolemaic stela) and 54 (amulet, from the Late period or early Ptolemaic).

but less flexible in use and location. Their usual location was probably the temple forecourt, relatively easy of access compared to the inner regions of the temple, but considerably removed from any domestic or working location in terms of both physical and metaphysical distance.

In Greco-Roman Dendera a stone block was found in situ in a building within the sanctuary to Hathor. It stood in a water channel that ran around three sides of that building.[211] The massive block was inscribed with a text that incorporated materials from several sources, among which can be detected some protective elements, including allusions to the Horus-Isis cycle used on *cippi*. It does not feature the usual *cippus*-image of the god victorious over his poisonous enemies, although there may have been a small statue on top of the block that has not survived. Daumas (p. 48) therefore viewed it as a healing *cippus* of unusual type, such that water did not collect in a basin but circulated through the water channel of the building itself.

Cippi are defined by the inclusion and centrality of Horus' sojourn in the marshes, although they often also include additional elements that reinforced the theme of defense against poisonous creatures, such as protective deities like Bes, Taweret and the eye of the sun. The textual extras of the Metternich stela included a spell against Apophis, a spell against poison, three spells to cure a cat bitten by something poisonous, a spell for protection of those traveling on water, another story involving Isis saving a child from poison in the marshes, and two more spells against scorpion sting and snakebite.[212] The Dendera block, as we have it, is thus rather atypical of the *cippus* genre in regard to both its text, in which the allusions to the Isis-Horus cycle are minimal, and its physical placement. Our view of its specific functionality ought perhaps to be refined, but some kind of protective use does seem implied.

As with amulets more generally, we cannot link any *cippus* specifically with individuals using Greek names or language, but the Isis-Horus cycle and its healing elements survived into the syncretic milieu of the Greek and demotic 'magical papyri.' The significance of the use of statues, amulets, and *cippi* for medicine and prophylaxis is that this kind of response to disease was largely independent of interaction with professionals: while the production of powerful images and texts ultimately depended upon

---

211 Daumas, F. (1957). 'Le sanatorium de Dendera', *BIFAO* 56, 35–57: discussed in more detail in 2.5, pp. 96–97.

212 See Allen, *Art of Medicine*, 51 and translation, 53–63.

access to the oral and written resources of the technically expert elite of the temples, subsequent mass production allowed for the co-optation, via objects, of religious, written and professional power for the patient. Within this arena, the close-focus diversity of artifactual medicine enabled personal and familial negotiation amongst a multiplicity of gods, artistic forms, authority claims and available materials, rather than choice between clearly distinctive ethnocultural forms. The self-conscious exclusion of the majority of amuletic materials on naturalistic grounds, a move familiar among but largely limited to Greek medical professionals, and its partial replacement by dietetic modes, would have been a rare choice on the part of most of their patients.

4.4. *Knife, Fire, and Bathing: How to Recognize Greek Medicine*

Herodotos' account of the sixth century physician Demokedes of Kroton includes the well-known episode of his enslavement in Darios I's court at Susa.[213] In Herodotos' words, the Persian king's physicians were Egyptian, because he considered them foremost in the art of medicine: νομίζων δὲ καὶ πρότερον περὶ ἑωυτὸν ἔχειν Αἰγυπτίων τοὺς δοκέοντας εἶναι πρώτους τὴν ἰητρικήν. But when Darios dislocated his ankle, their violent manipulations only succeeded in making it much worse: οἳ δὲ στρεβλοῦντες καὶ βιώμενοι τὸν πόδα κακὸν μέζον ἐργάζοντο. Demokedes, once brought to the king's attention, 'applied Greek remedies and used gentle means instead of their violent ones' (Ἑλληνικοῖσι ἰήμασι χρεώμενος καὶ ἤπια μετὰ τὰ ἰσχυρὰ), successfully eliminating the pain of the dislocation. He went on to prevent the Egyptian doctors from being impaled, and subsequently also cured Darios' wife Atossa, before escaping back to Kroton, a town in the far south of Italy.

This story is sometimes cited as further evidence for the high reputation of Egyptian medical practice in the ancient world, already well attested by Egyptian diplomatic correspondence. Egyptian physicians had long been a feature of non-Egyptian courts.[214] But Herodotos' version asserted the superiority of Demokedes over the previously acknowledged preeminent medical experts of antiquity: a very explicit claim that Greek and Egyptian medicine are not only different, but in an agonistic relationship in which the former is superior. This superiority is presented as being due, not simply

[213] 3.129.1–130.3.

[214] Ghalioungui, P. (1983). *The Physicians of Pharaonic Egypt*, 76–79.

to the better physician being a Greek, but to distinctively Greek remedies, Ἑλληνικοῖσι ἰήμασι.[215] Egyptian medicine, and consequently Egyptian practitioners, have been supplanted. It is interesting to note that although the story of Demokedes bears the hallmarks of a romanticized folk-tale, Artaxerxes II, Darios I's son, had a Greek personal physician: Ktesias of Knidos.[216]

Demokedes seems to treat the dislocation with topical remedies. These were a common alternative, in both classical Greek and Egyptian medicine, to mechanical treatments. The explicit characterization of violent and painful treatments as Egyptian, and Greek medicine as gentle is, however, a major surprise to anyone who has read Roman authors' depictions of Greek therapeutics as painful butchery, with an emphasis on surgery and cauterization.[217] Forceful treatments appear to have been something of a negative trope in Greco-Roman writings, in spite of the fact that surgery, in particular, underwent a rapid diversification in its techniques and functions during the Hellenistic era, one closely linked to the expansion in anatomical knowledge among physicians of Ptolemaic Alexandria. As we shall see, this trend differentiated 'Greek' from 'Egyptian' medicine, even while complex surgery was a minority option among practitioners of the former.

The word 'surgery' covers a variety of procedural responses to medical situations. In antiquity it included physical manipulation, as in the reducing of dislocations or realignment of bones; the excision or perforation of bodily externalities, from swellings to cataracts; cosmetic surgery and circumcision; the stitching and mending of wounds; and, most rarely, the invasive operations of internal surgery. Although minor incidents must have been dealt with regularly by laymen and through self-treatment, more complex forms of surgery required experience, expertise and a degree of specialization. Many of its forms were rare. It was a high-risk intervention utilized most frequently in high-risk circumstances including trauma and severe illness; and the obverse of low-risk, long-term, readily available health behaviors like amulet use or regimen.

---

215 Griffiths, A. 'Democedes of Croton: a Greek doctor at the court of Darius' in Sancisi-Weerdenburg, H. and A. Kuhrt. (1987). *The Greek Sources: proceedings of the Groningen 1984 Achaemenid History Workshop*, 37–51. Cf. Thomas, *Herodotus*, 41, on Herodotos' persistent use of *technê* to refer to Demokedes' style of medicine.

216 Ktesias: Diodoros 2.32. For the folk-tale nature of the story see Griffiths, 'Democedes'. Cf. 1.4.2, p. 41.

217 Especially Pliny *Natural History* 29.6.14 (quoting Cato).

Egyptian physicians knew the appearance of many traumatic injuries and means of treating them. This is attested to above all by the Smith papyrus, but also by cases in the Hearst, Carlsberg and Ramesseum papyri. Their methods included the excision or draining of swellings with the knife, amputation, cauterization, the setting of fractures with splints, the reduction of dislocations, the stitching of flesh wounds, and bandaging.[218] The skeletons of the pyramid workers of Giza, from ca. 2465–2323, often showed evidence of fractures; as most of these had healed in good alignment the use of splints was evidently standard procedure. One of the deceased still had a splint attached to his partially healed broken arm. In two probable amputations, success is indicated by the complete healing of the end of the bone.[219] Over 2500 years later, Galen, studying in Alexandria in about 155 CE, observed the amputation of a local peasant's finger by a physician after it was bitten by a snake.[220] Ebers 860, recommending the knife for removal of a swelling of fat on the neck, warns the practitioner to avoid cutting the blood vessels. (Details of the operation are not specified: a recipe for a topical application follows). There is a similar injunction at 871. Ebers 875 mentions a flint *ds*-knife (also used for snakebite at Brooklyn 72a) and a *s3s*-knife, there is a *ḥpt*-knife in Ebers 767 and some kind of reed-knife (Ebers 876). All were employed in the context of swellings or 'oozings', and apparently involved excision and drainage; knives were also used for snakebite and bites in general.[221] Cauterization was employed, again for swellings or sores.[222]

---

[218] Examples of most of these can be found in the Smith. Stitching: cases 3, 10, 14, 23, 26, 28, 47. Linen splints and braces of three different kinds are prescribed in cases 35, 36, 37. A mummy of 1065–740 from Thebes had a wooden toe, showing signs of use: Nerlich, A.G. et al. (2000). 'Ancient Egyptian prosthesis of the big toe', *The Lancet* volume 356 issue 9248, pp. 2176–2179 (http://www.thelancet.com/journals/lancet/article/PIISO140--673(00)03507--8/fulltext). A fracture is set in Smith case 12, cf. case 35. See below, p. 197, n. 237 for mechanical reductions.

[219] Hawass, Z. and A. Senussi. (2009). *Old Kingdom Pottery from Giza*, 17 note 25. For other possible examples of amputation and healed fractures from pharaonic Egypt: Macke, A. and C. Macke-Ribet. (1990). 'Les recherches anthropologiques. Vallée des Reines. Vallée des Rois. Vallée des Nobles', *Les Dossiers d'Archéologie* 149–150, 34–39.

[220] Galen *Affected Parts* 3.11 (8.197 Kühn). The ἄγροικος had bound his finger at the base as tightly as possible and run to the city for the doctor (δραμὼν ἐπὶ τὴν πόλιν πρὸς ἰατρὸν ...).

[221] *Brooklyn* 72a (flint knife); *Vienna Demotic Papyrus* XVI, 1 (*tk* -knife). For a full list of physicians' tools, see Westendorf, *Handbuch*, 487. The use of flint and reed-knives has sometimes been interpreted as evidence for an interest in (the empirical benefits) of sterile instrumentation: I join Bouchet-Bert, L. (1998). 'The question of *dḳr* and sterile blades in P. Ebers 875', *JEA* 84, 224–228, in being skeptical on this point.

[222] Smith 39 (pustular swellings); Ebers 856c (swellings of the *mtw*), 872. The first is one of three non-traumatic cases in the Smith text, the others being 45 and 46.

In southern Egypt, in the double temple of Haroeris and Sobek at Kom Ombo, the inner surface of the enclosure wall includes a Roman period depiction of craftsmen's tools that are often thought to be surgical ones. The identification is based on their similarity to instruments described in Greco-Roman medical texts. If correct, it suggests that Egyptian surgical instrumentation—and thus probably surgical procedures and goals—had evolved into a form similar to that of contemporary Greek-language medicine; or that this style of surgery and instrumentation represented an acceptable alternative to older forms, one with relevance to the religious expression of knowledge. Marie-Hélène Marganne suggests that priests here worked in a dual indigenous and Hellenistic tradition.[223]

This must, however, remain speculative, as there is no other indication that Egyptian physicians employed surgery as a method of treatment for non-traumatic internal illness in either the pharaonic or Greco-Roman periods. No certain surgical scars have been identified on over thirty thousand mummies examined in the last two centuries.[224] Examples of trepanation, a procedure that appears in the Neolithic period and as far apart as Europe and South America, are possible but not conclusive.[225] Even non-traumatic surgery that did not require an actual incision seems to have been rare. The still hotly debated evidence for surgical dentistry comes primarily from the period of the Old Kingdom, and the few examples of wired and bridged teeth known for this period may have been reconstructed during mummification or manufactured as charms.[226] Dental remedies in the extant medical papyri are non-surgical.[227] A large number of mummy remains attest to the practice of circumcision as common among the elite throughout antiquity; a scene in Ankhmahor's 24th century tomb at Saqqara clearly depicts the

---

[223] Marganne, M.-H. (1998). *La chirurgie dans l'Égypte gréco-romaine d'après les papyrus littéraires grecs*, 83. See also ibid. (1987). 'Les instruments chirurgicaux de l'Égypte gréco-romaine', *Archéologie et médecine. VII*[e] *Rencontres Internationales d'Archéologie et d'Histoire*, 403–412. The bibliography on Kom Ombo is collected by Nunn, *Egyptian Medicine*, 163–164.

[224] Rowling, 'Rise and decline', 316. Sullivan, R. (1996). 'The identity and work of the ancient Egyptian surgeon', *Journal of the Royal Society of Medicine* 89, 471, points out that mummification damaged and darkened the integument, reducing the chance of finding any iatrogenic incisions made.

[225] Distribution: Sullivan, 'Identity and work', 471. Possible case from pharaonic Egypt at Giza: Filer, J. (1995). *Disease*, 90–91. Trepanation in Greco-Roman Egypt: Pahl, W.M. (1993). *Altägyptische Schädelchirurgie*.

[226] Ikram, S. and A. Dodson. (1998). *The Mummy in Ancient Egypt*, 98.

[227] A special forceps (ῥιζάγραν) for extracting roots is attested for Greek medicine: Celsus 7.12.1.

procedure, but it is unclear whether the men making the cut are to be identified with physicians, as circumcision is never referred to in the extant medical papyri.[228]

Nor is any surgery prescribed as a treatment for gynecological conditions: the treatment is a local or oral application. This is in spite of the fact that gynecological problems are well represented in the extant Egyptian medical texts, especially in the Kahun papyrus, along with names for most distinctive female organs, including internal ones.[229] It also contrasts somewhat with Greek medicine, in which vaginal fumigations, pessaries and topicals were common treatments. Gynecology also included, as early as the classical period, the difficult and highly dangerous practice of embryotomy in cases of dystocia (the fetus was cut up in the womb and subsequently extracted).[230]

Similarly, there is no mention in the medical literature of eye operations, in spite of the high proportion of material and spoken remedies for eye conditions, including paragraphs 336–431 of the Ebers. The possibility remains that the compilers of these largely pharmaceutical *aide- memoires* did not record any surgical procedures that did exist; while the Smith text—of which only a small part dealing with the upper body survives—might have been composed for use in war.[231] Ebers 424 and 425, describing recipes for a 'twisting of eyelashes into the eye', make brief reference to the eyelash having been pulled out, but do not describe the procedure in any detail, unlike Celsus on the same topic.[232] There is however no other indication of

---

228 Mummies: Smith, G.E. and R. Dawson. (1924). *Egyptian Mummies*. Ankhmahor's tomb, with useful discussion: Kanawati, N. and A. Hassan. (1997). *The Teti Cemetery at Saqqara*, 49–50, plates 19, 55. Cf. a badly damaged scene in the temple of Mut-en-Ashara at Karnak: Pillet, M. (1952). 'Les scènes de naissance et de circoncision dans le temple nord-est de Mout, à Karnak', *ASAE* 52, 93–104, pl. 5. Diodoros 1.28.3: the Jews and the Kolkhi of the Pontos brought the custom of circumcision with them out of Egypt. Ankhmahor's tomb includes dialogue which names the operation as *sbt* (unattested in medical texts). Ebbell, B. (1937). *Papyrus Ebers*, 103 wrongly identified Ebers 732 (88.10–12) as an example of circumcision: the remedy is for a cut by acacia thorn: (Westendorf, *Handbuch*, 670; Bardinet, *Papyri médicaux*, 353).

229 Local and oral applications: e.g. Ebers 783.3, 784, 789, 800, Kahun 3, 4, 10. For the terminology of female genitalia, see Westendorf, *Handbuch*, 200–201.

230 *Superfetation* 7 and 9; cf. *Excising the fetus* 1; *Diseases of women* 1.70; Celsus 7.29, Soranos *Gynecology* 4.9–13 (*CMG* 4. 140–144). Herophilos used an instrument Tertullian calls a 'fetus-slayer' for such a procedure: von Staden, *Herophilus*, T247.

231 In Smith case 8 the *swnw* must have laid back a flap of skin on the skull, but the procedure is not described: Breasted, *Edwin Smith*, 208. War handbook: Allen, *Art of Medicine*, 10, 14, 71.

232 7.7.8. Trichiasis, in which eyelashes grow abnormally towards the eye, causing extreme irritation, has a number of causes, including infection by the endemic eye disease trachoma.

eye surgery within Egyptian medical literature.[233] In contrast, Greek surgical ophthalmology developed rapidly during the Hellenistic period, including cutting out cysts in the upper eyelid and even the removal of cataracts. According to Celsus cataract operations depended on a detailed knowledge of the anatomy of the eyeball, including the *arachnoeides* membrane (retina) named and probably observed for the first time by Herophilos in the third century.[234] Two ophthalmologic treatises survive among Ptolemaic Greek papyri (one from Hibeh and one from the Arsinoite nome), with several others known from the early Roman era. They include theories on the mechanism of vision and humoral explanations; the originals clearly derive entirely from a Greek medical milieu and its characteristic emphasis on debate and speculation.[235]

In this, developments in ophthalmology were typical of those in Greek intellectual medicine of the period, particularly in respect of surgical experimentation and anatomical knowledge. Alexandrian physicians played leading roles in this process, but innovations in tools and techniques diffused with relative rapidity from Alexandria to at least the Fayum, as in the case of the ophthalmologic treatises and several papyrus fragments on surgical techniques.[236] These describe Greek language surgery that included not only eye operations, cosmetic operations, ligatures, and mechanical dislocations—all of which, definitely or possibly, had parallels in Egyptian practice[237]—but also phlebotomy, a more extensive use of cauterization, embryotomy, and surgical interventions in the throat and in the pelvic area. Before the third century, Greek medicine had used cauterization and the knife primarily for wounds, and, more ambitiously, on visible structures

---

Their removal must have been one of the commonest operations in Greco-Roman medicine: e.g. Jackson, R. (1998). *Doctors and Diseases in the Roman Empire*, 121.

233 The pseudo-Galenic medical treatise *Introduction or, The doctor*, probably from the later 1st century CE (14.674–797 Kühn, cf. p. 198 n. 243) praises Egyptian advances in operations including eye surgery.

234 Celsus 7.7.6.

235 Cartonnage from Hibeh, MP3 2343.1 (early 3rd century BCE) and P. Ashm. Libr., MP3 2344 ((2nd century BCE). See the discussion of these as texts 1 and 2 in Marganne, M.-H. (1994). *L'ophtalmologie dans l'Égypte gréco-romaine d'après les papyrus littéraires grecs*, 37–105.

236 Marganne, *La chirurgie*, 157–159, 161; Eye operations: Marganne, *L'ophtalmologie*, 182–183.

237 Smith case 25 (with plate 6) describes the reduction of a dislocated jaw, which parallels both modern procedure and the method outlined in the Alexandrian Apollonios of Kition's first century text *Commentary on Hippocrates' On Joints* 2 (*CMG* 11.1.1, 48–50 with plate 14). Smith case 43 applies external remedies to a dislocation.

such as facial mutilations.[238] Nonetheless internal surgery in cases where there was no pre-existing break in the body's surface was practiced before the Hellenistic period: *Diseases* described an operation to remove pus in the pleural cavity which necessitated an incision between the ribs and the insertion of a draining tube.[239] By the first century CE, the encyclopedist Celsus could devote his entire seventh book to 'cases in which the practitioner does not find wounds but makes them.'[240] The examples listed include the removal of hernias from the inguinal region or the scrotum, the excision of tonsils, incisions into the bladder to remove stone, the replacement of prolapsed intestines, and, similarly to the *Diseases* procedure, the draining of water in dropsy through a tube inserted after deliberate perforation of the abdominal cavity.[241] In cases of liver ailments Erasistratos was said to have 'cut the skin and the membrane covering the liver and applied drugs extensively to the organ itself; then he drew aside the stomach and boldly laid bare the part that was affected.'[242] He was also credited with the invention of a catheter to drain the bladder.[243]

There is no evidence from either pharaonic or Late and Ptolemaic Egypt that indicates a corresponding interest in non-traumatic surgery among practitioners of Egyptian medicine. The topic is closely related to the growth in anatomical knowledge, and therefore to the methodological tool of animal or human dissection. This investigative procedure was employed by only a very few physicians during the Ptolemaic period, but its influence on Greek medical controversies and treatments was considerable.

It might be thought that Egyptian medicine had a routine, long-standing equivalent of human dissection as a result of embalming. The domains of embalmer, physician, and animal sacrificer were perceived as at least closely related in pharaonic Egypt. The Smith quoted a 'Treatise on what pertains to

---

238 For the latter see *P.Univ.Giss.* IV 44 (ca. 100 BCE) ed. Marganne, *La chirugie*, especially p. 186.

239 *Diseases* 2.47 (7.64–72 Littré).

240 Celsus 7 praef. 5.

241 Celsus 7.19, 7.12.2, 7.26.2, 7.20, 7.15. The operation to remove bladder stone was risky, killing Antiokhos VI in the second century: Livy 55; Josephus *Jewish Antiquities* 13.218. The pre-Hellenistic *Oath*'s apparent restriction of it to specialists suggests that the procedure was already known in the classical period. That Celsus' descriptions often go back to the Hellenistic period and sometimes before can be safely assumed not only by the similarity between some procedures but also by Celsus' highlighting of the work of Alexandrian surgeons of the Ptolemaic period in the preface to book 7.

242 Caelius Aurelianus *Chronic Diseases* 3.4.65 (*CML* 6.1, 2.716.29–32 Bendz).

243 Ps.-Galen *Introduction, or, The doctor* 13 (14.751 Kühn) (above, p. 197, n. 233).

the embalmer', and the grandson of one embalmer was a 'chief of physicians' (*wr swnw*) in the Middle Kingdom (ca. 2040–1650). By about 380 the same word, *swnw*, was used for the embalmer as well as the physician, and the term 'remedy' (*pḫrt*) was used for treatment of both the living and the dead.[244]

The complexity and degree of human dissection in embalming has, however, often been viewed as minimal: as a complement to knowledge gained from animal butchery, it would have produced an awareness of major internal organs within the body cavity, but not to the degree visible among the Alexandrian anatomists or that required for complex surgery. This view has been challenged, but however elaborate the dissection involved in the ritual preparation of the dead, it is not evidence that dissection was employed as a methodological tool within an investigative medicine.[245] We assume they are related because that is how modern research works. But human dissection for the sake of medical inquiry was throughout antiquity the exception not the rule. The question is not why such investigations were absent in Egyptian, Roman, Mesopotamian and most classical Greek medicine, but rather why the limited use of animal dissection, culminating in systematic human dissection and vivisection by a few physicians in third century Alexandria, came to be part of Greek medicine during the Hellenistic era.[246]

Using dissection for improving anatomical knowledge requires the assumption that one's current state of knowledge is inadequate for one's purpose, or even incomplete. Several Greek physicians in antiquity were certainly of the view that medicine and anatomical knowledge of the time was sufficient to the point of perfection, so long as it was correctly applied.[247] The replication of knowledge, let alone its revision, was not required. Although Egyptian texts were never so methodologically explicit, they appear to have similarly assumed that the information obtained from traumatic injuries

---

244 Priests of Sakhmet were not only *swnw* but also specialists in animal sacrifices: 5.1.1, p. 207; in general von Kanel, F. (1984). *Les Prêtres-ouâb de Sekhmet et les conjurateurs de Serket*. Treatise: Smith case 19 gloss A, cf. case 3 gloss A. Family: Ghalioungui, *Physicians*, no. 59. Same word: Ritner, *Mechanics*, 54–56.

245 Complex dissection: Pahl, W.M. and Parsche, F. (1991). 'Rätselhafte Befunde an anthropologischem Untersuchungsmaterial aus Ägypten: Addenda zu Herodots ⟨⟨Historie⟩⟩, Lib. II, 86–88 und zum ägyptischen Sparagmos?' *Anthropologische Anzeiger* 49, 39–48.

246 See von Staden, *Herophilus*, 139–153; and below, 6.3, pp. 254–258. Even then, dissection as a technique was employed by few physicians. Galen (*Anatomical Procedures*) has to defend the need for it in the second century CE, while the Empiricists and Methodists rejected its usefulness entirely.

247 *Art* 3 and especially *Places in Man* 46 (p. 84 Craik): 'In my view, medicine has all been discovered …'.

and embalming was sufficient both to treat such injuries and to explain physiology and disease. Such experiential knowledge was understood, transmitted and subsumed into a traditional, high status, 'secret' knowledge of experts.[248] The deliberate acquisition of information by investigation, or even innovative speculation, about the nature of the body and its workings was unnecessary, impossible or inappropriate, or all of these at once.

Diodoros of Sicily reported that the mummification attendant whose role it is to make the initial incisions was ritually abused by the other embalmers.[249] This suggests that there was a taboo against cutting up dead bodies, perhaps derived from one of Egyptian religion's central myths: the butchery of Osiris by the chaotic god Seth before Osiris' reconstitution and resurrection.[250] Such a taboo would certainly explain, if an explanation is required, the lack of any tradition of dissection and anatomical investigation beyond everyday observation. It is not, however, sufficient in itself to account for the absence of non-traumatic surgery. This kind of surgery had been undertaken in classical Greece on the limited and piecemeal foundations of accidental observation, some animal dissection, intense speculation, and empirical experience and training, and without embalming.[251]

The imputation of value to bodily wholeness might have been a contributing factor for the absence of internal surgery—the deliberate incision of the undamaged living body. Taboos, however, often fail to withstand potentially overwhelming advantages such as survival, once such an advantage is believed to exist.[252] The point at which a widespread dislike turns into a cultural taboo is also difficult to identify. Aristotle remarked on the revulsion inspired in himself by dissection, but this did not prevent him dissect-

---

[248] For secrecy as an explicit procedure and aim in Egyptian technical writings and practices, see Baines, 'Restricted knowledge'. Ebers 206 implies that medicines sometimes came under the heading of trade or family secrets: 'You shall prepare for him medicines, secret to who is under the doctor, except for your own daughter'. See 5.1.2, pp. 215–216.

[249] Diodoros Sikelos 1.91.4. The *ḳs* of *BM* 10390 (136) is rendered in some Greek texts by σκυτεύς, implying a role in the evisceration of the body.

[250] Supporting evidence may be visible in the use of mutilation by knives as a form of execration. See Ritner, *Mechanics*, 163–167.

[251] For a survey of the origins and early history of dissection in Greek medicine and philosophy see Lloyd, *Methods and Problems*, 167–193. Anatomy was rare in the Hippocratic corpus and where it did appear, as in *Fractures* and *Joints*, was usually limited to knowledge gained in the actual treatment of injuries. As for human dissection, this was non-existent until third century Alexandria.

[252] Modern examples include test-tube babies, post-mortem dissection, and organ transplants.

ing animals.[253] To account for the absence of non-traumatic operations and aggressive anatomical exploration from the repertoire of the *swnw* in terms of religious taboo is to assume that an explicit interdiction is necessary to prevent these developments. A culture which managed the violability of the body as an integral part of its religious system did not prohibit anatomical dissection or invasive surgery; but the conceptual framework of Egyptian medicine did not require that kind of approach.[254]

4.5. *Selecting Practitioners and Practices*

The actual number of physicians, especially outside Alexandria, who specialized in or attempted difficult surgical procedures was probably small. Such therapies were without precedent in either the professional or popular sectors of Egyptian society and quite possibly had negative religious implications. Estimating the level of uptake of available surgical options by inhabitants of the *chora*, or even the city, is impossible. Relevant factors in such decision making would have been the painfulness or morbidity of the condition, the availability of surgical practitioners in the region, cost, and experience with or preferences about alternative therapies (appeals to the gods, drug or regimen use).

Other kinds of practices are also exclusively associated with Greek-language medical works, or Latin authors' reports of Greek medicine. Phlebotomy was controversial even among Greek physicians, but arguments both for and against it were closely embedded in the biological-philosophical Greek medical discourse, utilizing humoral concepts or Erasistratos' model of fluids under pressure.[255] Within Egyptian medicine, the procedure was novel and free-floating within the semantic network, unanchored to any prior system of meaning.

The use of caustics and cauterization, not only for open wounds, but also for eye conditions and 'dropsical' swellings was also much more regular in Greek medicine than in Egyptian (or Roman) therapeutics.[256]

---

253 *Parts of Animals* 645a27–30.

254 It has been suggested that the sudden acceptability of human dissection among Alexandrian Greek physicians was partly based upon mummification as a local cultural norm. Against this view, von Staden, *Herophilus*, 149–150; but revived by Ritner, 'Innovations', 115. See 6.2–3, pp. 253–258 and above 4.4, p. 199.

255 Arguing that phlebotomy caused a catastrophic shift in this system, Erasistratos rejected its use altogether: Galen *Blood-letting, against the Erasistrateans in Rome* (11.196.13–197.12 Kühn). Other physicians disagreed over what constituted appropriate cases or amounts.

256 See *Places in Man* (13, 21, 24), ed. Craik, E. (1998). Craik's commentary points to possible

Dietetics, in combination with other elements of regimen such as instructions on bathing and exercise, were described in a significant proportion of medical texts of the classical period. Medical regimens emerged from Greek physicians' expansion of more basic dietary advice, in which foods, herbs and *pharmaka* were less distinct and far more readily available on a routine and local basis. Such systems allowed for equivalencies and exchange between Egyptian and Greek foodstuffs and medicines, but a more elaborate regimen seems to have been a Greek speciality, highly dependent upon professionalized advice and humoral/environmental models. Its more complex forms, as many have pointed out, were effectively applicable only to those with the freedom to apply them: a largely urbanized socioeconomic elite. Among health-care seeking behaviors, choice of a culturally distinctive form of Greek medicine, then, also implied socioeconomic status, again reinforcing the association between Hellenizing behaviors and the elite.

These kinds of treatments were probably only available from practitioners with Greek language capability, who had trained with specialists in surgery or were familiar with humoral models.[257] Patient choice of practitioner and therapy was thus partly defined by attitudes toward Greek medicine as an ethnocultural construct; and partly by the linked question of the perceived medical authority of Greek-language practitioners. In the first century CE, the elder Pliny accepted some Greek pharmaceuticals but ignored practices, like surgery, alien to his understanding of illness and medicine. Some patients might have perceived practitioners who presented themselves according to Egyptian medical forms as having a particular expertise with enemas, purgatives or intestinal complaints, in accordance with (Greek) perceptions of what was distinctive about Egyptian medicine.

Egyptian parallels for the eye disorder, but, as she notes, surgical or cauterizing remedies do not occur in the latter tradition. Cauterizing (with caustic drugs or hot iron): as a last resort, *Diseases* 2.12 (7.22 Littré); 12 cauterizations at different points on the body stops flow of harmful bile and phlegm around body, curing recurrent headache, *Internal Affections* 18 (7.212 Littré). Used for eye problem, *Vision* 3–5 (9.154–158 Littré); to fix dislocated shoulder, *Joints* 11 (4.106 Littré). Risk: *Joints* 11 (4.106 Littré). Death: *Epidemics* 5.7.1–4 (5.206–208 Littré).

[257] That some physicians might have attempted operations solely on the basis of reading surgical treatises cannot be ruled out, but seems unlikely to have inspired much success or confidence among patients. In the late nineteenth century, patients of low socioeconomic status and education had considerable agency in rejecting surgery or selecting preferred practitioners, and doctors had to work hard to persuade potential clients: Wilde, S. 'Submitting to surgery in the 1890s: four vignettes', in Bala, *Biomedicine*, 171–189.

In many cases, health care was sought primarily on the basis of factors that were not connected to ethnocultural constructs or ethnic identifications, or only very indirectly so. We should remember that in comparison to self-medication, lay assistance, and folk healers, the professionalized discourses standing in contrast were relevant to only a small proportion of illness events or health-care seeking behaviors. Much religious and non-material healing, moreover, involved systems in which different gods, drugs, and amulets could be employed in equivalencies and exchange under the same broad explanatory model and therapeutic familiarity: I buy painkillers in foreign drugstores in spite of unfamiliar branding. It is also clear that patients in the Greco-Roman world frequently resorted to multiple therapies, models, and practitioners when immediate responses failed: those in Egypt must have often done likewise. For example, phlebotomy in Greek medicine is often employed as a stronger alternative to enemas; while the late first century CE physician Heliodoros, possibly from Egypt, criticized the incompetence of physicians whose operations in the anal region caused incurable excremental incontinence.[258] The Egyptian enema-specialist and the *iatros* with his surgical and cupping tools were not always far apart.[259] In second century Alexandria, such an enema-specialist intersected with Greek-language speakers, apparently on a professional basis, although the exact form of the interaction in this singular example is difficult to establish.[260]

The interpenetration of medical systems within Ptolemaic Egypt offered its inhabitants alternatives in drugs, treatments, and ways of understanding both illness and health care.[261] The experience of illness was negotiated within the patient-practitioner encounter and between the individual and the cultural systems in which he was embedded; among the relevant factors were the preferences and understandings of a more generally negotiated social and cultural identity.

---

258 P. Münch. II 23, MP3 458.300, quoted by Marganne, *La chirurgie*, 157.

259 *Regimen in acute diseases* appendix, ch. 3 (2.394ff. Littré): if the patient is young and strong and the illness severe, treat acute illness with phlebotomy (τὰ ὀξέα πάθεα φλεβοτομήσεις); if weak or if too much blood has been taken, instead give an enema every other day. Cf. chapter 4: give enemas unless the disease is great and severe.

260 *UPZ* I 148 (second century): for full discussion and bibliography, see chapter 5, pp. 205–206.

261 Alternatives can be either complementary, subsidiary, or exclusive of others.

CHAPTER FIVE

IDENTIFYING MEDICAL PRACTITIONERS

In the second century, a woman wrote in Greek to a male member of her family, looking forward to the fact that he would soon be returning to the city of Alexandria and a new job there.

> Learning that you are studying Egyptian letters, I am happy for you and for myself, since now at least, on your return to the city, you will be teaching the boys in the establishment of Phalou..es the enema-doctor, and you will have a means of living in your old age.[1]

This document has been much discussed since its publication in 1893.[2] The commonest interpretation, advocated, among others, by Wilcken, Schubart, Préaux, and Rostovtzeff, is that a Greek mother is writing to her Greek son to congratulate him on having learnt to speak or write the Egyptian language, with the result that he will be able to teach Greek to the children, or possibly the slaves (the term τὰ παιδάρια is ambiguous), of an Egyptian physician specializing in enemas.[3] In 1964, Roger Rémondon argued that the letter's recipient would be teaching, not Greek to Egyptian 'boys', but Egyptian to Greek medical apprentices. That was why the letter's author identified his learning of Egyptian writing as the critical factor in his employment. From this Rémondon deduced that enema-treatments, and consequently enema-doctors, were popular among the Greek-speaking residents of (probably) Alexandria, and that this popularity created a demand for Greeks trained in this Egyptian specialty.

---

1 *UPZ* I 148 = TM 3540 (second century BCE): Πυθανομένη μανθάνειν σε αἰγύπτια γράμματα συνεχάρην σοι καὶ ἐμαυτῆι, ὅτι νῦν γε παραγενόμενος εἰς τὴν πόλιν διδάξεις παρὰ Φαλου.. *ἰατροκλύστηι* τὰ παιδάρια καὶ ἕξεις ἐφόδιον εἰς τὸ γῆρας.

2 Discussions: Mitteis, L. and U. Wilcken. (1912) *Gründzüge und Chrestomathie der Papyrusukunde*, 22, 162 and *UPZ* I, p. 635; Schubart, W. (1923). *Ein Jahrtausend am Nil*, 51; Rostovtzeff, M. (1941). *Social and Economic History of the Hellenistic World* 883, 1093, 1545; Préaux, Cl. (1929). 'Lettres privées grecques d'Égypte relatives à l'éducation', *RBPh* 8, 770. See also Bagnall, R.S. (1995). *Reading Papyri, Writing Ancient History*, 33–35.

3 For this reason τὰ παιδάρια is often translated as 'slaves' or 'slave-boys', e.g. Bagnall, R.S. and R. Cribiore. (2006). *Women's Letters from Ancient Egypt* 113 (no. 15 = A 2.9), but this might be an over-specific translation.

It is not clear to me why Rémondon supposes that such apprentices were necessarily all Greek, although obviously a bilingual teacher indicates that some or most of them were. The letter implies that not just fluency in the Egyptian language, but fluency in *written* Egyptian (γράμματα), was important for its recipient. Most speakers of Egyptian were entirely or largely illiterate in that language, especially its hieratic and hieroglyphic forms.[4] An Egyptian enema-specialist might well have employed someone else to teach medical texts to his apprentices or slave-assistants; and that someone might have trained speakers of Egyptian, speakers of Greek, and bilingual individuals in the written texts of Egyptian medicine, in addition to any oral translation required.[5] We need not, then, be exclusive about who was teaching what to whom, so long as we realize that this Alexandrian enema-doctor required a bilingual—probably biliterate—intermediary within his extended household.

5.1.1. *Defining the Egyptian Physician*

Iatroklystes, 'enema-doctor', might be the Greek translation of the Egyptian medical title 'shepherd of the rectum', attested twice in early pharaonic inscriptions.[6] Greco-Roman texts did not customarily identify physicians by such subsidiary titles related to particular areas of medical practice. Egyptian terminology, however, involved several such titles, which are usually added to the more common and general terms for 'physician' or 'healer'. These are the terms used in medical texts to designate practitioners, and they do not appear in non-medical contexts (with the qualified exception

[4] Baines, J. and C.J. Eyre. (1983). 'Four notes on literacy.' *GM* 61, 65–96: pharaonic Egypt's literate elite comprised under 1% of the population. John Ray tentatively estimates that about 0.25% of the total population of mid-fourth century BC Egypt was fluent in written demotic, with 7–8% having some degree of functional literacy in demotic: 'Literacy and language in Egypt in the late and Persian periods', in Bowman, A.K. and G. Woolf. (1994). *Literacy and Power in the Ancient World*, 64–65 with n. 31.

[5] Medical practitioners, like other ritualists, probably learnt their skills in temples, possibly in the 'house of life', the library-scriptorium of a sanctuary. See Gardiner, A.H. (1938). 'The house of life', *JEA* 24, 157–158; Westendorf, W. (1999). *Handbuch der Altägyptischen Medizin*, 476–477; below, 5.2.1, p. 221, n. 63. On literacy see also note 4 above.

[6] Ghalioungui, P. (1983). *The Physicians of Pharaonic Egypt* nos. 7 and 43, both from the Old Kingdom. The title is not subsequently recorded in Egyptian. *Iatroklystes* occurs twice in the Ptolemaic period: in the Greek letter above (*UPZ* I 148), where the physician has an Egyptian name, and in the fragmentary accounts of *P.Hib.* II 268.14–15, TM 5223 (ca. 260). It may identify from a Greek viewpoint a continuing feature of and specialization within Egyptian medicine, rather than an exclusive specialist in this practice.

of the *wʿb*-officials of Sakhmet), demonstrating that the category 'medical expert' existed in Egyptian culture. These titles also appear in biographical and funerary inscriptions, but here they are frequently accompanied by cultic or administrative titles. Thus, although medical expert was an Egyptian category, and medical expertise an identifiable branch of knowledge and skill roughly comparable to the Greek notion of the 'medical craft' (*iatrikê technê*), in many Egyptian cases it was not an individual's exclusive occupation or specialization. This was a medical culture in which a high-status medical identity was dependent on the rare, powerful and valued skill of scribal literacy. (For medical practice by the non-literate, or minimally so, see e.g. 5.1.3, pp. 217–219).

Egyptian medical texts have three designations for the expert in medicine. The Smith papyrus says: 'on which any *wʿb*-official of Sakhmet and *swnw* put his hands or his fingers ...'. A gloss in the Ebers is almost identical: 'If any *swnw*, any *wʿb*-official of Sakhmet or any *sꜣw* places his two hands or fingers ...'.[7] Autobiographical graffiti by physicians sent on government expeditions to the alabaster quarries at Hatnub not only use precisely these titles, but also the terminology of the diagnostic laying on of hands.[8]

These and other references, in medical papyri and biographical inscriptions, make it clear that *swnw* carries the meaning of physician: it refers exclusively to practitioners of healing. *Wʿb*-official ('pure priest') of Sakhmet also identifies healers. Although their chief role was the practice of medicine, there is some evidence that they were also involved in the process of cattle sacrifice. Their involvement in medical expertise probably developed from their role of intercessors with a goddess associated with epidemic disease and hostility.[9] All *wʿb*-officials of Sakhmet, then, could be identified as *swnw*, but not all *swnw* as *wʿb*-officials of Sakhmet. Several inscriptions identify their subjects by both titles.[10]

The third term employed by the Ebers text is the *sꜣw* (ritual expert, magician).[11] *Sꜣw* seems to refer to an expert in dealing with non-mortals, perhaps especially through protective ritual. So much of this field of action

[7] Smith case 1 gloss A, ed. and trans. Allen, J. (2005). *The Art of Medicine in Ancient Egypt*. Ebers 854a, trans. Nunn. J. (1996). *Ancient Egyptian Medicine*, 113.

[8] Below, 5.1.2, pp. 213–214, nn. 33–34.

[9] von Känel, F. (1984). *Les prêtres-ouâb de Sekhmet et les conjurateurs de Serket*, 240 argues *wʿb* here designates a special purity for interceding with the goddess, and not the basic purity required for cultic attendants (the usual meaning, e.g. Allen, *Art of Medicine*, who translates *wʿb Sḫmt* as 'lay priest of Sakhmet').

[10] Ghalioungui, *Physicians*, nos. 16, 64, 74, 62 and possibly 6.

[11] Faulkner, R.O. (1962). *A Concise Dictionary of Middle Egyptian*, 207.

concerned medical dangers as to make the term essentially equivalent to 'physician': any *s3w* could be described as a *swnw*, although in non-medical contexts it probably had a broader range of application. A very similar expertise was that of the cult officials of the god *Ḥk3* (Heka), 'creative force, magic'; and the high-status ritual specialists of all cults, the *ẖry-ḥbt* ('lector priest') best known for their funerary roles and protection of the king's person. Several known physicians (*swnw*) held these positions or other religious titles, including the title of *sš*, 'scribe', which encompassed both administrative and ritual functions.[12]

The term *swnw*, then, does not single out a particular type of healer, or associate them as individuals or as a group with any specific god. It identifies a specialist or expert in a particular field of operation (medicine) within a more general category of protective and defensive practices.

The translation and functions of the another specialist, the *ḫrp šrḳt*, are not entirely certain. The *ḫrp šrḳt* was an intermediary, or possibly an intercessor, with the scorpion goddess Serqet, in cases of poisonous bites or stings, one of the main nosological categories in Egyptian medicine.[13] The title was held by important individuals, sometimes in addition to other medical and religious positions, but could also apply on a part-time basis to artisans in the village of Deir el-Medina (below 5.1.2, pp. 212–213).

Within these general categories were many differentiations. Some of these were the apparent specialties in particular kinds of medicine (or rather, particular kinds of illness) mentioned above. 'Doctor of the eyes', with nine examples, is the commonest.[14] The phenomenon is most apparent among physicians known from early Egyptian history (2686–2055 BCE). No such specialists appear among the seventy-two physicians attested between

---

[12] Borghouts, J.F. 'Magie', *LÄ* 3, 1138–1151; on cultic titles and medicine see Nunn, *Egyptian Medicine*, 120.

[13] Opinions on the meaning of this title and the precise activities of its bearer vary somewhat. Gardiner, A.H. (1917). 'Professional magicians in ancient Egypt', *PSBA* 39, 31–44 viewed him as interceding with a dangerous goddess. But Serqet appears frequently in helpful and healing contexts in medicine's central mythic cycle of Isis and Horus, as do her scorpions: von Känel, *Les prêtres-ouâb*, 284 suggests she was rather invoked in support against venomous attacks.

[14] Physicians of the eyes: 7 from 2686–2055 (Old Kingdom and First Intermediate periods), 2 from 1069–332 (Third Intermediate and Late periods). Cf. Herodotos 3.1.1: the best eye-doctor in Egypt, at the Persian court of Kyros. Of the belly: 2 from the Old Kingdom, 1 Late period. Teeth: 3 Old Kingdom examples and 1 Late period, plus two Old Kingdom *jbh*, which seems to be a term for 'dentist.' Physician-supervisors of butchers: 3 in the Old Kingdom. The inspector of liquids in the *ntntnt*: 2 from the Old Kingdom. The meaning of the last remains unclear; it notably does not include the word *swnw* unlike all the other 'specializations' (except *jbh*, 'dentist'). Information collected by Nunn, *Egyptian Medicine*, table 6.1.

2055 and 1069, but there are subsequent examples. According to Herodotos, the Late period in Egypt featured doctors who specialized in conditions of the eyes, head, belly, and in invisible diseases.[15] Among the fifteen known physicians of that era, one is a specialist in 'the belly and eyes' and another is the chief of the 'dentists' of the palace; Greek-language records of the Ptolemaic period offer two enema-specialists.[16]

It is difficult to know what Herodotos meant by each physician being the healer of one disease; but his specialties of body area map quite well onto the Egyptian categories attested for that period: eyes, belly, and teeth. No evidence mentions 'specialists in the head', but many remedies listed by area are 'for the head.'[17] Herodotos' 'physician of non-visible diseases', i.e. internal disease, is clearly heavily interpreted on the basis of Greek medical categories.[18]

Nothing, in fact, suggests that this method of distinguishing among individual physicians, according to their reputation or specialization, corresponded to differentiations in medical procedure. The medical texts suggest a common form of expertise for the *swnw*, *w'b*-officials of Sakhmet and *s3w* and do not indicate that there was any further specialization either within or between these categories.[19] The use of specialist-subject titles similarly seems to advertize the reputation, skill and power of a physician in a particular area, but this use is not based on a distinction between different skills or kinds of medicine. We should not infer the existence of ophthalmology from the presence of the category 'physician of the eyes.' 'Specializations' accumulated for important doctors, as for Irenakhty, whose stele declared him to be an eye-doctor at the palace, doctor of the belly at the palace, shepherd of the anus, and interpreter of liquids in the *ntntnt*, as well as physician at the palace, inspector of physicians at the palace, chief of physicians at the palace, and *ḫrp šrḳt*. He was, one gathers, a successful physician and extremely important among those attached to the court.[20]

---

15 2.84. ἡ δὲ ἰητρικὴ κατὰ τάδε σφι δέδασται: μιῆς νούσου ἕκαστος ἰητρός ἐστι καὶ οὐ πλεόνων. πάντα δ' ἰητρῶν ἐστι πλέα: οἵ μὲν γὰρ ὀφθαλμῶν ἰητροὶ κατεστᾶσι, οἵ δὲ κεφαλῆς, οἵ δὲ ὀδόντων, οἵ δὲ τῶν κατὰ νηδύν, οἵ δὲ τῶν ἀφανέων νούσων. 'Medicine is specialized among them in this way: each physician is the healer of a single disease and not of any others. The whole country is full of physicians, some are doctors of the eyes, some of the head, some of the teeth, some of the abdominal area, and some of non-visible diseases.'

16 Ghalioungui, *Physicians*, nos. 114 and 122. Enema-specialists: above p. 206, n. 6.

17 *GdM* 5.59 ff. This point was made by Lloyd, A.B. (1976). *Herodotus Book II, Commentary 1–98*, 349 ad loc.

18 Thomas, R. (2000). *Herodotus in Context*, 41, pointing to the close parallel in [Hipp.] *The art* 10.1. For what Herodotos might have meant: Lloyd, *Commentary*, 350 ad loc.

19 Westendorf, *Handbuch*, 472–475.

20 Ghalioungui, *Physicians*, no. 7.

The examples of actual specialists, moreover, are not only very early, but like Irenakhty, were often associated with the palace, either through a specific title such as 'chief of the eye doctors of the palace' or through having other titles that assert a connection to the king or to the palace (Great House).[21] Westendorf, *Handbuch*, 474 therefore identifies the institution of the royal court and administration, with its high concentration of medical experts, as the unique context in which this differentiation between physicians emerged. It may have remained largely restricted to the court (until Ptolemaic rule) and to certain sanctuaries or concentrations of sanctuaries. There expert ritual specialists were common, as indicated by titles such as, 'one with authority over physicians of the temple of Amon', or the 'chief of physicians of the place of truth (necropolis)'.[22]

An institutional role is further implied by the titles that relate to the court, such as 'physician at the palace,' and perhaps particularly for the 'king's doctor' or 'doctor to the Lord of the Two Lands', which might designate his personal physician. Several inscriptions, furthermore, refer to physicians employed on official military or mining expeditions. These confirm that some title-holders were actively engaged in administration of medical posts, and probably in medical practice themselves. The *wr swnw* Harkhebi, probably from the delta town of Buto around 700, owned an alabaster jar inscribed with biographical information and the label 'special ointment', probably for his medical practice. The physicians belonging to 'the office of the king's physicians' who made up Rameses XI's (1099–1069) eye paint from ingredients like galena were evidently more than nominal experts.[23]

The other sub-set of medical titles, the largest group, indicated a position within various administrative hierarchies. The commonest term is *wr swnw*, chief physician; but also including 'one with authority over physicians', 'overseer of physicians', and 'controller of physicians'. These probably indicated status as much as functionality, having evolved, like the subject-specialist titles, within the manifold hierarchies and subtle distinctions of the court and leading temples. A hierarchy also existed for the *wʿb*-officials of Sakhmet and *ḫrp šrḳt*. Similar titles were in use during the Ptolemaic

---

21 About half the specialists on the former definition, two-thirds on the second. Of the two Late period specialists one is the chief dentist of the palace; the doctor of the eyes and the belly has no similar title.

22 Ghalioungui, *Physicians*, nos. 75 and 81. For other examples ibid., pp. 46–47.

23 Harkhebi: most recently Allen, *Art of Medicine*, no. 56. Physicians processing eye paint: Wente, E. (1990). *Letters from Ancient Egypt*, no. 35, cf. no. 36. Quoted in 4.2.4, p. 180.

period and may represent the survival, in some form, of these medical-administrative ranks and functions: below, 5.5, pp. 239–241.

Several VIPs with medical titles held other administrative or ritual positions. Of these, some, like the position of lector priest, an important ritualist, also implied medical expertise. Others were less closely associated with defensive and healing practices. These individuals might have been experts who had subsequently acquired a more general power and status; several Greek court physicians of the Hellenistic era similarly, if informally, converted their political access into roles as royal advisors, conspirators and ambassadors.[24] Nor was there a sharp distinction between medical expertise and other forms of social and conceptual authority. Egyptian physicians were experts in the use of the creative power of *ḥkꜣ* and in dealing with gods or dead people at least as much as they were trauma surgeons or makers of eye-paint. Status and acknowledged expertise were derived from a high degree of medical-magical knowledge, preserved in written form in the temples. Medical authority, like other forms of power, was associated with the state and the religious infrastructure of the society, the traditional sources of access to and power over the forces of entropy and restoration. The modern tendency to define Imhotep, the paradigm of the healer, as an 'architect' *and* a physician, is anachronistic. These are modern distinctions, applied to an individual with an encompassing expertise in managing significant aspects of the universe on behalf of the king and for the sake of cosmic order and local well-being.

It is possible that some high-ranking medical positions were chiefly honorific. These titles served more to highlight the recipient's pre-eminence and acknowledge the degree of his competence and knowledge, than to define his daily activities. In later periods, the number of positions implying administrative oversight or particularly high status seems to increase for some categories of healer, or emerge for the first time. Overseers (*jmj-r*) of *ḫrp šrḳt* are attested only in the Late and Greco-Roman periods, and attestations of this title among the *wʿb*-officials of Sakhmet are also more common in the Late period than earlier. Fréderique von Känel, in her analysis of cult officials of Sakhmet and the *ḫrp šrḳt*, calls this phenomenon 'grade inflation'.[25] It is not uncommon, among our examples, for individuals to be simultaneously identified as several 'kinds' and grades of healer at one and the same time.

---

24 Westendorf, *Handbuch*, 478–479. Greek court physicians: below 5.2.1, pp. 224–226.

25 von Känel, *Les prêtres-ouâb*, 245ff.: the only example of *jmj-r* (overseer) of *sꜣw* is from the Late period; attestations of overseers of *wʿb*-officials of Sakhmet are also much more common in extant sources at this time.

The multiplication of medical and other ritual or administrative positions enhanced the status of their owner. This places most of the known physicians of late Egypt as defined by their ranks within the court and temple administration, rather than differentiated according to the practice of specialist, exclusive kinds of medicine.

In the extant evidence for physicians in Egypt, then, the dominant features are official positions, status hierarchies, and the advertisement of expertise through 'specialization' (a genre of emphasis rather than a statement of distinctive medical technqiues). But only 130–150 physicians are known for the two millennia or so of the entire pharaonic era. The overwhelming majority of these, moreover, are from high-status official contexts—the temples or the court administration—and the socioeconomic elite of pharaonic Egypt. They constitute a small, possibly unrepresentative, sample of Egyptian medical expertise.

5.1.2. *Obtaining Medical Assistance in Pharaonic Egypt*

A different, if not necessarily more typical, point of view is provided by the desert village of Deir el-Medina; built and occupied during the 18th and 19th dynasties (1550–1186) as living quarters for the artisans building the tombs in the valley of the kings, and for their families. The workmen were supplied with a monthly stipend of basic rations—mainly grain, oil and dates—recorded on ostraka. These reveal that certain workmen also functioned as physicians (*swnw*) or as *ḫrp šrḳt*. The *swnw* Pephyrpide seems to have been given time off (on two recorded occasions) for the purpose of 'preparing medicines'; a rare insight into physicians' medical activities.[26]

The amounts distributed by the government to (a workman acting as) *swnw* or *ḫrp šrḳt* are small compared to the standard rations. As Janssen suggests, they probably supplemented the usual workman's payment. The accumulated salary and status of these part-time medical professionals would in that case have been just below that of the foreman or a scribe.[27] The income of those able to designate themselves as *swnw* was probably also

[26] *BM* 5634 ll. 21–22. The work crew of sixty men was divided into 2 'sides': a *swnw* might therefore have been responsible for treating either 30 or 60 men. The village numbered some 400 inhabitants.

[27] Janssen, J. (1997). *Village Varia*, chapter 2, 'Rations and Ranks', esp. 26–29. Wages of *swnw*: *O. Cair.* 25608; *O. deM.* 376, 1–9; O. Gardiner 184 (unpubl.) and six other texts (Janssen ibid., 26). Wage of *ḫrp šrḳt*: O. IFAO 1296 unpubl; O. Gardiner 21.4 unpubl.

supplemented by private fees charged for medical problems experienced by non-workmen, such as their women and children, or traders and others from outside the village. In ca. 1155 a physician received objects valued at 22 copper deben in payment from a named individual.[28]

The *ḫrp šrḳt* appears in narrative only once in the Deir el-Medina records; when he reads out the house-by-house list of village inhabitants before the oracle of Amenhotep III in a case of theft. The god, in response, identifies the culprit.[29] The *ḫrp šrḳt* was evidently literate—not unusual among the village artisans—and an important figure within the social dynamics of the community. Direct evidence of more routine behavior is lacking, but probably consisted primarily of healing those bitten by scorpions or snakes: on several occasions workmen were listed as off work for a few days due to scorpion bites.[30] In a letter, the *ḫrp šrḳt* Amenmose places an order for some remedial foods on behalf of another cult official, who is ill: he might be either acting simply as a letter-writer or is effectively prescribing the items selected.[31] The Late period (664–332) Brooklyn medical papyrus on venomous bites says:[32]

> Beginning of the collection of remedies to drive out the poison of all snakes, all scorpions, all tarantulas and all serpents, which is in the hand of the *ḫrp šrḳt*, and to drive away all snakes and seal their mouths.

Janssen thinks the *ḫrp šrḳt* was also responsible for catching venomous creatures, as a preventative measure. I doubt whether a scorpion population could be effectively managed in this way, but the *ḫrp šrḳt* might have helped in the warding off snakes or scorpions with incantations, incense or significant artifacts, and perhaps caught or drove off these animals when they were actually found in a home.

Other state projects also involved the official provision of physicians. Inscriptions from the alabaster quarries at Hatnub, in the eastern desert, name Aha-nakht, *wʿb*-official of Sakhmet, and Hery-shef-nakht, chief of the king's physicians, *wʿb*-official of Sakhmet, overseer of *sꜣw*.[33] From around

---

28 *Pap.Turin* 1880 vs. 5, 2–12, discussed further 5.3.2, p. 235, n. 113.

29 *O. Gardiner* 4, from the mid 20th dynasty (1196–1069).

30 Janssen, J. (1980). 'Absence from work by the necropolis workmen of Thebes', *SAK* 8, 136–137. Cf. above 1.1, p. 16 for scorpion bite at a Roman era Egyptian quarry.

31 *O.UCL* 31399 (1279–1213 BCE); Wente, *Letters*, no. 186, p. 142.

32 Sauneron, S. (1989). *Une traité égyptien d'ophiologie*, no. 39.

33 For both see Anthes, R. (1928). *Die Felseninschriften von Hatnub*, nos. 15 and 21 (cf. 25), pp. 33–35, 56–59, 89; von Känel, *Les prêtres-ouâb* no. 10, pp. 17–20. Hery-shef-nakht only, as 'chief of the king's physicians': Ghalioungui, *Physicians*, no. 64.

the same time (1985–1773), in a list of about 100 names from a quarry in the Sinai desert is a *wr swnw*.[34] Many of these expeditions in search of necessary or rare minerals, to remote places and requiring unskilled labor, were essentially those of the army.[35]

There were also medical texts in private hands, as at Deir el-Medina, where several belonged to the family of the scribe Qenherkopeshef.[36] 'Scribe' was a common additional title for physicians, as it formally acknowledged the capacity to read and use powerful written materials against illness or other dangers. It is therefore likely that Qenherkopehsef's family and other literate individuals in the village, especially those with access to medical or defensive texts, practiced medicine on their own behalf and possibly, for a fee, on behalf of others.

Among the category of medical practitioners is the *rḫt* or 'knowing one, knowledgeable woman'. This designation occurs on a few fragmentary hieratic ostraka from the area of Deir el-Medina, and an unpublished papyrus fragment.[37] In all known instances it has a feminine termination, describing a woman, who is consulted for information about various problematic incidents, apparently ones usually involving hostile action by gods or similar entities. In the longest of these cases, a man writes to a woman about the implications of a recent event, the deaths of two children, in which she had some role. He complains that she has not yet sought out the *rḫt*.[38] She should do so, and ask the *rḫt*, firstly, what is the situation and destiny of the two dead children; secondly, how he, presumably their father, and their

[34] Gardiner, A.H. et al. (1952). *The Inscriptions of Sinai part I*, no. 85; Ghalioungui, *Physicians*, no. 63. The Hatnub inscriptions might be slightly earlier, from the end of the eleventh dynasty (2055–1985).

[35] Quirke, S. (1990). *Ancient Egyptian Religion*, 84, 86.

[36] Chester Beatty papyri 6–8 and 11–16 (London, British Museum nos. 10686–10688, 10691–10696), published by Gardiner, A.H. (1935, 2 vols.) *Hieratic Papyri in the British Museum*. In addition one side of Chester Beatty 9; (BM EA 10689, TM 57068) and one side of Papyrus IFAO Deir el-Medina 1, translated by Černy, J. *Papyrus hieratiques de Deir el-Medineh* 1 (Nos. I–XVII), ed. G. Posener (1978). For the reconstruction of this group of Deir el-Medina papyri as the family archive of Qenherkopeshef, see also Pestman, P.W. 'Who were the owners, in the 'Community of Workmen', of the Chester Beatty Papyri?' in Demarée, R.J. and J.J. Janssen. (1982). *Gleanings from Deir el-Medina*, 155–172.

[37] O. Cair. 25674 recto; O. Gardiner 149 (unpubl.); above, n. 36; Pap. Bibliothèque Nationale 237, carton 1. Texts (nos. 15–16) and discussion: Borghouts, J.F. (1982). 'Divine intervention in ancient Egypt and its manifestation', in Demarée and Janssen, *Gleanings*. Cf. above 4.4, p. 200 n. 248.

[38] Letellier, B. 'La destinée de deux enfants. Un ostracon ramesside inédit', in Vercoutter, J. (1980). *IFAO: Livre du centenaire 1880–1980*, 127–133.

mother will now fare; and thirdly, the name of the entity responsible for the children's deaths, in case it attacks their parents as well. The three questions are obviously closely connected. J.F. Borghouts observes that the *rḫt* also appears more than once in the mythic cycle of Isis and Horus on the Late period Metternich healing stele, where she behaves in a similar manner to that documented by the earlier Deir el-Medina ostraka: as identifying the mysterious entities behind misfortunes. The context of these examples suggests that the misfortune in question often concerned the bites of venomous animals, and in one instance further implies that the *rḫt* was also capable, like the *ḫrp šrḳt*, of making such animals withdraw through the use of powerful words. The Deir el-Medina ostraka indicate that such proceedings were reasonably commonplace, and that the *rḫt* played a significant role in mediating between ordinary people and the otherworld, or, from a modern point of view, in helping individuals manage and understand dangers and difficult events.

In other cultures women often function as seers, or specialists in the non-evident. The *rḫt* might thus be placed in the 'folk sector' of unofficial expertise, but the evidence of the Metternich stele embeds her deep within elite ideological templates. The related terminology of *rḫt, rḫyt, rst* was a common Ptolemaic era epithet of Isis/Hathor. The *rḫt* of Deir el-Medina was at best a (female) member of the minor elite, but on the Metternich stele Horus is cured by a *rḫt* who is also described as 'noblewoman' (*rpyt*) in her district.[39] The *rḫt* should probably be seen as another part-time professional ritualist, without a government post, but often of relatively high social status and considerable community standing among both sexes; consulted frequently on situations involving illness and poison.

It is moreover possible, I think, that the position of *rḫt* represents women from families in which the males were trained in literacy and ritual performance at a temple's House of Life, or within the family, and who subsequently held related official positions as 'scribes', cult officials, or medical experts. On the Metternich stele, Isis-as-a-*rḫt* declares that her learning was acquired from her father. For Isis, this probably means Ra, but a mortal 'knowing woman' could likewise have acquired a relevant training in a private capacity. A physician's handbook might imply that the daughters of physicians were included within his professional life, but not in quite the

[39] *Rḫt*: Borghouts, 'Divine intervention', 26–27. Cf. Baines, J. (1987). 'Practical religion and piety', *JEA* 73, 93ff.

same way as official apprentices or attendants: 'You shall prepare for him medicines, secret to who is under the doctor, except for your own daughter.'[40]

Her gender, in the absence of a specific cult affiliation, foreclosed most official positions, but created a space of power for such women within local communities. Unlike the *ḫrp šrḳt*, she does not appear in public or official settings, but in a private sphere of interaction: an unofficial but respected professional in dealings with the otherworld.

5.1.3. *The Practitioner at Large in Ptolemaic Egypt*

In documents of Ptolemaic Egypt, the words *swnw* and *iatros* appear to be used co-extensively, in reference to the same category.[41] In extant official texts the *swnw/iatros*, which I translate as 'physician', is the only term employed for a medical professional, as in the listings of households by occupation (where it also includes female members of the household).[42] In addition, as we have seen, two private Greek documents, a letter and an accounts list, use the term *iatroklystes*, which may be a translation or equivalent to the rare Egyptian 'shepherd of the rectum' (not recorded for any physician after 2055).[43]

With this exception, any specialists within the category 'physician' are not identified as such in extant Ptolemaic evidence. Moreover, other medical designations known for Greek or Egyptian practitioners of medicine earlier and elsewhere, such as *kathartês, rhizotomos, s3w, ḫrp šrḳt*, or *wʿb*-official of Sakhmet, are not used, or not used with the meaning 'physician.' *Wʿb*-priests of Sakhmet are attested in religious contexts for the Greco-Roman period: they presumably still acted as medical experts, but were not separately identified as physicians by the administration.[44] *S3w* could be a similar case, or subsumed within official use of the term *swnw*. The terminology is standardized, but it also seems to be the case that some medical practitioners, including those who practiced healing as a subsidiary

---

[40] Ebers 260. Nunn, *Egyptian Medicine*, 130 also views this as indicating intra-familial transmission of knowledge.

[41] See further below, 5.3.3, pp. 236–238.

[42] Similarly the designation 'teacher' might also include other adult males in a family (presumably non-working and perhaps elderly): Cribiore, R. (1996). *Writing, Teachers and Students in Graeco-Roman Egypt*, 21.

[43] See this chapter, p. 205 with nn. 1–2 and p. 206, n. 6.

[44] von Känel, *Les prêtres-ouâb*, 248–249.

activity, were not recognized by the bureaucracy as relevant to its aims or definitions (below, 5.3.3).

The mentions of the enema-physicians, however, provide some confirmatory evidence for what we would expect: that these other kinds of practitioner, perhaps including other 'specialists', did not disappear from the scene, but only from official perceptions. Occasional or part-time healers would also have gone unrecorded. Thus to the glimpses we have of physicians within the cities, towns and villages of Ptolemaic Egypt, and to the oracles, ritualists, and (possibly) dream-interpreters of cults and sanctuaries—where medical experts such as lector priests and *wʿb*-officials of Sakhmet could still be found—we must add a silent population of other kinds of healer, dependent on local, unofficial recognition.

In Greek society, root-cutters and drug-sellers were crucial parts of pharmaceutical trade and the collection of medical knowledge. No known Greek text from Egypt mentions either, but a Ptolemaic handbook on drugs included instructions on finding and identifying plants in the wild.[45] Plant collectors and hunters must have supplemented the personal efforts of doctors. As we have seen in chapters three and four, most of the good evidence for interaction between Egyptian and Greek medicine, over the period between pre-Ptolemaic texts and the earlier Roman era, is in two areas.[46] One of these is pharmaceuticals. The other is the medical use of the gods, through supplication, oracular inquiry, and the incantatory or artifactual invocation of divine powers. Classical period *iatroi* had been unusual in their redefinition of how drugs work and what caused disease, which tended to exclude direct divine agency, and many elite physicians retained this approach; but other kinds of Greek healers had not ring-fenced their explanatory concepts in this way. These healers, probably including lower-status physicians as well as purifier and the like, remained—in general terms—closer to Egyptian types of explanation. Some other professions, like the Greek athletics trainer or the Egyptian lector priest, were experts in matters that touched on medicine and illness, without it being their primary focus, and hence could also be sought out for information, advice and assistance. Galen's numerous and varied sources for drug lore included a boxer.[47]

---

45 See 4.2.4, p. 178 with n. 157.

46 For evidence of interaction and synthesis see below 5.2.1, especially pp. 221–223, and 5.2.3, pp. 229–232.

47 *The composition of drugs according to place* 9.5 (13.294 Kühn).

In addition to individuals who spent most of their time, and derived most of their income, from medical activities—*swnw/iatroi, ḫrp šrḳt*, drug-sellers—were those for whom healing was a kind of occasional expertise, available when required, but required not often enough to provide a living within the confines of village life. Multiple occupations were usual in communities in which supplementary incomes were often necessary and the population too small to create the demand required for specialization in trade. One fragmentary village record lists 35 different occupations.[48] The workman who doubled as a *swnw* at Deir el-Medina was a high status example of this kind of individual (5.1.2, p. 212). Collectively, they formed the local reservoir of medically related knowledge and skills. As Vivian Nutton puts it, "Galen's treatise [*Recognizing the best doctor*] reveals the enormous range of expertises that could be classified as medical, and, above all, the extreme fluidity of any line separating a layman from a *medicus*."[49]

Female healers, or healers of women, or healers of women suffering women-specific problems, are particularly difficult to locate in Ptolemaic Egypt, although comparative evidence from all societies implies their presence. The Greek midwife (*maia*) was a significant person in Greco-Roman society. Their role was not limited to childbirth and pregnancy. The classical period text *Diseases of women* mentions women carrying out gynecological examinations and Plato takes female *iatroi* for granted.[50] The funerary monument of Phanostrate, from the mid fourth century, identified her as *maia* and *iatros*.[51] Stories circulated of girls disguising themselves as men and learning to become doctors; their popularity with female patients caused scandal before the truth was revealed. One of these stories involved the Alexandrian anatomist Herophilos in the teacher role.[52]

Many Greco-Roman physicians viewed female physiology and pathology as different from that of the male in many more contexts than reproductive events themselves. Soranos' *Gynecology*, written for literate midwives, included a section on this well-worn debate of whether there were such things as 'diseases peculiar to women'. The view of the female body as almost a different species from the human male was at least partially inter-

---

[48] *P.Count* 6, TM 4367 (ca. 232).

[49] Nutton. V. (1990). 'The patient's choice: a new treatise by Galen', *CQ* 40 (1), 256.

[50] *Diseases of women* 1.68 (8.142.13ff. Littré), apparently on instructions of a male physician; Plato *Republic* 454d2.

[51] *IG* II^2 6873. Demand, N. (1994). *Birth, Death and Motherhood in Classical Greece* 68, 132–133.

[52] Herophilos and Agnodike: Hyginus *Fabulae* 254. See King, H. (1986). 'Agnodike and the profession of medicine', *PCPhS* 32, 53–77.

nalized by contemporary understanding among women as well, and it may have strengthened a notion of separate medicine for that gender. The role of female practitioners in medicine, however, has probably more to do with female networks in a society of relatively strict gender separation.[53]

In Egyptian society, women associated with newborn infants are usually described as 'nurse': *ʿtjyt, mnt, ḫnmt.t.* The last usually refers to a divinity. As *mnt* can also be applied to men, the term must have implied a broader definition of care than wet-nursing alone.[54] Nurses might have been the women attendants helping during birth itself: a customary term for 'midwife' is unknown, and in fact we have no evidence for this as a category separate from nurses and/or older women of the family and community acting as helpers. Women at the birth probably took on the roles of the goddesses associated with childbirth, including Hathor, Taweret, and Nephthys. An Old Kingdom (2686–2125) inscription does identify a high-status woman, also an official in the cult of the king's mother, as the 'female overseer of female physicians' but the exact implications of this title are unknown: it might have been primarily honorific or administrative.[55] Female ritual experts were usually restricted to specific cults or roles, and it would probably have been among such ritualists that women who assisted in childbirth, pregnancy, or with female-specific illness were often located. Among the relatively wealthy, women who held the title *nbt pr*, household manager, might have been specialists in birth magic.[56] Another possibility sometimes suggested, particularly for village medicine, is the *rḫt*, 'knowledgeable woman' (above 5.1.2, pp. 214–215 with nn. 37–39).

5.2.1. *Numbers and Kinds of Healer in Ptolemaic Egypt*

As for the numbers of physicians in Ptolemaic Egypt, this is impossible to estimate with any degree of reliability. Even if adequate evidence were

53 E.g. Galen *Prognosis* 8.

54 The existence of wet-nurses is attested several times in Ptolemaic papyri, as well as from pharaonic period texts and the Greek world. See Clarysse, W. and D.J. Thompson. (2008). *Counting the People in Hellenistic Egypt*, 2.267–272.

55 Ghalioungui, *Physicians*, no. 19. The overseer Peseshet is definitely female; for a survey of views on whether the 'female physicians' (*swnw.t*) she supervises are a scribal error for male physicians (*swnw*) see Nunn, *Egyptian Medicine*, 124–125. Possibly the feminine ending was mistakenly applied to the doctors supervised instead of the person supervising, but the title appears in three places and would be a rare error: female physicians remain a strong possibility.

56 *Nbt pr* as a birth ritualist: Quirke, S. (2005) *Lahun: a town in Egypt 1800 BC*, 81–84.

available, this would also take no account of those healers who were not recognized as *iatroi* or *swnw* (physicians), such as non-specialized ritual experts, root-cutters, or female healers.[57]

Anecdotal evidence and comparative material from other pre-modern societies, however, suggests that physicians were rarer in rural areas, and that higher-status individuals and training were associated with urban locations, with their higher population density and larger numbers of the wealthier kind of client.[58] In Galen's story from second century CE Egypt, when a peasant farmer receives a venomous bite he has to self-medicate until he can reach a doctor, which in that case meant running ἐπὶ πόλιν: for those further away from a population center, the doctor must often have been several days out of reach.[59] Physicians in the Egyptian tradition, chiefly the *swnw* and priests of Sakhmet, are unlikely to have been more accessible, although their numbers are even more difficult to assess, even in the broadest of terms. Over the entire pharaonic period, over two thousand years, only about 150 individuals are attested as *swnw*.[60] These are invariably officials of the court, employees assigned to the army, or experts from the temples: in other words *swnw* associated with the elite and hence most likely to appear in existing monumental and other written records. The term *swnw* is also applied to a lower status individual—the Deir el-Medina craftsman who also supplied medical care to other workmen, for an additional salary.[61] He

[57] A tax register from a region of the Fayum (*P.Count* 2), for instance, has 11 or 16 physicians in a total population of 18,065 people., but this record might be partial or atypical. Clarysse-Thompson, *Counting*, 2.109–110 note that village populations in these early Ptolemaic registers fluctate drastically, indicating either extensive internal migration or a problem in the demographic reliability of what records survive. There are about 30 instances of *iatros* in Greek-language documents of the Ptolemaic period, when H. Harrauer compiled his list of *iatroi* in *CPR* XIII (1987), *Griechische Texte* XI, 89–91, s.v. ἰατρός. For Harrauer's no. 20, see now *P.Count* 27 fr. 1, line 8 and note ad loc., p. 385. For Harrauer's no. 23, now of Roman date (after CE 162): Bataille, A. (1951). *Les inscriptions grecques du temple de Hatshepsout à Deir el-Bahari*, no. 65; Lajtar, A. (2006). *Deir el-Bahari* no. 94. Cf. 2.4.2, p. 89.

[58] Compare the teaching of letters. In about CE 100 a student complains that a prospective teacher of Greek letters and literature is not of the quality one expects in a town: 'I am so distressed because he, who taught in the country (ἐπὶ τῆς χώρας), thinks he can compete with the other teachers': *P.Oxy.* XVIII 2190, TM 25933. Trans. Cribiore, *Writing*, 16. Urban teachers charged higher fees: the same would have applied to physicians.

[59] Galen *Affected parts* 3.11 (8.197 Kühn).

[60] For comparison, a summary of occupations appearing in documentary papyri (those available up to 1987) of Greek-ruled Egypt from the Ptolemaic thorugh the Byzantine period, includes 154 *iatroi*: Harrauer, *CPR* XIII, 89–100; cf. Hanson, A.E. 'Doctors' literacy and papyri of medical content', in Horstmanshoff, M. (2010). *Hippocrates and Medical Education*, 190.

[61] Above 5.1.2, p. 212, n. 26.

might nonetheless have been literate to some degree in hieroglyphics, like many of his colleagues, since their work required a facility with inscriptional decorative programs. If *swnw* also designated healers who were non-literate in hieroglyphics, or in other forms of written script as well, we have no evidence for this use of the term. If, on the other hand, *swnw* indicated the ability to read and use written sources, like temple ritualists such as the lector priests to whom the term *swnw* was sometimes applied, then it must have been restricted to a small proportion of the population.[62] As, moreover, a specialty within larger ritual positions, it is more likely to have been a phenomenon of the training and resources available in the larger temples and scribal schools.[63]

We can therefore conclude, unsurprisingly, that higher-status healers, i.e. those recognized as 'physicians' (*iatroi* or *swnw*), were not a readily accessible resource for many, especially outside the major cities and towns. The genre of *euporista* or 'easily available medicines' testifies to the importance of self-medication and the fact that access to experts was often difficult or prohibitively expensive. An early example of this genre was by the late first century BCE Alexandrian physician Apollonios Mys, a member of the Herophilean *hairesis*.

Medical texts might also be used by people who were literate but not specialists in medicine.[64] Some of the pottery shards and papyri from Greco-Roman Egypt that contain recipe collections are probably by laymen.[65] The survival of Greek as well as Egyptian medical works in the private

---

62 See above 5.1.1, p. 206, n. 4.

63 The sparse evidence about schools in earlier periods of Egypt demonstrates that gatherings of children for the purpose of being taught their letters certainly existed. A temple setting is implied in at least some instances. By the Ptolemaic period, basic instruction was probably only for demotic in most cases, with hieratic and hieroglyphics reserved for a privileged few: Tait, J. (1997). 'Aspects of demotic education', *Akten des 21. Internationalen Papyrologenkongresses*, 931–938; Williams, R.J. (1972). 'Scribal training in ancient Egypt', *JAOS* 92, 214–221; also the brief analysis by Morgan, T. (1998). *Literate Education in the Hellenistic and Roman Worlds*, 274. Van Minnen, 'Boorish or bookish?' (below, n. 66) 110, identifies demotic school texts found in the Fayum villages of Karanis, Tebtynis, and Soknopaiou Nesos as from scribal schools for the sons of cult officials. There seems to have been a school, probably teaching Egyptinan letters, in the second century Sarapieon: in an account of one of his dreams the recluse Ptolemaios (see 1.3.2, p. 31 n. 124) mentions the *didaskalion* of Tothes: *UPZ* I 78.9–14, TM 3469; see Cribiore, R. (2001). *Gymnastics of the Mind: Greek education in Hellenistic and Roman Egypt*, 19.

64 For non-specialist cult officials as *swnw* in pharaonic Egypt, see 5.1.1, p. 211.

65 A possible example is MP3 2410.11, a late first-century prescription for colds and breathing problems, badly copied by a writer of the later first century CE on a papyrus that otherwise dealt with poetic subject matter (in a different hand): see Hanson, 'Doctors' literacy', 197.

collections of ritualists at Tebtynis in the Greco-Roman Fayum suggests these ritualists offered medical assistance that drew to an extent on both traditions, particularly as they were often written rapidly on the back of reused papyri, indicating texts for use rather than display.[66] The family of priests at Sobek's temple in Tebtynis probably owned the illustrated Greek herbal found there; fragments of a demotic herbal may have come from the same location.[67]

Interestingly, Greek and Egyptian texts overlap for only some genres, as van Minnen observes (p. 178): medical-botanical texts and astrological-astronomical ones are found equally often in both languages, but the same does not apply to dream interpretations, lexica, and legal texts (exclusively demotic). This may be a statistical accident: most of the genres represented at Tebtynis only in demotic are known from Greek versions at other sites (Roman period). Alternatively, if this division represents something about the particular interests of cult officials at Tebtynis, it would seem that medicine, astrology, and botany were areas where Greek expertise was felt to be relevant to the demands of their local community. The medical texts in question comprise both treatises and lists of prescriptions.[68]

Although there are no direct translations of demotic and Greek texts into those of the other language among papyri found at Tebtynis, examples from elsewhere in the Greco-Roman Fayum show translation and combination of medical information from different linguistic traditions, some of which persisted into written form. An ostrakon found at Narmouthis, perhaps from the second or third century CE, contains a combined Greek and demotic list of pharmaceutical ingredients under the demotic heading 'remedies'.[69]

---

[66] Van Minnen, P. (1998). 'Boorish or bookish? Literature in Egyptian villages in the Fayum in the Graeco-Roman period', *JJP* 28, 99–184, especially 157–180 (Tebtynis); Hanson, A.E. 'Greek medical papyri from the Fayum village of Tebtunis: patient involvement in a local health-care system?' in van der Eijk, Ph. (2005). *Hippocrates in Context*, 387–402. Greek literary papyri (including technical literature) is also found in similar contexts in other Fayum villages, i.e. Karanis and Soknopaiou Nesos; the latter is a likely if not certain source for the demotic medical papyri now in Vienna: van Minnen, 'Boorish or bookish?', 152.

[67] For these herbals see chapter 4.2.4, pp. 178–179 with nn. 157, 161.

[68] *P.Tebt.* II 272 (TM 60048); ibid. II 449 (TM 63407); ibid. II 679 with *P.Tebt.Tait* 39–41 (TM 63596); *PSI Congr.* XXI 3 (TM 65525), first century BCE; *P.Tebt.Tait* 43 (TM 63282); ibid. 44 (TM 63283); *PSI* X 1180 (TM 63458); *P.Tebt.* II 273 (TM 63789); ibid. II 689 (TM 63232); ibid. II 678 (TM 63409). Listed by van Minnen, 'Boorish or Bookish?', 156–165.

[69] OMM no. 155, unpublished: see M.-H. Marganne. (1996). 'La médecine dans l'Égypte romaine: les sources et les méthodes', *ANRW* 2.37.3, 2709–2740; van Minnen, 'Boorish or bookish?', 137; cf. *O. Stras.* I 619, TM 63705, again a mixture of Greek and demotic substances

Greek loanwords appear in Egyptian medical-magical texts of the Greco-Roman period.[70] This is discussed in more detail below, 5.2.3, pp. 229–232.

Where local temples were absent altogether, cult officials rotating through villages on a part time basis offered a solution to local shortages in expert personnel, and could have represented an occasional medical resource.[71] Midwives, amulet men (*s3w*), and others with relevant medical, magical and pharmaceutical skill supplemented self-medication and the assistance of family and friends. The knowledge and attitudes of many of these practitioners evolved primarily through oral and experiential channels as part of the 'folk' medicine of the community in general. As ethno-cultural and linguistic divisions became increasingly fluid and complex in the later Ptolemaic and Roman era, the combining, non-exclusive approach to medical knowledge may have developed in this context first—residents who offered care to their friends and neighbors within a particular village or group of villages. Temple ritualists, or even the rare specialist physicians, would then have found themselves responding to expectations of such bicultural medical care (and were in any case usually members and potential patients of such communities themselves).

A slightly different picture emerges from considering the evidence for Greek physicians at an earlier point in the Greco-Roman era in Egypt. Where Greek physicians were to be found in the Ptolemaic *chora*, they tended to be people of significance. Several appear in the Zenon archive, which chiefly concerns personages and events of importance in the region of Philadelphia in the Fayum, many of whom also had close connections with Alexandria. Artemidoros, the physician of Apollonios the *dioketes* (the chief financial officer of the Ptolemaic administration) appears on six occasions in the Zenon papyri, buying expensive items.[72] In local society physicians were influential and wealthy men who often acted as witnesses in legal documents: a result and demonstration of both literacy and their reputable standing within local communities. For example, the physician Theopompos of Thessaly, son of Ariston, appears as a witness in several legal

(of which only the Greek items have been published). I am grateful to Ann Ellis Hanson for drawing my attenton to OMM no. 155 and allowing me to see her copy of its text.

[70] See Dieleman, J. (2005). *Priests, Tongues, and Rites. The London-Leiden Magical Manuscripts and Translation in Egyptian Ritual (100–300 CE)* 117–118, 312. Cf. above 3.4, pp. 135–136 with nn. 127, 129–130; 4.2.3, p. 167, nn. 107–108.

[71] Priests in rotation: Frankfurter, D. (1998). *Religion in Roman Egypt*, 100.

[72] Harrauer, *CPR* XIII, 89–91 s.v. ἰατρός nos. 3–9; discussed by Gorteman, Cl. (1957). 'Médecins de cour dans l'Égypte du IIIe siècle avant J.-C.', *CdÉ* 32, 332–334.

documents of the Philadelphia region.[73] The same six witnesses appear in two of these documents: five of these (including Theopompos) are using Greek names and appear in other papyri as local VIPs with ties to the government and the *dioketes* Apollonios.[74] The sixth witness is Amosis, the Egyptian *komogrammateus* of Philadelphia. Village scribes, the leading interface between that community and the centralized bureaucracy, and people of considerable local importance, were necessarily literate in Greek.[75] And in general Zenon—the deputy of the *dioketes* and therefore the most important person in earlier third-century Philadelphia—and his associates of similar status were highly Hellenocentric.[76] There is no indication that Zenon himself spoke or read Egyptian.

The highest-status physicians in Ptolemaic Egypt were those of Alexandrian intellectual life, who were often significant members of the court and related social circles. Thus physicians were often influential and high-status persons in Alexandria, as at other Hellenistic courts.[77] The career of Andreas of Karystos, the personal physician of Ptolemy IV, who was eventually assassinated in an attempt on the king's life, is a good example of this type of individual and their activities, connections, and background. The author of several works on medical and other topics, he was accused of plagiarism by another intellectual, Eratosthenes, who held the post of Librarian.[78] Andreas had been a student of the third-century physician Herophilos; another Herophilean, Bakkheios of Tanagra, wrote what was probably the first Hippocratic lexicon in the late third century, with the assistance of lemmata provided by Eratosthenes' successor as Librarian, Aristophanes of Byzantion.[79] Herophilos himself is shown in this kind of

---

[73] Θεόπομπος Ἀριστίωνος Θεσσαλὸς ἰατρός: *P.Col.Zen.* I 54, TM 1770 (ca. 250), line 26; and *SB* XIV 11659, TM 4205 (ca. 256). Theopompos: *PP* 16609, with a list of ten additional papyri (but not including *SB* XIV 11659) in which a person of this name occurs in the Philadelphia area in the mid-third century BCE.

[74] Two of these also have ethnics from outside Egypt (Magnesia and Kyrenaia); the two sons of Kleon are 'Elenians': probably the island of Elenion near Kanopos.

[75] The best known village scribe in the Ptolemaic era is Menkhes: see chapter 1.3.1, p. 28, nn. 112–113.

[76] For Greek literature and Greek music in the lives of Zenon and his correpondents: van Minnen, 'Boorish or bookish?', 145; Clarysse, W. (1977). 'De Griekse cultuur in het Zenon-archief', *Kleio* 7, 61–63.

[77] Other Hellenistic courts: Antiokhos III's physician Apollophanes gave strategic advice on the invasion of Koilê-Syria (Polybios 5.58); Eumenes of Pergamon sent his physician Stratios, 'a man of good sense and persuasive power', to reason with the king's brother Attalos (Polybios 30.2).

[78] von Staden, H. (1989). *Herophilus. The Art of Medicine in Early Alexandria*, 472 (*An.* 2).

[79] Vallance, J.T. (2000). *The Lost Theory of Asclepiades of Bithynia*, 101 ff.

intellectual and social context, during the visit of the logician Diodoros Kronos to Philadelphos' court.[80] Hellenistic poets utilized contemporary ideas from Alexandrian medicine, as well as Egyptian myth and ritual.[81]

Ptolemy III made a dedicatory inscription in honor of his personal physician, Xenophanes(?) son of Sosikratos of Heraklea.[82] In early 242, a letter of the Zenon correspondence mentioned that the Alexandrian physician Neon—anxiously awaiting the delivery of some cushions and carpets—is in favor with the king.[83] A couple of years earlier, another of Zenon's correspondents, discussing efforts by several people to assist their mutual friend Hermokrates, currently imprisoned on various charges, described one such person as particularly influential: Kaphisophon, son of Philippos the physician. C.C. Edgar identified him as probably the Kaphisophon sent as a θεωρός to Kos, by Ptolemy II or Ptolemy III, in order to honor the cult of Asklepios there.[84] Kaphisophon's father, the physician Philippos, might have been the doctor Philippos of Kos to whom Kallimakhos addressed his epigram on medicine.[85] Poseidippos wrote an epigram to the physician Medeios of Olynthos, who held the prestigious post of eponymous priest of Alexander and the *Theoi Adelphoi* under Ptolemy II Philadelphos, and also seems to have been concerned with the official administration of the medical tax, the revenues of which were distributed to physicians (below 5.3.3, p. 237 with

---

[80] Kallimakhos fr. 393 Pfeiffer; Diogenes Laertios 2.111–112. Diodoros one day went to Herophilos with a broken shoulder, and Herophilos borrowed one of Diodoros' own arguments against motion to prove to him that it could not be dislocated. Sedley, D.N. (1977). 'Diodorus Cronus and Hellenistic philosophy', *PCPhS* 23, 79, notes that 'the story is an obvious Hellenistic fabrication', but it indicates the shared social and intellectual milieu of well-known philosophers and physicians. See 6.4, p. 260.

[81] For the use of medical ideas by Hellenistic poets see also Most, G.W. (1981). 'Callimachus and Herophilus', *Hermes* 109,188–196; but with von Staden, *Herophilus*, 394–395. Apollonios Rhodios *Argonautika* 3.761–765 applies to Medea the work on the nerves by the Alexandrian anatomists: Solmsen, F. (1961). 'Greek philosophy and the discovery of the nerves', *MH* 18, 150–197; Hunter, R. (1989). *Apollonius of Rhodes: "Argonautica" Book 3*, 180. Cf. Lang, P.M. (2009). 'Goats and the sacred disease in Callimachus' *Acontius and Cydippe*', *CP* 104, 85–90; and in general Stephens, S. (2003). *Seeing Double: intercultural poetics in Ptolemaic Alexandria.*

[82] *SEG* XVIII 640, TM 6084 (246–221 BCE). The name (alternatively Xanthippos) and patronymic were read by Fraser, P.M. (1958). 'Bibliography: Graeco-Roman Egypt. Greek Inscriptions (1957)', *JEA* 44, 112, no. 26.

[83] *P.Cair.Zen.* IV 59571 ll. 7–14 esp. 12–14: γίνωσκε δὲ καὶ Νέωνα εὐημεροῦντα παρὰ τῶι βασιλεῖ.

[84] Kaphisophon: *OGIS* 42. Identifcation with the Kaphisophon of *P.Mich.Zen* 55, TM 1955 (240) proposed by Edgar, C.C. (1931). *Zenon Papyri in the University of Michigan Collection*, 126.

[85] Philippos of Kos (*PP* 6.16640): Kallimakhos *Ep.* 46.

n. 119).[86] Physicians might take on other official roles as trusted members of court society: the Herophilean Demetrios Phakas went on diplomatic missions for Ptolemy XII.[87]

This is a very small and select group. Those known from this kind of context for Ptolemaic Alexandria have Greek names and patronymics: they also have city ethnics from outside Egypt. They had received an appropriate formal education in reading, writing, famous works of Greek literature, and mathematics; to which was added medical training with a well-reputed physician.[88] Herophilos, for example, is said to have been a student of Praxagoras of Kos. They worked within a culture in which ideas on naturalistic, ontological, epistemological, moral and political problems were part of elite discourse; hence the poets' use of contemporary and past medical thought (p. 225 with n. 81) and the mutual significance of medicine and philosophy.[89] Several Alexandrian physicians of the Ptolemaic period wrote extensive treatises, usually on medical or related subjects, sometimes working within the developing literary interest in the grammatical and critical analysis of texts. Erasistratos' views on anatomy indicate a close study of contemporary work in mechanics and physics; Herophilos' ideas suggest an interest in the role of mathematics in medicine, an approach later employed by Galen.[90]

---

[86] Poseidippos' epigram: *P.Mil.Vogl.* VIII 39, 14.30–37. Eponymous priest: *BGU* VI 1227, TM 2661 and others. Connected to the *iatrikon* and its revenues: *P.Cair.Zen.* I 59036, TM 696. See Bing, P. (2002). 'Medeios of Olynthos, son of Lampon, and the "Iamatika" of Posidippus', *ZPE* 140, 297–300; and below 6.4, p. 261.

[87] Caesar *Civil Wars* 3.109.3–6. Cf. Makhaon, physician of Kyzikos, an envoy of the Greek states to the Roman embassies: *IGR* 4.134.

[88] Self-taught physicians were possible but rare: Asklepiades of Bithynia is the first well-known example. Autodidacticism fitted into his and later the Methodists' self-presentation as independent iconoclasts. The lengthy and complicated education of Galen is at the other end of this spectrum. For the importance of well-reputed teachers (often from Kos) in assessing a physician, see 5.3.3, especially p. 237.

[89] Aristotle *Respiration* 480b26ff. cf. *Sensation* 436a17–b2. 'The more subtle and inquisitive doctors speak about nature and claim to derive their principles from it, while the more accomplished investigators of nature generally end by a study of the principles of medicine.'

[90] Erasistratos does not appear in extant reports of Alexandrian society of the time—one of the reasons why his presence there has at times been doubted—but according to Diogenes Laertios 7.186, the son (or grandson: he has the same name) of Erasistratos's teacher, Khrysippos of Knidos, was court physician to a Ptolemy. Cf. Pliny 29.3. But at *Scholia on Theocritus* 17.128, the younger Khrysippos is said to be of Rhodes, not Knidos. Discussed by Massar, N. (2005). *Soigner et servir*, 61–62; see also 6.4, pp. 261, 264.

5.2.2. *Inclusive and Exclusive Medicine*

The success of the Alexandrian physicians described in 5.2.1 demonstrates the success of the brand of medicine they had in common: naturalistic, highly theoretical, and closely related to philosophy. In the fourth century Aristotle defined the category of *iatros* as consisting of three groups: 'Physician means both the ordinary practitioner, and the master of the craft, and thirdly, the man who has studied medicine as part of his general education.'[91] The implication of this is that the educated layman counted as one of the *iatroi* not because of what he did, but because of what he knew: and in Aristotle's terms this represented an adherence to the naturalistic model of the cosmos and its constituents. Aristotle's well-educated man could be a better doctor than the 'ordinary physician', and an actual example of this trope is provided by a story from Aulus Gellius' *Attic Nights*. The Roman aristocrat Calvisius Taurus, travelling in a rural area of Attica during the second century CE, met a local doctor whom he discovered to be ignorant of the distinction between veins and arteries, unlike Calvisius Taurus himself and his equally well-educated friends. (A systematic differentiation between veins and arteries had been articulated by Herophilos at the latest, in the mid-third century BCE.)[92]

This naturalistic, intellectualized, initially Hellenocentric form of medicine, or, in Kleinman's terms, this particular semantic network, became an integral part of the aristocratic lay culture of Hellenic or Hellenizing social elites. This was the case not only in Greece and the islands, but in the Hellenistic kingdoms and even in late Republican and imperial Rome, the elder Cato's objections notwithstanding.[93] One consequence here is so familiar that it usually goes unmentioned: by the end of the fourth century it was the expert specialist in this kind of Greek medicine—Aristotle's *arkhitektonikos*—that had become the natural choice for kings, tyrants and emperors across the Greco-Roman world. The shift is dramatized by Herodotos' tale of Demokedes of Kroton, who replaced the Egyptian doctors

---

[91] *Politics* 1282a3–4.: ἰατρὸς δ' ὅ τε δημιουργὰς καὶ ὁ ἀρχιτεκτονικὸς καὶ τρίτος ὁ πεπαιδευμένος περὶ τὴν τέχνην. Cf. Cicero *Duties* 1.150–151 on the social status of medicine and other occupations for free Roman gentlemen.

[92] Aulus Gellius *Attic Nights* 18.10.

[93] E.g. Pliny's citation of Cato on the dangers of Greek physicians at *Natural History* 29.7.14. See Nijhuis, K. 'Greek doctors and Roman patients: a medical anthropological approach', in van der Eijk, Ph., H.F.J. Horstmanshoff, and P.H. Schrijvers. (1995). *Ancient Medicine in its Socio-Cultural Context*, 1.49–67.

at the court of Dareios I, king of regional superpower Persia, in spite of their reputation as the best physicians in the world.[94] Other medical models and practitioners were, within the Greco-Roman social elite, effectively marginalized.

The practitioners of this kind of medicine are often explicit that they operate within an exclusive explanatory model. Their reception of alternatives, such as remedies and ideas taken from Egyptian medicine, is conditioned by this. In the second century CE, for instance, Galen recognized remedies and ingredients such as the plants and minerals used in amulets, or recipes for drugs from Ptah's temple in Memphis, but disallowed the attendant explanatory model.[95] Medicine which involves such 'magical' thinking was not accepted by naturalistic practitioners even when elements from it, such as ingredients, recipes or possibly even ideas were appropriated. (Potential patients often took a less rigorous view; and non-naturalistic practitioners remained competitive).[96] It is therefore amongst the sociopolitical elites of Egypt that Greek medicine was most likely to have been a preferred and even exclusive alternate, strongly linked to naturalistic models and defined as a linguistic-cultural specialty. The Greeks of Zenon's archive would fit this profile: as a group they seem to have operated entirely within a Greek-language semantic network and its associated performance of a Hellenic identity; and many had access to elite-status physicians, making a choice between 'Greek' forms of medicine and others a viable one in practical terms. In general, the domination of Greek practitioners and medicine among the political elite may have encouraged perceptions of medicine as a cultural choice; whether the primary criterion was its association with the performance of Greekness or simply its association with the rich and powerful. (See below, 5.3.3, pp. 236–239).

But the characteristics associated with elite Alexandrian medicine are not widely replicated outside the nexus of the court and Alexandrian intellectual strata. These include its emphasis on methodology and epistemology, the rival medical schools with their fiercely articulated differences, the competitive innovation and internal distinctiveness.[97] Results in anatomi-

---

[94] Herodotos 3.129.1–130.3. See 4.4, p. 192, and 1.4.2, p. 41.

[95] See, respectively, 4.2.2, pp. 156–157 with n. 63 and 2.3.3, p. 73 with n. 107.

[96] E.g. Thessalos, who supplied the converse reaction by accepting the explanatory model of Greco-Egyptian 'astrological medicine' and consequently the religious authority of Egyptian cultic institutions. By his time, Egyptian religious thought was significant in several areas of Greek philosophy and magic. See below 5.2.3, pp. 230–231 and nn. 100–102.

[97] See von Staden, *Herophilus*, part 2 and 'Hairesis and heresy: the case of the "haireseis iatrikai"', in Meyer, B.F. and E.P. Sanders. (1982). *Jewish and Christian Self-Definition in the*

cal understanding, radical forms of surgery, new explanatory models and increasingly complicated drug therapies circulated through or filtered down to the peripheries of Alexandria's intellectual hothouse. A guide to the Methodist medical sect, for example, is among the medical texts being read in Oxyrhynkhos in the Roman era.[98] Many *iatroi* working in the *chora* were probably conservative or parochial as to techniques and ideas. The rural Attic *iatros* encountered by Calvisius Taurus was either employing an anatomical model several centuries out of date, which did not distinguish between veins or arteries; or had an understanding based solely on local knowledge and his own experience of treating the body, without access to the ideas—old or new—to be found in written texts or among physicians from further afield.

Thus, for physicians peripheral to the nexus of Alexandrian influence, the definition of what it was to be a reputable practitioner was somewhat different to the exclusive elitism of the *arkhitektonikos*: driven by the needs of local clients and the alternative available resources of Egypt, including the knowledge and skill of *swnw* and other healers. Over time, this mutually appropriative process proved successful, at least within the Fayum (above 5.2.1 and below, 5.2.3). Elite practitioners continued to adapt Egyptian information to their own explanatory models, but Egyptian defensive medicine also became integrated into a different strand of Greco-Roman culture; the religious-philosophical approach.

5.2.3. *Evolving Perceptions and Medical Choices in the Greco-Roman Fayum*

The evidence from the Greco-Roman Fayum, described briefly in 5.2.1, shows that by the end of the second century CE, a considerable amount of medical knowledge from both Greek and Egyptian linguistic traditions had been translated, combined and utilized. Egyptian ritual specialists included Greek medical works within their private collections, implying that they were integrating practices or even ideas from an originally Greek medical system into traditional forms of treatment. That this was not the isolated eccentric interest of a few individual officials is demonstrated by the

---

Graeco-Roman World, 76–100, 199–206, on this tendency of the medical *haireseis*, e.g. subtle but polemicised differences on pulse theory between Herophileans.

98 MP3 2360.2 (two papyri fragments combined by I. Andorlini (1992). 'Papiri e medicina: POxy II 234 + POxy LII 3654', in El-Mosalamy, A.H.S. *Proceedings of the 19th International Congress of Papyrology* 1.375–390); Hanson, 'Doctors' literacy', 192–193.

fact that Greek loanwords appear in medically relevant texts of the earlier Roman period; while unpublished ostraka show the act of recipe translation, enabling them to be used by a speaker of either language.[99] The appearance of such texts among the very small proportion of ostraka published or described suggests that there are many more such examples in the mass of those excavated but not yet examined. Appropriating alternative expertise in this fashion expanded available medical resources and resources and gave practitioners access to patients whose expectations were guided by experience of different traditions.

The roots of this outcome can be seen in the Ptolemaic period as early as the third century. People with Greek names and using the Greek language, including those in Zenon's circle of Hellenocentric and influential individuals, visited Egyptian healing sites, stayed in their vicinity, and accepted dream instructions from gods there (chapter 2). Pharmaceutical exchange, albeit divorced from its original explanatory context, is visible in the medical recipes of the Alexandrian physician Herophilos, an influential figure in medical theory and practice throughout the Greco-Roman world (4.2.3, p. 175). A parallel to cultural interaction in medicine can be seen in the developing magical and religious synthesis that emerged as Hermeticism and the combined resources of the *PDM* and *PGM* (cf. 2.2.1, pp. 59–60). This is also the process that produced the autobiographical narrative of Thessalos that serves as the introduction to *The virtues of plants*, a text which has been variously dated from the second to the sixth centuries CE. Its author supplies an account of his search among the temples and priests of Egypt for medical wisdom in the mode of the treatises of 'Nechepso' on astrological medicine (themselves a fixture of Roman-period Hermeticism), eventually receiving a vision of Imhotep-Asklepios in Thebes. As Fowden observes, this emphasis on the Egyptian cultic milieu is a characteristic of both philosophical and technical Hermetic works.[100] The early Herodotos-style respect, among those from the Greco-Roman world, for Egypt's venerable religious institutions became, in the later Hellenistic and Roman eras, an idea of Egyptian temples and their officials (one partially created by those officials) as exoticized, arcanely powerful sources of authority

---

99 Ostraka: 5.2.1, p. 222, n. 69 above. Loanwords, p. 223, n. 70.

100 Fowden, G. (1986, pb. repr. 1993). *The Egyptian Hermes*, 162–166; Moyer, I.S. 'Thessalos and the limits of empire', in Moyer. (2011). *Egypt and the Limits of Hellenism*. The name 'Thessalos' may be meant to invoke the late first century Methodist physician Thessalos of Tralles. Some of the manuscripts omit Thessalos' authorial claims and ascribe the text to Hermes Trimegistos.

that also carried meaning within Greek intellectual thinking, notably philosophy.[101] 'Egyptian priests' came to represent an alternative, synthesized knowledge paradigm applicable to all forms of manipulating the natural cosmos, including medical outcomes; a trend reinforced by astrological medicine and its supposed Greco-Egyptian origins.[102]

The evolution of a bi-cultural medical system took place because of choices made by patients and practitioners during the Ptolemaic and Roman periods. But these would not always have been choices that regarded Greek and Egyptian practitioners, or their techniques and ideas, as equivalent to each other. Patients' expectations of medical practitioners were derived from familial and local culture, including prior experience. Linguistic capability might also have been an issue on practical grounds. As in the roughly contemporaneous encounter between Greek medicine and Roman society, selecting between different kinds of practitioners or idea was sometimes a means of expressing identity, either between, or within, a particular community.[103]

A large proportion of the socio-economic elite of Ptolemaic Egypt, especially in the third and much of the second century, employed Greek names, a Greek linguistic capability, and often ethnically-linked elements of culture, such as gymnasia. In this stratum of society, including the upper levels of the court and bureaucracy, the medicine recorded is of a particular kind: the *iatrikê technê* embedded within Greek literary and intellectual culture, and exclusive of other kinds of healing. This association of the dominant elite with Greek practitioners and particular medical forms rendered medicine in both the cities and the *chora* a potential arena for the expression, or declaration, of aspirational social identity. Galen supplies an insider's take on this attitude:

> I write this neither for the Germans, nor for other wild or barbarian people, nor for bear, lions, wild boars or other wild animals, but for Greeks and those who may have been born barbarians, but who strive to attain the qualities of Greeks.[104]

---

[101] E.g. the Egyptian Stoic and cult official Khairemon: see Fowden, *Egyptian Hermes*, 54–56. For contacts between Egyptian cult officials and Greek philosophy during the Roman, rather than the Ptolemaic period, cf. van Minnen, 'Boorish or bookish?', 113.

[102] For astrological medicine and its invented Egyptian (as opposed to Greco-Babylonian) origins, see Barton, T. (1994). *Ancient Astrology*; Fowden, *Egyptian Hermes*, 67–68, 167. Some of the extant Hermetic corpus is derived from astrological texts circulating, possibly as early as the second century BCE, under the names of the Egyptian priest 'Petosiris' and the Egyptian king 'Nekhepsô'.

[103] For the Roman reaction to Greek medicine, above 5.2.2, p. 227 with n. 93.

[104] Galen *Maintaining health* 1.10 (6.51 Kühn).

This is not a simple equation by which medical positioning or choice automatically follows ethnicity, not least because perception of personal ethnicity is partly developed through such choices. The Alexandrian *iatroklystes* (this chapter, pp. 205–206) requiring some kind of bilingual teacher in his household provides empirical support for Greek-speakers using a treatment that was particularly associated with Egyptian medicine. Questions of choice, however, relate to how different medical practitioners were perceived, as either a matter of status and competence, or in terms of the kinds of medicine they offered. These perceptions are related to issues of social status, language use, and ethnic designations. In this context, the early-Ptolemaic institution of the 'medical tax' is potentially revealing of the concerns and preferences of local elites in regard to medicine.

5.3.1. *The Medical Tax*

The *iatrikon* or 'medical tax' was a relatively short-lived phenomenon in Ptolemaic Egypt, which is only mentioned in some thirteen documents between ca. 310 to ca. 175, and thus seems to have died out in the early or middle second century.[105] It seems not to have existed in the three Greek constitutional cities (*poleis*) of Egypt, indicating that it developed in response to conditions in less urban or less Hellenized areas of Egypt. It does appear in Halikarnassos, a city in Karia under Ptolemaic rule, and this may also have been the case for other overseas possessions garrisoned or governed by the Ptolemies.[106] Another *iatrikon* tax is also attested at Delphi and Teos, as a means of funding the salary of a public physician.[107]

The medical tax was levied on certain sectors of the population. These appear to have been various local elites, especially the military. Its revenues were eventually distributed to some or all physicians: that is, to at least some of the individuals defined as *iatroi* in Greek papyri and *swnw* in demotic ones (for the extent to which these terms are co-extensive, see below 5.3.3, pp. 236–237).

We are concerned with two related questions. Firstly, what was the *iatrikon* for? Secondly, what were the criteria for being a recipient, as a

---

[105] Papyri collected by Nanetti, O. (1944). 'TO IATRIKON', *Aegyptus* 24, 119–125, together with *PSI* IV 371, TM 2056 (250 BCE); *P.Hamb.* II 171, TM 4325 (246 BCE): below 5.3.3, pp. 236–237 with nn. 118, 121.

[106] Halikarnassos: *P.Cair.Zen.* I 59036, TM 696 (257 BCE). Cf. p. 226, n. 86; p. 235, n. 114; p. 237, n. 119.

[107] Stimolo, P.A. (2002). 'Lo iatrikon', *Epigraphica* 64, 17–27.

'physician', of the tax's revenues, and what does this tell us about perceptions of what constituted a reputable medical practitioner?

The *iatrikon* was not a universal tax. The two groups definitely known to have supplied the revenues of the medical tax are both from a military context: those on active service and the reserve force represented by the cleruchs, settler families whose initial allotment of land had been a reward from the Ptolemies for military service. All known examples of the medical tax's payment involve individuals from one of these categories. A third possible group of contributors comprises the larger group of individuals defined for fiscal purposes as 'Greek': the so called tax-Hellenes.[108]

The payers of the tax thus comprised relatively affluent, Greek-dominated sections of society—wealthy cleruchs and military forces; possibly 'tax-Hellenes'—perceived as valuable to the Ptolemaic government. The fact that the *iatrikon* was levied on this influential sector of society suggests that its function was closely related to these individuals' needs and preferences. This is further supported by what is known about the *iatrikon*'s possible precedents in pre-Ptolemaic Egypt and contemporary Hellenistic *poleis*.

5.3.2. *The Medical Tax: Precedents*

The Greek civic institution of the public physician (*dêmosios iatros*) dates back to the fourth century BCE, and was common among city-states of the Hellenistic period, where it is often attested by civic decrees in honor of the physicians concerned. The *dêmosios iatros* (or two *dêmosioi iatroi* in the case of Athens and Kos)[109] was hired by the civic authorities of a *polis* for a regular salary, which guaranteed not free treatment but an assured degree of competence. The physician gained official recognition, reputable publicity, and a minimal salary in addition to the fees charged to patients.[110]

---

[108] In fiscal papyri the designation *Wynn* (demotic) or *Hellene* (Greek) identifies people who were exempt from the universal tax of one obol per year. The largely symbolic tax-status may have involved non-fiscal privileges as well. In spite of the terminology, people with Jewish or Egyptian names could hold 'Hellene' tax-status. In the early Ptolemaic period the obol-tax seems to have been subsumed within the salt-tax. Clarysse-Thompson, *Counting*, 2.71–72.

[109] *IG* II^2 1772 ll. 9–13; *Syll.*^{3} 943 ll. 7–9; see Massar, *Soigner*, 32 with n. 5.

[110] Cohn-Haft, L. (1956). *The Public Physicians of Ancient Greece*. Several inscriptions honor public physicians for forfeiting their salary or treating certain groups of people without charge. Such instances are recorded precisely because they represent displays of euergetic

There is also an Egyptian precedent and model for the payment of physicians from state revenues. According to Diodoros Sikelos, in his section on Egyptian *nomoi*:

> On their military campaigns and their journeys in the country they all receive treatment without the payment of any private fee; for the physicians draw their support from public funds and administer their treatments in accordance with a written law which was composed in ancient times by many famous physicians.[111]

This Egyptian law or custom has been seen as a precedent for the *iatrikon*.[112] This may well be correct, but it is important then to be clear about what precisely Diodoros' report (based on Hekataios of Abdera's late fourth or early third century *Aigyptiaka*) implies. The passage has been read as an assertion of government-funded provision of medicine to civilians not directly engaged upon state affairs, but this is not what it says. Diodoros explains quite clearly that only those directly involved on military and other official business are entitled to free treatment.

Diodoros' remarks, however accurately they may or may not report Hekataios' idealizing rendition of unknown sources of information about medicine in the Persian and earlier periods, can easily be read as describing what we already know from pharaonic era inscriptions and other records (above, 5.1.1). Physicians formed part of the state-salaried workforce on army expeditions to remote desert quarries, and presumably also on campaigns. Medical provision was also made for government projects closer to home: an additional salary was paid to a Deir el-Medina workman for his work as a *swnw* (5.1.2, p. 212). The title-carrying physicians of the palace and administration were no doubt also salaried. But there might have been other

behavior above and beyond the contractual call of duty: they do not articulate the normal role of the public physician. War was another special circumstance: the physician Onasilos and his brothers were hired by a Cypriot king and *polis* for the free treatment of those wounded in the seige of the city. Masson, O. (1961 repr. 1983). *Inscriptions chypriotes syllabiques* no. 217 (before 270 BCE); cf. Massar, *Soigner*, 34–37. For inscriptions relating to physicians of the Hellenistic world: Samama, E. (2003). *Médecins dans le monde grec: sources épigraphiques sur la naissance d'un corps médical*, especially 37–45.

[111] 1.82.3. Amundsen, D.W. and G.B. Ferngren, (1978). 'The forensic role of physicians in Ptolemaic and Roman Egypt', *Bulletin of the History of Medicine* 52, 338 think the passage refers to the Ptolemaic period, but in a section on Egyptian customs Diodoros is more likely to be describing earlier practice (cf. Lippi, 'Breve note', n. 112 below). The view that all physicians in pre-Ptolemaic Egypt were paid by the state seems to have gone unchallenged for a century: Préaux, Cl. (1939). *L'économie royal des Lagides*, 45, 401; Clarysse-Thompson, *Counting* 2.162.

[112] E.g. Lippi, D. (1983). 'Breve nota sullo "iatrikon"', *BASP* 20, 135–136.

swnw, drawing salaries from temple revenues, and the same individuals could act in a private capacity.[113]

This Egyptian practice of direct employment of doctors on state business is similar to Greek cities' contracts with physicians in times of warfare.[114] The *dêmosios iatros* arrangement was slightly different: it did not pay directly for medical care, but guaranteed its availability, in a reputable form, for those whose tax revenues paid the physician a basic or supplementary income, possibly with priority over other potential clients. Private fees normally supervened.

The innovation of the medical tax is not quite the same as either, but has similarities with both. It echoes the pharaonic payment in its apparently close relationship to the military sector, although its remit was more extensive: cleruchs, and certainly tax-Hellenes, were not serving military, although they did have a considerable stake in Ptolemaic rule and represented a *de facto* security resource. Like the public physician in Greek city states, but on a larger scale, the *iatrikon* seems to have been intended, by granting official recognition and some minimal salary, to maintain numbers of acceptable medical practitioners in certain areas of the Ptolemaic empire; just as in Teos and Delphi it provided the salary of the public physician. Ensuring that the expectations of Greek settlers and soldiers were met was the principal focus of the arrangement, and it seems probable that cleruchs and soldiers had first call upon the services of local doctors (for a fee). A secondary useful effect was an extension in medical provision for all residents of the region, including not only other Greek settlers, but also, potentially, people who defined their identities in all kinds of ways.[115] If its purpose was to guarantee the presence of physicians in rural areas, this explains the

---

113 Pharaonic example of *swnw* receiving private payment (objects valued at 22 copper deben): *Pap.Turin* 1880 vs. 5, 2–12, above 5.1.2, p. 213, n. 28. Janssen, *Village Varia*, 26–29 thinks this example is puzzling in view of the Diodoros passage, but that is because he thinks Diodoros is describing free treatment for all in the manner of the British National Health Service (the comparison is explicit). The problem with inserting this modern concept into antiquity is cogently expressed by Cohn-Haft, *Public Physicians*, 3.

114 See Onasilos' contract, n. 110 above. In his 1997 Ph.D. thesis, 'Ethnic designations in Hellenistic Egypt', Csaba La'da argues strongly for 'Greek' physicians being miliary personnel. He seems to envisage a situation in which such army doctors provided free treatment for soldiers, and possibly their families. Bagnall, R.S. (1976). *The Administration of the Ptolemaic Possessions Outside Egypt*, 94–98, argued the revenues of the *iatrikon* might have been used in Halikarnassos (*P.Cair.Zen.* I 59036, TM 696; cf. above pp. 225–226, 235, 237, nn. 86, 106, 119) for the payment of army and navy physicans stationed there.

115 Cf. the exemption from the salt tax for various categories of person and occupation, including 'physicians'.

absence of evidence for the *iatrikon* in the three *poleis* of Egypt, where medical experts were concentrated.

5.3.3. *The Medical Tax: Reputable Recipients*

The revenues from the tax were paid to physicians. The few extant papyri referring to this process are all in Greek, and so the word employed is *iatros*. In other official documents of the period, *iatros* and the Egyptian word *swnw* are used as equivalents.[116] The semantic extent of *swnw* as used in these contexts is not entirely clear, but pharaonic era evidence suggests a literate ritualist specializing in medicine. *Swnw* would thus translate *iatros* directly and vice versa, but its use also implies that such ritualists could be identified as *iatroi*; and Greek physicians as *swnw* in demotic documentation. This indicates an official lack of differentiation between medical systems and practitioners in favor of simply recognizing those identified within various sectors of Egyptian society as professional healers. This would seem to exclude those practicing healing on a more occasional basis, as a secondary aspect of their principal occupational designation (cult ritualists without a specialization in medicine) or through an alternative paradigm—in Greek terminology *iatros* does not include drug-sellers, purifiers and root-cutters (5.1.3, p. 217). The exclusion, however, is only bureaucratic: *iatros* and *swnw* act as place-holders for those identified as reputable healers by the society in which they operate.

The revenues of the medical tax, then, were paid to those identified as *iatroi*/*swnw*. In practice, this identification might have been made by other physicians as part of an administrative network, although the mechanism by which payments were made is not completely transparent. Usually the amounts collected were paid to a bank, from which the individual disbursements were made.[117] On a mid-third century papyrus, the physician Demetrios acknowledged receipt of a sum received from the banker Nikanor, of a bank in Oxyrhynkhos, drawn from the account of the medical tax, for the month of Khoiak. Some of the phrasing in this receipt suggests Demetrios might have been an intermediary in the process, who distributed

[116] The translation 'physician' might be glossed as 'reputable medical practitioner practising within a dominant cultual paradigm'. For *iatroi*/*swnw* in Ptolemaic documents, see Clarysse-Thompson, *Counting*, 2.162–164.

[117] Other Ptolemaic officials were similarly paid a monthly salary through a royal bank: Préaux, *L'economie*, 45.

the sum given to him to other physicians in the area.[118] In the case of the city of Halikarnassos, another doctor, Medeios of Olynthos, is probably also involved in administering the *iatrikon*, but in this case the revenues from the tax held were also used, on a temporary basis, for emergency funds in other areas.[119] On another occasion, however, the revenues passed directly from tax-payer to physician.[120] This last instance reinforces the impression that the criteria were casual, and based upon personal and local knowledge of individual reputation. In this case the *iatrikon*'s function as a reciprocal arrangement between the tax-payer and the service provider is particularly clear, since the intermediate network of administration has been bypassed except for record-keeping.

What remains unclear is how broad were the (unofficial) criteria used by administrating doctors and other officials, or the payers of the medical tax, to identify suitable recipients of the tax's revenues. The overall fiscal administration, as we saw above, seems not to have distinguished between different medical models: *swnw* as ritualists would count as *iatroi*. The interests of the largely Hellenic social elites of the early Ptolemaic period, however, might have been more specific.

It might be useful here to compare the institution of the public physician in the wider Hellenistic world. Such an individual was also selected, like the recipients of the *iatrikon*-funded salary, on the basis of his reputation for competence or even expertise at providing medical care for citizens of the *polis* that employed him, and, secondly, to its other residents. In several cases public physicians were head-hunted from Kos, the island city-state famous for its medical practitioners in the culturally dominant naturalistic paradigm. An alternative criterion was the reputation of the physician's teacher.

Recipients of the *iatrikon* payments were much more numerous and necessarily less well-connected.[121] In Egypt, the students of famous teachers

---

118 *P.Hamb.* II 171, TM 4325 (246 BCE): τοῖς κατὰ τόπον | [ἰατροῖς πρὸς τ]ὸ λθ (ἔτος), ὃ συνέχω | [παρὰ τραπεζίτου ... ἰατρι]κὸν | [τοῦ Χοιάχ] τοῦ λθ (ἔτους).

119 *P.Cair.Zen.* I 59036, TM 696 (257 BCE). For Medeios cf. 5.2.1, pp. 225–226, n. 86; and 6.4, p. 261.

120 *P.Hib.* I 102, TM 8237 (248/47 BCE).

121 The similar use of a medical tax in Teos and Delphi (see n. 107), as a means of funding the salary of the public physician, was sufficient for only one high-status physician in each location. (The only known example of such a salary is the 1000 drachmae paid annually to Apollonios of Perge by Pamphylia in Seleukia: *I.Perge* 12 ll. 25–26; cf. four less clear examples in Massar, *Soigner*, 9). Although the pool of tax-payers of the *iatrikon* in early Ptolemaic Egypt is larger, it also had to provide for many more physicians. One of the *iatrikon* papyri from Egypt, *P.Hamb.* II 171, TM 4325 (above n. 118) includes a figure of 8 or 80 drachmae for

lived and worked in Alexandria. But the preferences and concerns of the group concerned with the payment and identification of suitable recipients is likely to have been similarly influential. The physicians who received payment from the medical tax may thus be a more narrowly representative group than those in fiscal or official papyri overall. Dorothy Thompson and Willy Clarysse have argued that the exemption from the salt-tax for teachers can be understood as an exemption for teachers of Greek language and letters only, while among other early exemptions from the tax were athletic victors and artists of Dionysos.[122] These exemptions privilege the culture and sense of identity of early immigrants and families in the Egyptian *chora*, and as such represent the Ptolemaic administration's efforts (possibly inconclusive) to respond to the demands of this group. The later exemption from the salt tax for physicians would have reinforced the *iatrikon*'s function of ensuring adequate access to reputable medicine outside Alexandria, Naukratis and Ptolemais, but perhaps in the non-culturally specific terms of other official documents concerning 'physicians.' The *iatrikon*, however, in this reconstruction, would have enabled the Hellenic or Hellenizing social elite of the early Ptolemaic *chora* to define medicine and its practitioners according to their own sense of what was acceptable—a sense that changed over generations of intermarriage and acculturation.

5.4. *In Conclusion*

Even if the *iatrikon* does indicate, as suggested above, that medicine could be a subsidiary part of the performance and identity of Hellenism, its disappearance after little more than a century suggests that this function became

the amount paid to Demetrios from the account of medical tax in one month, but he may have distributed this figure among other doctors: Massar (38) accepts the reading of 80 and calculates an annual salary of 960 drachma, assuming that it was for Demetrios alone. Several examples supply the tax levy as 2 artabae (ca. 4 drachmae). I have made various calculations on the basis of unsafe estimates of the number of tax payers and physicians within a region of the Fayum: the results, for what they are worth, suggest an income of 300–700 drachmae, depending on whether tax-Hellenes as well as cleruchs paid the levy. This kind of amount is comparable with the income of *technitai in* other Hellenistic cities, although well-known artisans could command more: Cohn-Haft, *Public physicians*, 38; Massar, *Soigner*, 37.

[122] On the salt tax, a universal levy on adults, see Clarysse-Thompson, *Counting*, 2.52–89. The initial grant of immunity, first recorded in 263, isolated professions distinctive to Greek culture: teachers, athletic coaches, artists of Dionysos, and victors at the Alexandrian games. *P.Hal.* 1 ll. 260–265, TM 5876 (after 259). For teachers as teachers of Greek, Clarysse-Thompson, *Counting*, 128–129. A second wave of exemptions for certain occupations including the police, several priestly groups, and physicians followed (probaby from 254).

irrelevant to those dwelling in the villages and towns of Egypt. Instead, certain Roman period ostraka show that another early tendency evolved into a widespread pattern: remedies and practices were translated and used as equivalents or additional resources. Those deriving from one linguistic tradition were not perceived as exclusive or inferior. This applies at least to materials and their preparation, although it remains unclear what explanatory models were in play when an Egyptian temple ritualist made use of a Greek medical text. Recipes could be divorced and reappropriated, just as Galen does with 'magical' amulets. It is also not clear if internal surgery or phlebotomy, initially Greek techniques, became widespread among those trained in Egyptian traditions of medicine. Certainly Egyptian defensive magic and its medical applications became authoritative elements in those strands of Greco-Roman thought associated with Hermeticism and non-naturalistic medicine. Some such differences in medical culture were probably still visible in Greco-Roman Egypt: an apprenticed *iatros* and the temple lector priest or scribally trained *swnw* were not identical sources of medical expertise. As practitioners reacted, however, to the needs and expectations of their clients, cultural concepts of what counted as authoritative medicine also evolved and became more inclusive: alternative remedies, ideas and terminology a resource to be investigated, mined, and sometimes appropriated.

The early Ptolemaic era was a period in which, for Egypt's inhabitants, notions of what constituted identity and status, including what counted as medical expertise, were under considerable and countervailing pressures. Medicine, among both practitioners and laymen, was potentially a means by which Hellenism could be displayed and preferred; or Egyptian tradition asserted. The invention of the *iatrikon* and, in particular, the absence of any demonstrable impact of Egyptian ideas upon the intellectual elite of Alexandrian medicine, is evidence that this was partially the case. But this situation also encouraged a fluidity in the creation of social identity and an adaptive, interactive cultural synthesis: the hybrid and alternative forms that medicine took in Greco-Roman Egypt reflect this process as well, and suggest that it was, over time, the dominant trend.

5.5. *Appendix: Ptolemaic Physicians and Official Positions*

In addition to physicians associated with the *iatrikon*, there are three unique and rather cryptic instances of other medical titles. These titles hint at the existence of a bureaucracy with specifically medical concerns.

An inscription from Delos describes Khrysermos as 'in charge of the physicians' (ἐπὶ τῶν ἰατρῶν), as well as holding the prestigious non-military titles *exegetes* and *epistates of the Museum*.[123] Such a post may derive from pharaonic precedent: Khrysermos' title is similar to the Egyptian *wr swnw* (chief physician). This was the title held by Udjahorresnet under Dareios I, when it indicated some kind of oversight of Egyptian medicine and training.[124]

Athenagoras the *archiatros* orders the undertakers and religious officials at the temple of Amenemhat III at Hawara to deliver free of charge the body of his assistant Herakleides, who had been wrongfully buried in their necropolis, to other associates of his.[125] The most likely meaning for *archiatros* is that Athenagoras was the personal physician of the king, since in Egypt the term does not supplant *dêmosios iatros* as the term for public physician until the fourth century CE.[126] None of the known personal physicians of the Ptolemies are in fact called *archiatros* in extant texts, but this is not conclusive. A Seleucid court physician is named *archiatros* in an inscription but merely *iatros* by Polybios (5.56.1; 5.81.6.2). But again, *archiatros* could also translate *wr swnw* and identify a physician of status, reputation, and perhaps an official medical role. Athenagoras' apparently numerous group of attendants testifies either to a large household, probably including apprentices, or to an important administrative position.

There is only person with a non-Greek name and a medical title attested in our evidence. This is Tatas, the *basilikos iatros* (royal physician, king's physician).[127] His title is paralleled by the better-known *basilikos grammateus*, the Greek translation of Egyptian 'king's scribe'; and again his position may derive from pharaonic and Persian antecedents. There were forty such king's scribes in the Ptolemaic administration, and the post was often held by people with Egyptian names, but it is unclear how far we can stretch the parallel of this title to the *basilikos iatros*. The document Tatas appears in is a letter from the *strategos* Aineas to the *epistates* Ptolemaios, and it concerns a complicated case of property law from the Theban necropolis in the later second century BCE, in which the ownership of a house in Thebes by an

---

[123] *OGIS* 104 (after ca. 150 BCE). For the position of *exegetes* see Strabo 17.12.6–9.

[124] For Udjahorresnet see 1.3.2, p. 34 n. 133.

[125] *SB* I 5216, TM 5636. Cf. Pestman, P.W. (2nd rev. ed. 1994). *The New Papyrological Primer*, 94–95 (text 12).

[126] Nutton, V. (1977 repr. 1988). 'Archiatri and the medical profession', in Nutton. (1988). *From Democedes to Harvey*, chapter V.

[127] *P.Tor.Choach.* 12 ii 25–26, TM 3563 (117 BCE). Translated by Bagnall, R.S. and P. Derow, (2004). *The Hellenistic Period: historical sources in translation*, no. 132.

association of libation pourers (*choachytai*) is being contested. Tatas has ordered the embalmers (*taricheutai*) to move their residence from Thebes to the west bank, in accordance with a royal decree, and the libation pourers' lawyer is contesting the claim that this decree also applies to them, as a group involved in caring for the dead. Tatas reported his action to the *strategos* Aineas, who cites it in his letter to the *epistates*.

The obvious interpretation, unless this report is atypical of Tatas' activities, is that the *basilikos iatros* was involved in state oversight of the funerary professions; enforcing and supervising royal decrees on the subject. The people who actually mummified the body were called in Greek *taricheutai*; in the Ptolemaic period *swnw* (physician) was often the demotic word for them. Rostovtzeff suggested that Tatas' function was 'to supervise from a sanitary point of view the functions of the priests in connection with burials.'[128] This is anachronistic, but there may be something in the concept that the masters of protection against decay—i.e. physicians and embalmers, for the living and dead respectively—were two closely related professions, specializing in different aspects of essentially the same expertise. In this context an administrative role over the embalmers of the necropolis might easily have become the province of a physician, acting on behalf of the king and hence the *basilikos iatros*.

[128] Rostovtzeff, M. (1941). *Social and Economic History of the Hellenistic World*, 2.1092–1093.

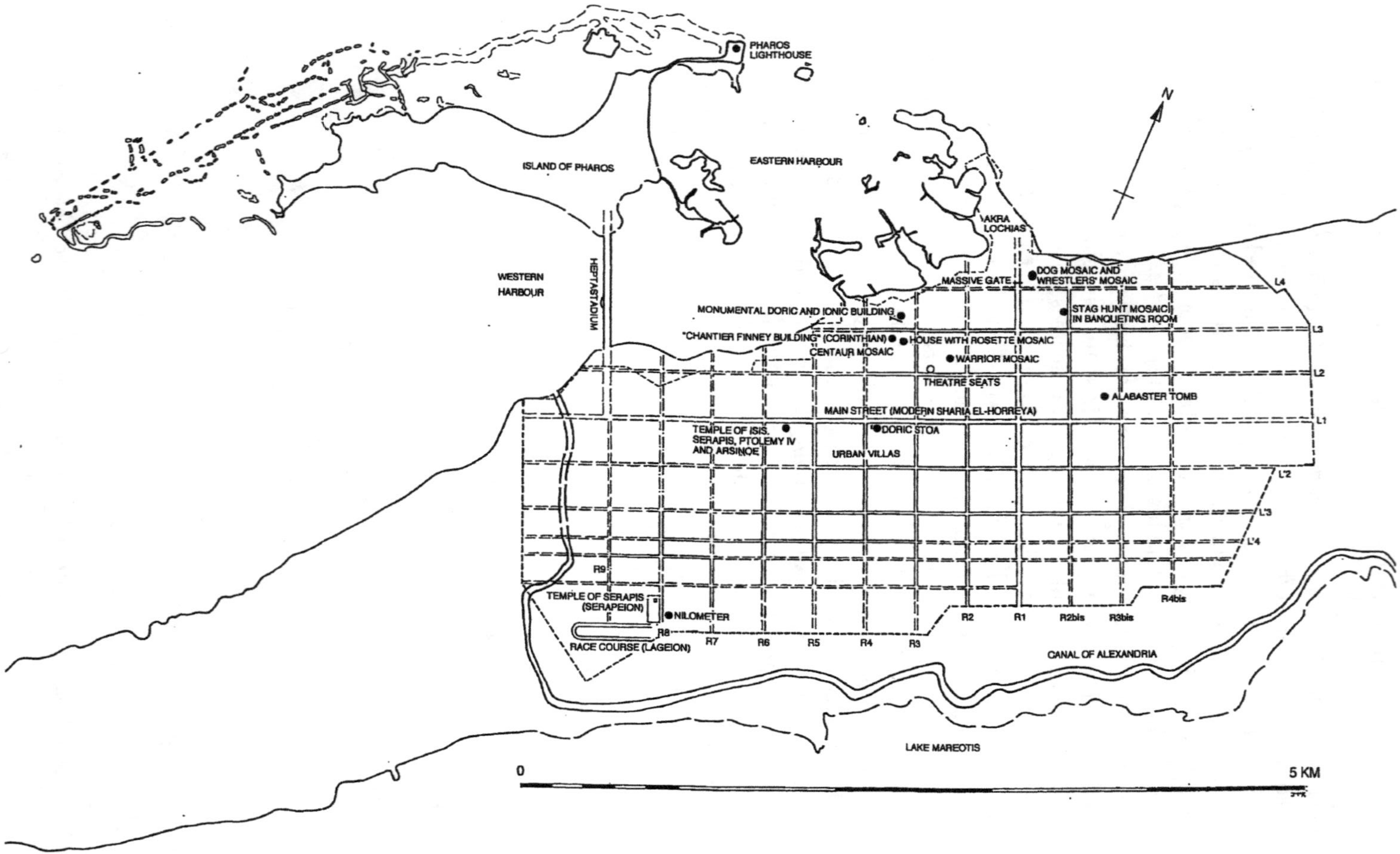

Figure 3. Ptolemaic Alexandria.

CHAPTER SIX

MEDICINE IN ALEXANDRIA

The seizure of Egypt by Ptolemy son of Lagos in 323 meant a return for Egypt to direct internal rule by the king, after the lengthy interregnum of satrap government.[1] Their fortunes were dependent solely upon the success and stability of Egypt itself. The Ptolemies were now better placed than the Persian emperors or even Alexander to occupy the traditional religious and nationalistic roles of the Egyptian king, and thus to embed themselves, with the support of Egyptian cult officials, within this ideological template.[2]

6.1. *A Greek City in Egypt*

Ptolemy originally established his government at Memphis, a pharaonic royal capital, but by 311 he had moved his residence to the new coastal city on a site selected by and named for Alexander of Macedon.[3] Alexandria was laid out according to the usual form of the Greek city grid, with water supplied through underground channels.[4] Other distinctively Hellenic features of the city were the Lageion hippodrome and athletic stadium, which almost certainly dates back to Soter's reign, and the agora, also established by the middle of the third century.[5] The palace seems to have been on the el-Silsila

---

[1] He was the effective king of Egypt as soon as he seized Egypt from the satrap Kleomenes following Alexander's death earlier that year, although he ruled formally in the names of Philip Arrhidaios and Alexander IV until 306, when he took the title *Basileus*.

[2] On the question of whether the earlier Ptolemies were crowned as Egyptian kings in Memphis, see 1.3.1, p. 27 n. 107.

[3] The Satrap Stele: Egyptian Museum, Cairo, no. 22182; translated by Rowe, A. (1955). 'A contribution to the archaeology of the Western desert III', *Bulletin of the John Rylands Library* 38, 156–158.

[4] For the geography and topography of Alexandria, see the discussions of textual and written sources by Fraser, P.M. (1972). *Ptolemaic Alexandria*, 1.3–37; Tkaczow, B. (1984). 'Remarques sur la topographie et l'architecture de l'ancienne Alexandrie dans les textes antiques', *Archeologia* 35, 1–25; McKenzie, J. (2007). *The Architecture of Alexandria and Egypt*, 19–79.

[5] McKenzie, *Architecture*, 47–48. As with the Library and Museion, such buildings are the physical fabric of Greek cultural institutions.

promontory and the area south-west of this, where excavations show buildings with expensive mosaic floors and Greek Doric and Ionic architecture.[6] Strabo's account of the area in the early Roman period mentions a theater near the palace, which may have been the 'great theater' of the third century. Athletic, musical, equestrian and dramatic contests were held as early as the 270s, early in Philadelphos' reign.[7] Such culturally specific activity and architecture integrated Alexandria, and to a lesser extent Egypt, within the Greek world, in competition not only with the important cities such as Pergamon or Ephesos within the other Hellenistic kingdoms, but also with older loci of cultural prestige such as Athens and Olympia.

The Library of Alexandria, located within the royal estate, was probably completed under Philadelphos, although most accounts of its origin involve one of Soter's leading administrators, Demetrios of Phaleron. Estimates of the number of papyrus rolls it contained tend to be in the hundreds of thousands, although the actual number could well have been much smaller than later accounts suggest.[8] But even on a smaller scale, the Library was a significant cultural statement. It had Greek and in particular Aristotelian antecedents, through both Demetrios of Phaleron's history as a member of the Lykeion and the bequest by Aristotle of his considerable private library to Theophrastos and hence in a sense to the Lykeion.[9] The Alexandrian Library, moreover, linked the power and prestige of the monarchic government to the reification of knowledge in textual form. Leading Greek scholars and writers were appointed to the post of Librarian, and anecdotes from later periods represent the Ptolemaic government as using its power to seize consignments of books or trick Athens out of the originals of its classic dramatic texts.[10] State patronage of such libraries rapidly emerged as

---

[6] McKenzie, *Architecture*, 68–69, who notes that second century mosaics in this area 'reflect the role of Alexandrian workshops in the development of this art' (69). The palace's location is described only for the end of the first century: Strabo *Geography* 17.1.9, cf. Julius Caesar *Civil Wars* 3.112.

[7] Strabo 17.1.9; Athenaios 14.620d (and see McKenzie, *Architecture*, 385 n. 98). Dramatic festivals in ca. 276–271: Theocritus *Idyll* 17.112–114; McKenzie, *Architecture*, 33, 48, 67–68.

[8] Bagnall. R. (2002). 'Alexandria: Library of dreams', *ProcAmPhilSoc* 146 no. 4, 348–362, reprinted in Bagnall. (2006). *Hellenistic and Roman Egypt*, 348–362. See also Fraser, *Alexandria*, 1.320–335; McKenzie, *Architecture*, 50–51 with a very complete bibliography in 385 n. 129.

[9] Demetrios' role in the Library's foundation: Diogenes Laertios 5.11–16. Aristotle leaves library to Theophrastos: Strabo 13.608, Diogenes Laertios 5.52. The subsequent history of this collection is disputed: according to Athenaios (1.3a–b) Theophrastos' legatee Neleos sold it to Philadelphos, *contra* Strabo and Plutarch (*Life of Sulla* 26).

[10] Galen, *Commentary on Hippocrates' Epidemics* 3 (*CMG* 5.10.2.1), who cites as his source

an arena of competition for prestige among Hellenistic kingdoms, and later within the Greco-Roman world, demonstrating the increased centrality of the written form to Greek *paideia*, and thus the continuing performance of Greek cultural forms in new contexts by members of the Hellenistic world's highly mobile Greek-speaking intelligentsia. The chief cities of the Successors became centers for Greek literary culture, technical subjects, philosophy and textual scholarship.

In Alexandria, the Museion seems to have been a focus for Ptolemaic patronage of such an intellectual literary community. Its philosophical and specifically Lykeion antecedents co-opted not only the Muses to the display of Ptolemaic wealth and prestige, but also the intellectual institutionalization that had emerged in the shape of the classical era philosophical schools.

Herodas' third century poem suggests that it was one of Alexandria's most famous places, but very few details survive.[11] Strabo's description of it in the 20s BCE locates it within the palace complex, with a covered walkway, lecture hall, and a large house with a common dining room for 'the learned men who share the Museion.' A priest of the Muses was appointed by the kings.[12]

The focus of these kinds of institutions is thus strongly Hellenocentric: a form of competitive display couched according to Greek criteria.[13] In this contest the status of Egyptian culture—its monumentalism, mythology, iconography, artistic techniques and forms—gave the Greeks of Egypt an advantage and a resource. The public space of Alexandria seems to have been dominated by obelisks, sphinxes and monumental statuary commissioned for earlier kings, such as the unusually massive obelisk made under one of the last Egyptian kings in the mid-fourth century that Philadelphos is said to have moved to the precinct of the Arsinoeion.[14] Similar monuments, including five obelisks and thirty-two sphinxes, have been found

---

the Alexandrian physician Zeuxis, who probably lived in the early 2nd century BCE; Ps.-Aristeas 9–10. Athenaios 1.3b also records the Ptolemies buying books.

[11] *Mime* 1.31. Mime 8 probably also refers to the Museion.

[12] Strabo 17.793–794. Posidippos' poem might refer to the erection of his statue in the Alexandrian Museion's garden under Philadelphos: *P.Mil.Vogl.* VIII 309 Ro, TM 62665 (third century), col. X 16–25, cf. LDAB 3852 with bibligraphy; ed. Bastianini, G. et al. (2001). *Epigrammi: P.Mil.Vogl. 8. 309*.

[13] See also Erskine, A. (1995). 'Culture and power in Ptolemaic Egypt: the Museum and Library of Alexandria', *G & R* 42.1, 38–48.

[14] Pliny *Natural History* 36.14.

underwater in what was the area of the Pharos lighthouse and the city's harbors; many were taken from the deserted sanctuaries of Heliopolis. Divorced from their original context, such monuments nonetheless expressed a degree of continuity with Egypt's past. This was reinforced by the Ptolemies' commissioning of statues of themselves in the apparel and style of earlier pharaohs: six red granite colossal representations of Ptolemaic kings and queens in Egyptian dress and style were also found near the Lighthouse site. Both kinds of monument served to impress tourists and traders, as well as displaying the power and wealth of the king and country to its own inhabitants. They represented the Ptolemaic attempt to present themselves as kings acceptable to indigenous elites, while simulataneously capitalizing, in relations with the wider Hellenistic world, on Egypt's image of power and antiquity.[15]

The Pharos lighthouse itself, built in the early third century, was a statement that relied partly on size, and consequently on implicit claims to wealth and state authority. But it was also a mark of Greek technical capacity, directed towards the nautical interests of the trading Greek world.[16] There is little we can say definitely about the original structure, except that it was original, impressive, complex, and expensive—Pliny claims it cost 800 talents, an enormous sum by the standards of the time, even in wealthy Egypt. The Heptastadion, the engineered causeway that connected the Pharos island to the coast and created two well-protected harbors rather than the natural one, was also a highly visible monument to both Alexandrian engineering and the Egyptian tradition of gigantic public works.[17]

In other ways the city utilized a mixture of Greek and Egyptian elements more directly, if sometimes subtly. Local knowledge has been detected in the choice of the site, in the orientation of its streets to catch the summer winds from the north-east; indigenous craftsmanship or influence is visible

---

[15] For these and other finds of underwater archeology in the former harbor area, including both Greek and dynastic columns and bases, see McKenzie, *Architecture*, 43; Empereur, J.-Y. (1998). *Alexandria Rediscovered.*

[16] The earliest evidence is an epigram by the third century poet Posidippos: *P.Louvre* 7172 (161 BCE), ed. and trans. Austin, C. and G. Bastianini. (2002). *Posidippi Pellaei quae supersunt omnia*, no. 115; Strabo 17.1.6. Pliny 36.18.83 records an epigram inscribed on the building itself that named the designer as Sostratos of Knidos, though this might refer to the dedication of the statue of Zeus Soter rather than the lighthouse tower itself: Bing, P. 'Between literature and the monuments', in Harder, M.A. et al. (1998). *Genre in Hellenistic Poetry*, 22–23.

[17] For a summary of the evidence on both the Lighthouse and the Heptastadion, see McKenzie, *Architecture*, 41–47.

in the probable use of Egyptian measurement units by the city's builders. The breadth of the city's chief thoroughfare, about 30 m, is reminiscent of the wide entranceways into Egyptian temples.[18] The enormous area of the royal palace included gardens, a feature also of older Egyptian palaces and temples.[19]

Such echoes are more likely in view of the number and importance of buildings in which Greek and Egyptian features were deliberately combined, or in which Egyptian elements were utilized somewhat differently from the past, as in the single rather than traditional double obelisks erected in Philadelphos' Arsinoeion. Arrian attributes the intention of building a temple to 'Isis the Egyptian' to Alexander, in addition to temples to Greek gods. Roman coins depict this temple as Egyptian in style, and it could well have been like this from the beginning.[20] The structures of the Sarapieon built under Euergetes I—after an earlier phase and possibly a pre-existing Egyptian sanctuary—are however almost entirely Greek, including its orientation and placement. Its foundation plaques, however, are an Egyptian standard; numerous statues carved in the traditional style and dating in fact from both the pharaonic and Ptolemaic periods, were probably placed there during the Ptolemaic, rather than the Roman, period of rule.[21] Some of the temples built in the next generation by Philopator obviously took inspiration from both traditions, and the ways in which Egyptian architectural features expanded the repertoire of Greek architecture in new ways is more generally visible in what remains of the city's buildings.[22] Philadelphos' pavilion, set up for a feast apparently connected with the great procession described by Athenaios, was an eastern and Egyptian custom previously utilized by Alexander. On an impressive scale, it had room for one hundred dining couches, was decorated with curtains, paintings, and sculptures, and featured a colonnade around three sides.[23]

---

18 Diodoros 17.52.3; Strabo 17.1.8; McKenzie, *Architecture*, 32, 38. Eratosthenes' estimate of the circumference of the earth (Pliny 12.53) may well have used an Egyptian value for *stade*. See Engels, D. (1985). 'The length of Eratosthenes' stade', *AJPh* 106.3, 298–311.

19 See e.g. Wilkinson, A. (1998). *The Garden in Ancient Egypt*.

20 Arrian *The Expedition* 3.1.5. Roman coins: McKenzie, *Architecture*, 39.

21 Egyptian temple: Tacitus *Histories* 4.84, and for a summary McKenzie, *Architecture*, 40, 53–55, with notes. Memphis Serapieion: see above 2.3.1, pp. 67–69 ff.

22 McKenzie, *Architecture*, 34–35.

23 McKenzie, *Architecture*, 49. Athenaios' version was based on the lost account by Philadelphos' contemporary Kallixenos of Rhodes: Rice, E.E. (1983). *The Grand Procession of Ptolemy Philadelphus*.

The incorporation of the history, reputation and imaginative resources of other peoples is similarly visible in the concept behind the Library: to maintain a text of every work in the world, but with the assumption that that text was either originally written or translated into the Greek language. Hence both the second-century account of the translation of the Septuagint for Philadelphos in the 'letter of Aristeas', and Manetho's Greek history of Egypt, written under Soter. It is a worldview in which the knowledge, works and beliefs of other societies become, via this linguistic prism, a part of Greek awareness and understanding of the world.

In the last few decades, scholarship on the Hellenistic period Greek literature has revealed much of the 'intercultural poetics' of the period; highlighting the subtle use of Egyptian themes and symbols within their allusive, compressed rendition of the accumulated semiotics of Greek thought, art and literature. The Library is arguably itself an echo of the *pr ʿnḫ* (house of life), the scriptorium-repository commonly attached to Egyptian sanctuaries, which institutionalized written culture among the Egyptian elite and formed a vitally authoritative part of the performance of ritual action. Soter's and Philadelphos' court administrations included an unknown number of important Egyptians, fluent in the negotiation of political and aesthetic power. The use, both obvious and subtle, of Egyptian styles or actual objects, in the physical, poetic and praxic cityscape thus forms part of a mutual, or at least mutually contested, expression of the resources of both cultures.

There is no need for this process to have been Greek-led, although it is plainly responsive to Ptolemaic aims. Criteria of aesthetics, theology and royal ideology had always driven change and variation in the works of Egyptian architect-officials and craftsman. In some cases this resulted in, for instance, novel architectural forms in temples and houses, of the kind described above, in which both Greek and Egyptian traditions were expressed rather than silenced, and this kind of architectural symbiosis offers an interesting example of how technical experts, motivated by political patronage, used two sets of traditions as a joint resource for the creation of a civic identity. The ancient obelisks brought from Heliopolis, however divorced from their original location and meaning, were both an appropriation of Egyptian symbol for Ptolemaic-Macedonian interests, and an acknowledgment and continuing display of that cultural power. The development of novel artistic forms within a process of mutual discovery and cultural expansion can also be glimpsed in more personal choices and social trends: most obviously in the mixture of Greek and Egyptian elements in the architecture and decoration of tombs found as early as the second century;

and, most famously, in the Roman period Greco-Roman funerary portraits from the Fayum and elsewhere.[24]

In some arenas, however, Egyptian materials seem to have been either excluded or translated so thoroughly as to be essentially transformed and subsumed into Greek systems of thought, practice and expression. The Library and Museion exemplifies this strand of Alexandrian life, and the Library at least is very closely connected to the best-known and most influential forms of medicine in Alexandria: that of the anatomists, the subsequent 'sects', and the court physicians. The majority of arguments for Egyptian influence on medicine have been made in relation to Alexandria's elite practitioners, chiefly Herophilos and Erasistratos, or dating back to the classical period. An alternative interpretation is that offered by Heinrich von Staden, whose detailed study of the fragments of Herophilos placed the Herophileans firmly in the context of history of Greek medical discourse, but who also partially attributed the unique practice of investigatory human vivisection to Alexandria's third-century BCE 'frontier' society.[25] The phrase is somewhat underdetermined, but it implies, in its evocation of a novel social situation, that factors peculiar to Alexandrian society and government produced equally distinctive approaches to medicine.

6.2. *Urban Pluralism*

Alexandria's diverse population grew rapidly, to become one of the greatest in the Greco-Roman world.[26] It was a principal trade center and Mediterranean port, but also the gateway of the Nile Valley and its agricultural wealth. The high population density offered its healers the concentration of disease to be found in ancient urban environments, as well as a sizeable proportion of clients with disposable income. In comparable societies, these conditions result in a higher ratio of doctors to the rest of the population than in rural areas or smaller towns. In such a center of linguistic,

---

[24] McKenzie, *Architecture*, 71; for a more detailed analysis Venit, S. (2002). *Monumental Tombs of Ancient Alexandria.*

[25] von Staden, H. (1989). *Herophilus: the art of medicine in ancient Alexandria*, 28–29.

[26] Diodoros Sikelos 17.52.6 gives a figure of over 300,000 'free men' for the city in the mid first century, not that this is notably reliable. *P.Yale* II 107, TM 58940 (CE 150–250) supplies 180,000, possibly the adult male citizens of Alexandria in the 30s CE. The city is unlikely to have numbered more than 500, 000 in total in the Roman period, and fewer in the Ptolemaic: Rathbone, D.W. (1990). 'Villages, land and population in Graeco-Roman Egypt', *PCPhS* 36, 120. Cf. above 1.2.1, p. 21 with n. 83.

demographical and cultural diversity, with a large transient population, medical systems could proliferate into specialist niches or offer some kind of eclectic synthesis, not unlike the contemporary invention of astrology.[27]

The case of the bilingual assistant to an Egyptian 'enema specialist' or *iatroklystes*, discussed in chapter five (pp. 205–206) gives us an example of the potential effects of this medical pluralism. Patients in the rest of the Greco-Roman world often seem to have responded eclectically when choice of not only individuals but different therapeutics or theories were available.[28] This occurred even when practitioners defined themselves against alternative approaches, implying that from within the professional standpoint there were systematic differences between certain physicians, epistemological schools, and the use of certain contested domains and words, notably the use of amulets, incantations, or other non-naturalistic therapies and explanations. Such alternatives were not necessarily oppositional and could be complementary, as in the case of naturalistic physicians and Asklepieian sanctuaries. In both complementary and oppositional approaches there was also a degree to which certain assumptions, diagnoses and therapies could be shared: dreams might be diagnostic in naturalistic medicine as well as in incubation, albeit with variant rationales or significance. But it was drugs and regimen which offered the greatest degree of overlap, and large cities offered the greatest opportunities for the development of pharmaceuticals.

Galen identified the defining moment in the invention of compound drugs as the work of Mantias, a Herophilean of the second century, but this was only the culmination of a longer trend, much of which is visible in the works of Alexandrian physicians and in particular the Herophileans.[29]

The drug recipes of the classical period were part of the Library's codification of knowledge. As such, they were accessible both through access to the library or the growth in the private book trade, in which Alexandria was an important center. But in this respect, as in others, the texts attributed to Hippokrates were not canonical; they marked tendencies and origins which other physicians diverged from or developed. This allowed, again, for an eclectic form of medical pluralism, this time on the part of medical practitioners.

---

[27] Barton, T. (1994). *Ancient Astrology*.

[28] On the question of whether Erasistratos can be located in Alexandria, see below, 6.4, p. 260 and 5.2.1, p. 226 n. 90.

[29] Galen *The composition of drugs by kind* 2.1 (13.462 Kühn) = von Staden, *Herophilus*, fr. *Ma.* 1.

As a whole, Alexandrian medicine of the Ptolemaic period was a large part of the transformation of Greek pharmacology from its representation in the Hippocratic recipes, which involved few ingredients and even fewer exotica, to the elaborate compound drugs dependent on international trade and multicultural exchange of the later Hellenistic and Roman eras. Some of the factors relevant to this transformation would have applied to all large cities of antiquity, although it is worth noting that Alexandria was one of the largest. Such cities produced a concentration of competition combined with the *capacity* for development produced by the combination of urban economics, environmental variation accessible through trade—from Mediterranean sea routes, upcountry Egypt, the spices and silks of India and China,[30] and even sub-Saharan Africa—and multicultural medical traditions. The result was diversification as well as complication: not only in the recipes themselves, but in the innovation of written genre. In the second century Krateuas, the beneficiary of patronage at another Hellenistic court, produced the first herbal in Greek writings to be accompanied by drawings. In Alexandria, Andreas of Karystos and Apollonios Mys, both Herophileans, wrote works aimed at a presumably expanding market of professionalized self-help for the literate, the former with a work on drugs or cosmetics entitled *Narthex* and the latter with *Readily available drugs*.[31] Recipes and regimens became increasingly identified with specific approaches, authors and physicians.

The role of Egyptian practitioners and medical culture in Alexandrian and thus Greco-Roman pharmacology has left less evidence behind. As discussed in 4.2.3 (pp. 175–176), pharmaceutical recipes of Herophilos show that local knowledge and resources were being exploited by Greek language physicians, including those of the mobile elite who had access to ingredients from all over the world. But there is little otherwise to suggest that Egyptian practitioners and practices had much impact on the physicians associated with the Ptolemaic court and intellectual environment.

Praxagoras of Kos, with whom Herophilos studied, is the first known Greek physician to have distinguished systematically between arteries and veins, and to have noted that pulsation is unique to the arteries.[32] Herophilos extended and revised the anatomy and physiology of this distinction, but

---

30 See e.g. Peppard, M. (2009). 'A letter concerning boats in Berenike and trade on the Red Sea', *ZPE* 171, 193–198.

31 Andreas: von Staden, *Herophilus*, 472–477. Apollonius Mys: ibid., 540–554.

32 Galen *Doctrines of Hippocrates and Plato* 6.7 = Steckerl, F. (1958). *The Fragments of Praxagoras and his School*, fr. 28.

his emphasis on the pulse as a clinical tool, subsequently a major feature of most Greco-Roman medicine, is more novel. It may have been inspired or encouraged by the very long-standing instruction to practitioners in Egyptian medical texts on the subject of the heart 'speaking' through each 'vessel' (*mt*) the substance-carrying vessels of the body.[33] Hippocratic writers use the word 'channel' (ὁδός) frequently (for Egyptian and Greek theories of medicine, see chapter 3).

One report attributes to Herophilos a theory that food gone bad leads to problems of the heart and hence the pulse, a notion not dissimilar from remarks made about the disease entity *wḫdw*, in much earlier Egyptian medical texts; one could say the same about Erasistratos' theory of too much food causing inflammation and blockages within the body.[34]

Surviving Herophilean texts show that eye conditions were a major concern; Egyptian medical texts contain a similarly high proportion of ophthalmological conditions and remedies. Eye conditions were often treatable and rarely fatal, and as such represented an excellent opportunity for the exercise of medicine to the satisfaction of both patient and physician.

But there are also well-attested antecedents for all these views within Greek medical history, and it is just as easy to concoct a plausible story for their emergence at this period that leaves out Egyptian 'influence', as it is to include one. This is not to argue the latter is thus disproven, but merely to assert that correspondence between theories is not in itself sufficient evidence of such influence. Moreover, such similarities are isolated elements within Erasistratean and Herophilean systems: the former in particular depended on work from contemporary, Alexandrian, mechanics and physics on the behavior of air and liquids under pressure. The principal cause in Egyptian disease theory, invasive entities, does not appear at all within Alexandrian elite medical discourse. The anatomists' findings would have ruled out much of Egyptian physiology and anatomy as we have it in Egyptian texts; although many of these date to early periods of Egyptian history, those from the Late or Greco-Roman period seem to assume a similar conceptual framework as earlier Egyptian material.

---

[33] Ebers 854a and Smith case 1 gloss A: *GdM* 4/2, 1, 172; 4/2, 24–25, 140; 5, 1, 299. For Herophilos see von Staden, *Herophilus*, 267–288.

[34] See above 3.2.3, pp. 123–124. Caelius Aurelianus *Acute Diseases* 2.39.225 (*CML* 6.1.1, 282.5 ff.) = von Staden, *Herophilus*, T214. Our main source for Erasistratos' theory is Galen: see Hankinson, R.H. (1998). *Galen on Antecedent Causes*.

Von Staden proposed that Egyptian mummification of the dead improved the prospects of the human dissection employed by Herophilos and Erasistratos (to an extent rarely seen subsequently), in a kind of social detoxification or Egyptianizing legitimization along the lines of the Ptolemaic adoption of marital incest.[35] If so, it seems probable that any such justification rather misunderstood the meaning and ritual of mummification, in which invasive incision of the body was minimalized and involved the ritual abuse of the attendant responsible.[36] But human dissection, animal dissection and the more rare human vivisection, all carried out for purposes of investigation rather than restoration of the body for its life in the otherworld, are again entirely explicable in terms of Greek medical and philosophical trends at the time. (On Alexandrian dissection and vivisection see below, 6.3, pp. 254–258). I have argued earlier (4.4. pp. 195–197, cf. pp. 153–154) that Egyptian medicine does not seem to have, at any point in its ancient history, engaged in the practice of invasive internal surgery; and that the emergence of dissection as an investigatory medium and invasive surgery as a therapeutic one in Greco-Roman medicine is an outlier in ancient systems of medicine generally, one unusually dependent on a particular set of contingent circumstances.

In conclusion, in the domain of therapeutics or possibly diagnostic methods, and perhaps in a concern with locally prevalent conditions (such as eye problems), the evidence is limited but suggests an eclectically adaptive approach. Hence Herophilos' use of crocodile dung, or the appearance of Mediterranean materials in Egyptian texts of the Ptolemaic period.[37]

On the other hand, in theoretical medicine, we have a lack of evidence for either one-way or two-way influence between Egyptian and Greek nosological and philosophical belief systems, defining these as the ideas and explanations to be found in medical texts and employed by a professional and technical elite. The extant texts instead appear to reflect relatively closed theoretical systems, in which internal innovation or difference was negotiated within a well-established discourse.

One alternative way to look at it is to suggest that there was a greater interchange and interest between physicians of Greek and Egyptian background than the absence of evidence, on a conservative reading, suggests, particularly in situations where ideas seemed confirmatory or

---

35 von Staden, *Herophilus*, 29.

36 Diodoros Sikelos 1.91.4.

37 See above 4.2.3, pp. 167–177, especially 174–177.

complementary; but that this exchange was a discourse of adaptive performance. (The Greek patients or apprentices of an Egyptian *iatroklystes* in Alexandria (ch. 5, pp. 205–206) possibly hint at such a situation). By the time any such assimilation, such as the diagnostic uses of the pulse, or Greek ingredients in Egyptian pharmaceutical texts, reached the written texts of which our evidence now consists, it had effectively been fully incorporated and rewritten into an apparently exclusive, linguistically delimited, system of thought.

This would explain the lack of visible engagement in Greek sources with Egyptian ideas, which contrasts so noticeably with the highly explicit contestation of concepts in internal naturalistic discourse. A close parallel would be the way in which Asklepieian medicine related to that of *iatroi* in the classical Greek world: an absence of direct polemical analysis and apparently complementary, distinct approaches to diagnosis and cure, but a visible overlap nonetheless in patients, therapeutics, and even specific concepts. I will return to this issue in 6.4.

6.3. *Only in Alexandria*

One reason why Egyptian influence has often been proposed as a factor in Alexandrian medicine is because Alexandria produced a number of unique and significant innovations in medical methodology, theory and therapeutics. I have already briefly discussed the compound drug tradition. Other notable items include the practice of human vivisection, which in antiquity occurs only, as far as we know, in third century Alexandria; the use of human dissection and animal dissection and vivisection, all of which was unusual in its extent and the first of which was a new domain of exploration; the theories of Herophilos of Khalkedon and Erasistratos of Keos; the appearance of works about works about medicine and a growing apparatus of medical scholarship as a literary genre; and the emergence of medical *haireseis*, in particular the Herophileans, Erasistrateans, and Empiricists.

Heinrich von Staden's often quoted description of Ptolemaic Alexandria as being a 'frontier' society highlighted the experimental, boundary-pushing nature of much literary and scientific activity in the city.[38] He coined the phrase partly in an effort to explain how human vivisection

[38] von Staden, *Herophilus* 28–29; above 6.1, p. 249 n. 25.

became, uniquely and temporarily, part of medical work and scientific patronage in mid-third century Alexandria. The first century CE medical encyclopedist Celsus reports in his preface that 'kings' had supplied Herophilos and Erasistratos with criminals from the prisons, and that dissection and vivisection had been carried out upon these individuals.

> [Theory-minded physicians say that] Herophilus and Erasistratus did this [dissection and examination of human internal remains] in the best way by far when they cut open men who were alive, criminals out of prison, received from kings. And while breath still remained in these criminals, they inspected those parts which nature previously had concealed, also their position, colour, shape, size, arrangement, hardness, softness, smoothness, connection, and the projections and depressions of each, and whether anything is inserted into another thing or whether anything receives a part of another into itself ...[39]

It is certainly a dramatic heuristic, and Celsus' discussion of the arguments for and against the practice several centuries later confirm that it was controversial on both ethical and epistemological grounds: '... nor is it cruel, as most people maintain, that remedies for innocent people of all times should be sought in the sacrifice of people guilty of crimes, and of only a few such people at that.'[40]

The term 'frontier society' implies, among other things, a shift from social norms or religious observance found elsewhere, i.e. in other, longer-established Greek societies, and a willingness to take risks and extend boundaries. The assumption is that human vivisection, or even human dissection, would not have been acceptable in, for example, fourth century

---

39 Celsus *Medicine* 1 pro. 23.6–25.1 = von Staden, *Herophilus*, T63a: '... longeque optime fecisse Herophilum et Erasistratum, qui nocentes homines, a regibus ex carcere acceptos, vivos incididerint, considerarintque etiamnum spiritu remanente ea, quae natura ante clausisset, eorumque positum, colorem, figuram, magnitudinem, ordinem, duritiem, mollitiem, levorem, contactum, processus deinde singulorum et recessus, et sive quid inseritur alteri, sive quid partem alterius in se recipit ...'. Translation by von Staden.

40 Ibid. 26 (T 63a): '... neque esse crudele, sicut plerique proponunt, hominum nocentium et horum quoque paucorum suppliciis remedia populis innocentibus saeculorum omnium quaeri.' The easiest assumption is that the 'kings' in question are the Ptolemies, since the sources are confident that Herophilos worked in Alexandria. Lloyd, G.E.R. 'Alcmaeon and the early history of dissection', repr. in Lloyd. (1991). *Methods and Problems in Greek Science*, 164–193, argues that it is improbable that both the Ptolemies and the Seleucids were generous in this fashion, though a case could perhaps be made for it as an another example of rivalry between the Successor kingdoms. If the plural refers neither to two dynasties, nor reflects a simple temporal uncertainty on the part of Celsus, it probably refers to the supply of criminals continuing through the change of kings from Soter to Philadelphos in 282/83.

Athens; that something about Alexandria in general or the Ptolemaic court in particular enabled it to occur. In the case of human vivisection, this freedom was apparently temporary.

One might suggest that an important element in the creation of such a 'frontier' ethos, among intellectuals at least, was the fact that Ptolemaic patronage, as that of the Seleucids or Attalids, involved a more absolute power than was the case in oligarchic or democratic societies. Human vivisection's brief appearance in the middle decades of the third century would seem to correlate with the power of rulers to transgress social norms or more specifically with societies in which political power was ultimately individual, arbitrary, and hierarchical: other Greco-Roman kings are said to have made a similar use of low-status humans by testing poisons on slaves.[41] The incestuous marriage of Philadelphos to Arsinoe II attracted at least some adverse comment from within the Greek world, although the Ptolemies could have pointed to both Greek and Egyptian precedent.[42]

But it is not entirely clear that human vivisection—in the quite limited circumstances that Celsus' account specifies—was as controversial as is often assumed from a modern perspective; nothing suggests that the majority of people in Alexandria either knew or cared about the fate of a few criminals. Celsus represented his own pro-dissection, anti-vivisection position as that of the moderate, but it is notable both that in the intervening centuries there had still been physicians prepared to argue (against the 'majority' view of its cruelty) that 'remedies for the innocent in all eras should be sought by the sacrifice of criminals, and only a few of those', and that even among its opponents the objections are as much epistemological, and informed by Empiricist and Methodist attitudes to the non-apparent, as ethical. Nor we can we be completely sure that either human dissection or vivisection would always have been unthinkable in classical Greece, or in non-monarchic societies. Aristotle's advocacy of animal dissection dated to only the fourth century, when it was itself a novel approach that required justification, not least that the insights it granted into the intellectual beauty

---

[41] Attalos III and Mithridates VI Eupator: Galen *Antidotes* 2.1 (14.2 Kühn), cf. *The powers and mixtures of simple drugs* 10.1 (12.252 Kühn). Kleopatra VII: Plutarch *Antony* 71.6ff.; *P.Hercul.* 817. A seventh century king of Assyria is also said to have tested poisons on slaves: Keyser, P. 'Science and magic in Galen's recipes', in Debru, A. (1997). *Galen on Pharmacology*, 180 and n. 27.

[42] The poet Sotades' famously critical remark, and its alleged repercussions for him, are reported by Plutarch *The education of children* 1a–14c. Zeus and Hera, however, supplied a Greek model, as Theokritos indirectly noted in his *Encomium of Ptolemy Philadelphus*, lines 33–34, ed. Hunter, R. (2003).

of nature's designs was adequate compensation for the sheer ugliness of the act and its immediate findings.[43]

Animal vivisection and dissection, like human dissection, seem never to have become common practices, even among physicians. Galen's adoption of these techniques, for which he repeatedly argued, was rare. Human vivisection assumed the usefulness of this kind of investigation and extended it to a dehumanized and possibly very small group of individuals.[44] It was therefore vulnerable to the same issues that beset such techniques as a group: the expense and organization required to obtain suitable subjects, especially difficult in the case of obtaining a regular supply of human corpses or living individuals, and the gore, disgust and empathy sometimes involved.[45] It is possible that it was these more pragmatic difficulties, rather than a social or moral resistance to interference with the human body, that required active government support.

The noticeable decline in dissection as a research or learning tool among later generations, and the complete disappearance of human vivisection, must be partly due to the increasingly disputed nature of Aristotelian-style empiricism among physicians and philosophers of subsequent generations.[46] Human vivisection and dissection produced no agreement among physiology, pathology or therapeutics amongst even its leading exponents: Herophilos, Erasistratos, and their followers. They had greater agreement on anatomy—as for instance in the proof, almost certainly accomplished by vivisectory work on the nerves as well as by dissection—that the *hegemonikon* was located in the head. Nonetheless, these anatomical discoveries failed to transform medicine. They did not always achieve widespread recognition even among physicians, and other intellectuals, including most members of the Hellenistic philosophical schools, disputed their epistemology and the relevance or accuracy of their findings. Given dissection's

[43] *Parts of Animals* 645a27–30.

[44] It is possible that the criminals so vivisected were not Greek, distancing them even further from a largely Greek socio-economic elite. I made this suggestion in a Cambridge Ph.D. thesis of 2001; and it has been independently articulated by Flemming, R. 'Empires of knowledge: medicine and health in the Hellenistic world', in Erskine, A. (2003). *The Blackwell Companion to the Hellenistic World*, 449–463.

[45] In *Anatomical Procedures* Galen advises against using a Barbary ape (macaque) as a subject for brain vivisection, because of the expression on its face during the procedure, which his audience did not care for: (9.11; 15 Kühn). Rocca, J. (2002). 'The brain beyond Kühn', *BICS* 45, 91 n. 36.

[46] This summary analysis largely follow von Staden, H. 'Hairesis and heresy: the case of the haireseis iatrikai', in Meyer, B.F. and E.P. Sanders. (1982). *Jewish and Christian Self-Definition*, 76–101.

failure to demonstrate medicine to the point of certainty, its epistemological attraction waned, and its continuation became very much a minority practice.

The corresponding disappearance of Ptolemaic support after Philadelphos is often supposed to be part of a loss of interest, among the members of the dynasty, in support for Greek intellectual and literary culture generally. This trend culminated in the expulsion of the intelligentsia by Ptolemy VIII Euergetes II in 145–144.[47] Aggressive modes of investigation, however, may have had an even briefer window for the support they required, before changes in intellectual fashion reduced dissection's epistemological prestige. Thus the association of human vivisection with early Ptolemaic Alexandria seems to have had less to do with a Ptolemaic indifference to Greek social norms, and more to do with short-term interest, peculiar to the political aims of Soter and his immediate successor, in this type of form and field of investigation, or simply in their support for intellectuals, among whom, in medicine, aggressive investigation was temporarily ascendant.

6.4. *Elite Medicine As an Exclusive System*

Nothing directly connects the anatomists or any other physician with either the Museion or the Library, although the number of commentaries and lexica produced by Herophileans and Empiricists suggests an acquaintance with the latter. If this apparent distinction was a real one, it probably reflected medicine's role as a professional occupation with paying clients—among whom, of course, were the Ptolemies themselves. The kind of physicians known to us for such methodological and theoretical work, from whose ranks came the court physicians and others employed by the social elite, were part of the Greek world's itinerant intelligentsia. This was a long-standing phenomenon, which, combined with Hellenistic period patronage, ensured concentrations of intellectuals in large urban centers, particularly those of the Successor kingdoms.[48]

---

[47] For this expulsion see Fraser, *Alexandria*, 1.86–88.

[48] Demokedes' career as reported by Herodotos 3.125–137 is an early example of the trade in prestigious physicians, and in how lucrative a skill medicine could be. In the Hellenistic era city-states requested public physicians from Kos (5.3.3, p. 237). The movements of an Apollonios of Perge or an Arkhimedes of Syrakuse, and the very fact that most third century Alexandrian intellectuals are from elsewhere in Greece and the Greek islands, testify to the mobility of elite thinkers and skilled specialists.

The surviving fragments of Herophilos and Erasistratos reveal that both used sophisticated, philosophical-style arguments in issues of epistemology and causation, while the biographical tradition also places them in the same intellectual milieu as philosophers. According to report Erasistratos studied with Theophrastos, and might have been influenced, directly or indirectly, by the theories of Straton of Lampsakos (at one point Philadelphos' tutor) on physics and the void.[49] Certainly his conception of human physiology made extensive use of mechanical systems designed and built by the mechanists of Alexandria. Mechanist writers like Heron argued that these systems demonstrated the existence of the kind of void or microvoid for which Straton had argued, a theory strongly opposed by most philosophers, including Aristotle.[50]

One would assume Herophilos was familiar with the society of the Museion, Library and court. Practitioners of elite medicine were members of the well-educated upper Greek social strata almost by definition, as a remark of Aristotle suggests: 'But 'physician' means both the ordinary practitioner, and the master of the craft, and thirdly, the man who has studied

[49] Diogenes Laertios 5.57, cf. Galen *Is blood naturally contained in the arteries?* 7 (4.729 Kühn): '[the Erasistrateans say] ὡς Θεοφράστῳ συνεγένετο.' Straton as Philadelphos' tutor: Diogenes Laertios 5.58; for his theories see Gottschalk, H.B. (1965). *Strato of Lampsacus: some texts.*

[50] In spite of frequent claims that Erasistratos had a Stratonesque theory of interstitial void existing in between particles of matter, all that can be securely said is that according to Galen he denied the existence of massed, continuous void: *The use of respiration* 2 (4.474 Kühn). Indeed this polemical text, which presents Erasistratos as in dialogue with 'opponents,' implies that Erasistratos also denied the possibility of interstitial void. See Furley, D.J. and J.S. Wilkie. (1984). *Galen on Respiration and the Arteries*, 32–35; Vallance, J.T. (1990). *The Lost Theory of Asclepiades of Bithynia*, 62ff. But von Staden, H. 'Body and machine', in (1996). *Alexandria and Alexandrianism*, 92 and n. 47 asserts that Galen's description of an experiment which demonstrates the existence of void was carried out by Erasistratos (*Natural faculties* 2.1 = *Scripta Minora* 3.154–155). He points out the similarity of this experiment to that carried out by early Alexandrian mechanists and cited in Peripatetic writers, cf. Gottschalk, *Strato*, 129. But the actual text does not seem to me to definitely indicate that Erasistratos carried out this experiment, which might have been added by Galen in order to illustrate the criticism of Erasistratos, or more probably by Asklepiades of Bithynia whose argument Galen is describing. Von Staden, H. 'Teleology and mechanism', in Kullmann, W. and S. Föllinger. (1997). *Aristotelische Biologie*, 183–208, further accepts that the suggestion that Erasistratos was directly influenced by Straton is a plausible one. On the connections between philosophy, medicine and mechanics in the third century see Vegetti, M. 'L'épistemologie d'Érasistrate et la technologie Hellénistique', in van der Eijk, Ph. et al. (1995). *Ancient Medicine in its Socio-Cultural Context*, 2. 461–471; von Staden, 'Body and machine', 83–206, and Tybjerg, K. (2000). *Doing Philosophy with Machines.*

medicine as part of his general education.'[51] Thus an apocryphal anecdote gives Herophilos a philosophical victory over the logician Diodoros Kronos, who was in Alexandria some time between the years 275 and 250: the physician is said to have used Diodoros' own arguments against motion to prove to the philosopher that either his shoulder was not in fact dislocated or there was something wrong with his arguments.[52] In the next generation acrimonious public accusations of plagiarism were leveled at Andreas of Karystos—Herophilos' former student and Philopator's physician—by the Librarian, geographer, and literary critic Eratosthenes.[53]

The most common variation of a story told by several Roman era sources places Erasistratos in the Seleucid court at Antioch. Its historical verity is inaccessible and certainly not unassailable, given that the story in question is a romance of the physician as detective. Other versions have different physicians or an astrologer in the medical role, while a very similar anecdote is told by Galen of himself.[54] It assumes, however, the plausibility of this role for Erasistratos, and it is certainly quite possible that he did spend at least some time at Antioch or even the Seleucid court, as well as at Alexandria.[55] Elite physicians were a highly mobile group, like other intellectuals and indeed ordinary itinerant doctors of the later classical and Hellenistic ages. Other parts of the biographical tradition place Erasistratos in Athens, learning from Aristotelian philosophers; he might also have spent an early period in Knidos, the home of his teacher Khrysippos.[56]

Various other references suggest—albeit never conclusively—that Erasistratos had family and other relationships in both capitals. His brother

---

[51] *Politics* 1282a3–4. Cf. ibid., *Respiration* 480b26 ff.: 'The more subtle and inquisitive doctors speak about nature and claim to derive their principles from it, while the more accomplished investigators of nature generally end by a study of the principles of medicine.'

[52] Sextus Empirikos *Outlines of Pyrrhonism* 2.245; see Sedley, D.N. (1977). 'Diodoros Cronus and Hellenistic Philosophy', *PCPhS* 23, 74–120, esp. 79. Other references to Diodoros Kronos in Alexandria: Kallimachos fr. 393 Pfeiffer; Diogenes Laertios 2.111–112.

[53] von Staden, *Herophilus*, fr. *An.* 2.

[54] The physician is Erasistratos according to Valerius Maximus *Nine books of memorable deeds and sayings* 5.7.3. ext. 1, with the astrologer Leptines as an alternative candidate; Plutarch *Life of Demetrius* 38; Appian *Roman history* 11.10; Lucian *How to write history* 35; Pliny *Natural History* 29.3; Julian *Beard-Hater* 347; *Suda*. s.v. *Erasistratos* no. 2896. References from Pinault, J.R. (1992). *Hippocratic Lives and Legends*, 105.

[55] See e.g. Lloyd, 'Alcmaeon', against the view of Fraser, P.M. (1969). 'The career of Erasistratus of Ceos', *Rendiconti del Istituto Lombardo* 103, 518–537. In addition to Celsus' anonymous kings, Caelius Aurelianus *Chronic Diseases* 5.2.50 (*CML* 6.1.2, 88.4–5) claims that Erasistratos 'promises king Ptolemy a soothing plaster'. Galen *Prognosis* 6 (*CMG* 5.8.1, 100.16 ff.)

[56] For Erasistratos' apprenticeship with Khrysippos see Diogenes Laertios 7.186, Pliny *NH* 29.5, Galen e.g. *Blood-letting, against Erasistratos* 7 (11.171 Kühn).

Kleophantos and the son of his teacher Khrysippos may both have worked in Alexandria; one report identifies the latter as personal physician to one of the Ptolemies.[57] In later generations the Erasistratean Apollophanes, himself from Seleukia, was at the court of Antiokhos III, while Apollonios of Memphis, a pupil of Erasistratos' medical associate Straton, is said to have worked in Alexandria.[58] A variant on the lovesickness story identifies the physician not as Erasistratos but as his father Kleombrotos.[59]

Such anecdotes and associations are often doxographic constructions; defining and organizing philosophy and other subjects through ideological lineages. The ways in which these relationships are portrayed, however, reveals the common intellectual world of the Hellenistic elite to be a relatively small pool of individuals, most of whom were known to each other personally or by repute. These individuals were similar in education, social status and modes of thought. Kallimakhos' and Theokritos' poems present a world in which physical and philosophical knowledge and inquiry, including that of medicine, was part of educated discourse. Kallimakhos satirizes Diodoros Kronos' logic, while both poets refer to physicians known to them by name and moving in the same circles: the spheres of the Museion, the Library and the court were not discrete but overlapping. The poet Poseidippos of Pella opened his *Iamatika* with an epigram on the dedication of a statue to Apollo by the physician Medeios of Olynthos. This Medeios can be identified as an important Ptolemaic official, holding the position of eponymus priest of Alexander and the *Theoi Adelphoi*. He also seems to have acted in an official capacity in the organization of the medical tax (*iatrikon*) and its disbursement. Poseidippos, however, emphasizes his medical skill—his discovery of a cure for the bite of the Libyan asp.[60]

The Ptolemies themselves were part of this small and personal intellectual community. Philadelphos was taught by the Aristotelian Straton,

---

[57] Galen *Commentary on Hippocrates' Epidemics III* 2.3 (*CMG* 5.10.2.1, 77.20) and Rufus *Diseases of the bladder and kidneys* 4.1 (*CMG* 3.1, 128.55); Khrysippos' son as Ptolemaic physician: Diogenes Laertios 7.186 cf. *Scholia in Theocritum* 17.128, although here the younger Khrysippos is said to be from Rhodes, not Knidos.

[58] Caelius Aurelianus *Acute Diseases* 2.33.173 (*CML* 6.1.1, 248.9–11) with Polybios 5.56, 5.58; Ps.-Galen, *Introduction, or the doctor* 10 (14.699–700 Kühn). *Pace* Fraser, *Alexandria*, 1.347, who argues that no Erasistratean can be located in Alexandria.

[59] Kleombrotos: Pliny *Natural History* 7.12 (in his first reference to the story, which he gives twice, the second time featuring Erasistratos).

[60] For the *Iamatika*, *P.Mil.Vogl.* VIII 39, 14.30–37. Eponymous priest: *BGU* VI 1227, TM 2661 and others. Connected to the *iatrikon* and its revenues: *P.Cair.Zen.* I 59036, TM 696. See Bing, P. (2002). 'Medeios of Olynthos, son of Lampon, and the "Iamatika" of Posidippus', *ZPE* 140, 297–300; and chapter 5.2.1, p. 225, and 5.3.3, p. 237.

Philopator is said to have tricked the Stoic philosopher Sphairos with wax pomegranates in a debate over the cognitive impression, and the astronomer Konon named a constellation for queen Berenike.[61]

The Library, as discussed in 6.1, was crucial to Alexandria's creation as a Greek cultural nexus, as Ptolemy I and Ptolemy II attempted to position themselves as Alexander's true successors and the natural leaders of the Greek world. It reified the Greek understanding of themselves and their position in the world through the appropriation and control of the world's texts. This can be seen not only in the concept of a complete collection itself, but also in the concern to establish the notion of an authoritative, singular, correct text against which variant copies, new works, or interpretations could be compared; and similarly in the commentaries and lexica that similarly assigned meanings to particular words. This textual aspect of elite medicine is also very marked in the emergence of the medical 'sects'. This is not the place to discuss either the positions of the sects or the process by which they emerged; such studies have already been accomplished and in what follows I have generally followed von Staden's *Herophilos* (1989) and his 'Hairesis and heresy' (1982).

The creation of Empiricism's identity as an *hairesis* began with polemical attacks on individuals who employed other, rival methods. Philinos of Kos attacked non-Empiricist physicians, writing a six-book treatise against a contemporary student of Herophilos, Bakkheios of Tanagra. There is no evidence that this was not an attack by one individual upon another, in the usual form of Greek medical debate. But it was a short step from criticizing individuals who used non-Empiricist methods to criticizing non-Empiricist methods full stop, and thus to identifying non-Empiricists as a group. That this was the next move is suggested by the title of Sarapion's *Against the sects*, written not long after Philinos' work.[62] The term *hairesis* does not seem to have been applied to such intellectual groupings before it was adopted for the medical ones.[63] Sarapion's title is its first known application to this purpose and his work identified non-Empiricist figures as members of rival groups rather than as individuals. Thus Sarapion presented non-Empiricist

[61] Diogenes Laertios 7.177 and Athenaios 354e; Kallimachos *Koma Berenikes* (fr. 110 Pfeiffer).

[62] Caelius Aurelianus *Acute Diseases* 2.6.32 (*CML* 6.1.1, 148.21–25). Philinos fl. ca. 250; Sarapion fl. ca. 225 making him a younger contemporary of Bakkheios, fl. ca. 275–200: von Staden, H. 'Hellenistic reflections on the history of medicine', in van der Eijk, Ph. (1999). *Ancient Histories of Medicine*, 160.

[63] von Staden, 'Hairesis and heresy', 80.

medicine as a set of (incorrect) choices between doctrinal options, while Empiricism was not in fact itself a choice between equally bad alternatives and guesses, but a way of doing medicine without commitment or decision one way or the other.

Hairesis, on this reading, began its technical life as an insult, but by the first century at the latest—and probably before—it was a means of self-identification. Heraklides of Tarenton wrote a book, 'The empiricist sect' and this apologetic tendency was echoed by the Herophileans. Again, it is not entirely clear at what stage certain physicians began to be identified or to identify themselves as followers of Herophilos. The term *hairesis* in Sarapion's polemical attack in the third century presumably referred *inter alia* to Herophileans. They are not however known to have defined themselves as a distinct group before the first century, when no less than three Herophileans write treatises entitled *The sect of Herophilos*. In the third century, however, Herophilos' former student Bakkheios of Tanagra wrote a book called 'Memories of Herophilos and those from his household'.[64] This description of the first generation of Herophileans as those 'from the house of Herophilos' expresses the transient and informal nature of the relationship between an expert and his apprentices.

The Erasistrateans appear to be a slightly different case from the Herophileans, and perhaps at first constituted even less of an identifiable group. Von Staden remarks on the absence of treatises by and on the members of the Erasistratean *hairesis*. References to any exegetical works by Erasistrateans in later authors are also lacking, although numerous Hippocratic commentaries and lexica by Herophileans and Empiricists are cited.[65] On the other hand polemical interaction is said to have taken place not only between Erasistratos himself and members of other sects but also between other sects and Erasistrateans.[66] Galen refers to Erasistratos' criticisms of Empiricism, while Erasistrateans attacked Bakkheios of Tanagra on the subject of the pulse, presumably in a contemporary debate.[67] Apollonios of Memphis was probably the first Erasistratean to define the pulse, in what looks like a reaction to the Herophilean emphasis on this topic. Of course attributions by later authors do not necessarily mean that these physicians were in fact identified at the time as Erasistrateans, and again the known

64 von Staden, *Herophilus*, fr. *Ba.* 78.
65 von Staden, 'Hellenistic reflections', 186–187.
66 See e.g. Galen *The sects* 5 (*Scripta Minora* 3.1.9).
67 Galen *The difference of pulses* 4 (8.733 Kühn).

interactions are specifically related to individuals rather than *haireseis*. But there is no reason to suppose that physicians with views broadly similar to those of Erasistratos were not identified as his followers, in the same way that followers of Herophilos were. That such physicians existed in the third century is suggested not only by the report of their opposition to Bakkheios, but also by Galen's explicit citation of Erasistrateans for this period.[68]

The Erasistrateans seem, however, to have been rather more scattered than members of the other Hellenistic sects. Seven such physicians are known. Apollophanes of Seleukia, who became personal physician to Antiokhos III; Erasistratos' apprentice Straton; Straton's apprentice Apollonios of Memphis; Khrysippos; Hikesios the founder of the Erasistratean school at Smyrna; and possibly Xenophon.[69] If Erasistratos did spend a relatively limited part of his career in Alexandria, it would not be surprising to find his ex-apprentices and followers spread more thinly and widely, without the geographical *locus* that seemed to be essential for the formation of an *hairesis*.

In this case the explanation for the absence of apologetic or polemical literature among the Erasistrateans is that the term 'Erasistratean' refers to Erasistratos' scattered ex-apprentices, who to some extent followed his teachings and theories but did not perhaps feel any need to identify themselves as members of a group. Later authors used the term 'Erasistratean' for these physicians as they used it for contemporary followers of Erasistratos. Some later Erasistrateans did form a recognizable and possibly more doctrinally coherent group, probably from around the time that Hikesios founded the Erasistratean school in first century Smyrna. This might also explain why the early Empiricists, while they target Erasistratos, do not do the same for 'Erasistrateans'.[70]

All the early medical *haireseis* should be seen as loosely identified sets of individuals for the first two hundred or so years of their existence. While philosophers had for some time formed groups of doctrinally similar indi-

---

[68] Galen *Natural faculties* 1.17 (*Scripta Minora* 3.150–151). Erasistratos' student Straton is said to have written 'I am of the household of Erasistratos': *Blood-letting, against the Erasistrateans in Rome* 2 (11.197 Kühn). As with Bakkheios' memoirs, this might refer to either an intellectual association or a literal location, or both.

[69] Diogenes Laertios 5.61; *PP* 16577; Diogenes Laertios 7.186; *PP* 16611; *PP* 16625 and Galen *Anatomical Procedures* 8.10 (14.699 Kühn). There is no reason to suppose that the Ptolemaic court physician Khrysippos, the son of Erasistratos' teacher, was himself an Erasistratean. According to Galen 'Khrysippeans' and 'Erasistrateans' disagreed: *Blood-letting, against Erasistratos* 2 (11.151 Kühn).

[70] von Staden, 'Hellenistic reflections', 186–187.

viduals, schools like the Academy, Lykeion, Stoa and Garden required a deliberate act of foundation and were strongly associated with a place. The medical sects not only took longer to become established, but even then followed a slightly different pattern. Only the emigration of some Herophileans to Asia Minor in the first century seems to have involved the foundation of a formal institution and a cult association.[71] Similarly, the Erasistratean Hikesios provided a centre for like-minded physicians at Smyrna at the beginning of the first century.[72]

The story of the emergence of the medical sects demonstrates, and is defined by, three features of elite medicine in this period, and in particular in Alexandria. In the first place, it has a strong textual component, not only through apologetic and polemical literature but also in the ways in which both the sects and individuals presented themselves in relation both to each other and to earlier medical literature and personalities. The second characteristic is closely related to the first. Medical texts wrote the performance and reputation of elite physicians; they defined the terms with which they related to each other and to other aspects of elite Greek culture. But the discourse thus produced was an internal, if somewhat schizophrenic debate that locked the medical practitioners of the Hellenistic elites into an exhaustive dialogue of methodological and theoretical difference. It was a discourse that demanded an individualized relationship to a common written past and contested present, producing an intertextualized, multiplying diversification of theoretical and epistemological positions within a relatively small area; as in the Herophilean differences on the pulse.[73] Hence the third feature of Alexandrian elite medicine: the small numbers of people involved in this intertextual, inter-theoretical and self-referencing performance of medical status.

There is, then, a crucial set of differences between the medicine practiced by an exclusive intellectual elite in the upper social strata of Alexandria, and that of the rest of the city. If Egyptian ideas or drug ingredients were utilized by physicians like Herophilos, they were transformed beyond recognition. Their place in the conceptual space of Greek medical texts existed only insofar as individual ideas or persons could be accommodated within the Greek models; Egyptian medicine is a creation of the hierarchical anthropological viewpoint of Greek writings on the Other. Historians are the only writers

---

71 von Staden, 'Hairesis and heresy,' 80, 93–94.

72 Cadoux, C.J. (1938). *Ancient Smyrna*,150–151.

73 As analyzed by von Staden, *Herophilus*, 446–449.

who describe it. The anatomists and their successors within the sects did not *explicitly* reference or engage with Egyptian medicine as a system, as an alternative, or as a useful system of knowledge—or with any individuals who self-identified in Egyptian terms. Elite medicine in Alexandria and subsequently was a deliberate expression of Greek identity, recognized and reinforced by royal patronage, not through racial markers or even solely linguistic ones, but through an exclusive performance of *paideia* that differentiated the uninitiated or uncooperative from a shared assertion of cultural authority. This added another barrier between the medicine of the elite, confirmed by their access to and employment at court, and practitioners of other kinds of healing or lesser status.

The medicine of the elite physicians of Alexandria existed firmly within a particular politico-cultural context: the Ptolemaic project to make Alexandria the capital of the Greek cultural world. It was outside the court, the Library, the Museion, and other such identity claims, that boundaries between practitioners and practices were less distinct, and where adaptation to changing cultural conditions and the necessity of functioning in more than one socio-cultural environment encouraged more eclectic forms of knowledge.

Thus Alexandria encapsulates the plurality of engagement at its most manifold and commonplace, as Jewish, Egyptian and Greek forms of medical practice, and related systems of knowledge, interacted through competion, trade and adaptation. The city's most famous institutions, however, represent Greek cultural exclusivity at its most extreme: the attempt to define knowledge and its canon through an excluding framework of heuristics, demonstration and textual control.

BIBLIOGRAPHY

Africa, T.W. "Herodotus and Diodorus on Egypt." *Journal of Near Eastern Studies* 22 (1963): 254–258.

Aleshire, S.B. *The Athenian Asklepieion: The People, Their Dedications, and the Inventories*. Amsterdam: J.C. Gieben, 1989.

———. *Asklepios at Athens: Epigraphic and Prosopographic Essays on the Athenian Healing Cults*. Amsterdam: Gieben, 1991.

Allen, J.P. *Genesis in Egypt: The Philosophy of Ancient Egyptian Creation Accounts*. New Haven, Conn.: Yale Egyptological Seminar, 1988.

———. "The Egyptian Concept of the World." In *Mysterious Lands*, edited by D. O'Connor and S. Quirke, 23–30. London: UCL Press, 2003.

———. *The Egyptian Coffin Texts. Volume 8, Middle Kingdom Copies of Pyramid Texts*. Chicago: Oriental Institute of the University of Chicago, 2006.

———. *Middle Egyptian: An Introduction to the Language and Culture of Hieroglyphs*. 2nd ed., rev. ed. Cambridge: Cambridge University Press, 2010.

———. with an essay by D.T. Mininberg. *The Art of Medicine in Ancient Egypt*. pbk. ed. New York and New Haven: Metropolitan Museum of Art; Yale University Press, 2005.

Amigues, S. *Théophraste. Recherches sur les plantes*. Paris: Les Belles Lettres, 1988–1993.

Andorlini, I. "Riflessi e applicazioni della terapia ippocratica nella testimonianza dei papiri." In *Aspetti della terapia nel Corpus Hippocraticum*, edited by I. Garofalo, 431–446. Firenze: L.S. Olschki, 1999.

———. ed. *Greek Medical Papyri I*. Firenze: Istituto Papirologico G. Vitelli, 2001.

———. ed. *Greek Medical Papyri II*. Firenze: Istituto Papirologico G. Vitelli, 2009.

Andrews, A.C. "The Opium Poppy as Food and Spice in the Classical Period." *Agricultural History* 26, no. 4 (1952): 152–155.

Angel, J.L. "Osteoporosis: Thalassemia?" *American Journal of Physical Anthropology* 22, no. 3 (1964): 369–374.

———. "Porotic Hyperostosis or Osteoporosis Symmetrica." In *Diseases in Antiquity: A Survey of the Diseases, Injuries, and Surgery for Early Populations*, edited by Don R. Brothwell and A.T. Sandison, 378–389. Springfield, IL: Charles C. Thomas, 1966.

———. *The People of Lerna: Analysis of a Prehistoric Aegean Population*. Princeton, N.J.; Washington: American School of Classical Studies at Athens; Smithsonian Institution Press, 1971.

———. "Ecology and Population in the Eastern Mediterranean." *World Archaeology* 4 (1972): 88–105.

———. "Health as a Crucial Factor in the Changes from Farming to Developed Farming in the Eastern Mediterranean." In *Paleopathology at the Origins of Agriculture*, edited by M.N. Cohen and G.J. Armelagos, 51–70. Orlando, FL: Academic Press, 1984.

Anthes, R. "The Legal Aspect of the Instruction of Amenemhet." *Journal of Near Eastern Studies* 16 (1957): 176–191.

Arnold, D. *Temples of the Last Pharaohs*. Oxford: Oxford University Press, 1999.

Arnold, D. ed. *The Encyclopaedia of Ancient Egyptian Archaeology*. London: I.B. Tauris, 2003.

Arnold, D. "A Chronology. The Later History and Excavations of the Temple of Hatshepsut at Deir El-Bahri." In *Hatshepsut. From Queen to Pharaoh*, edited by C.H. Roehrig, R. Dreyfus and C. Keller, 290–293. New York; New Haven: Metropolitan Museum of Art; Yale University Press, 2005.

Ashton, S.-A. "The Ptolemaic Royal Image and the Egyptian Tradition." In *'Never Had the Like Occurred': Egypt's View of Its Past*, edited by J. Tait, 213–223. London: UCL, 2003.

Bagnall, R.S. "The Origins of Ptolemaic Cleruchs." *Hellenistic and Roman Egypt: sources and approaches* 21 (1984): 7–20.

———. *Reading Papyri, Writing Ancient History*. London: Routledge, 1995.

———. "Decolonizing Ptolemaic Egypt." In *Hellenistic Constructs: Essays in Culture, History, and Historiography*, edited by P. Cartledge, P. Garnsey and E.S. Gruen, 225–241. Berkeley: University of California Press, 1997.

———. "The People of the Roman Fayum." In *Portraits and Masks: Burial Customs in Roman Egypt*, edited by M. Bierbrier, 7–15. London: British Museum Press, 1997.

———. "Archaeological Work on Hellenistic and Roman Egypt." *American Journal of Archeology* 105 (2001): 227–244.

———. "Alexandria: Library of Dreams." *Proceedings of the American Philosophical Society* 146 (2002): 348–362.

———. "Dioskourides: Three Rolls." *Bulletin de la Societé Archéologique d'Alexandrie* 47 (2003): 11–25.

———. *Hellenistic and Roman Egypt: Sources and Approaches*. Aldershot, UK and Burlington, VT: Ashgate/Variorum, 2006.

———. *Everyday Writing in the Graeco-Roman East*. Berkeley: University of California Press, 2011.

Bagnall, R.S., and B.W. Frier. *The Demography of Roman Egypt*. Cambridge: Cambridge University Press, 1994.

Baillet, J. "La stèle de Menschieh." *Revue Archéologique* 13 (1889): 70–83.

Baines, J. "Literacy and Ancient Egyptian Society." *Man: The Journal of the Royal Anthropological Institute* n.s. 8, no. 3 (1983): 572–599.

———. "Practical Religion and Piety." *Journal of Egyptian Archaeology* 73 (1987): 79–98.

———. "Restricted Knowledge, Hierarchy and Decorum: Modern Perceptions and Ancient Institutions." *Journal of the American Research Center in Egypt* 27 (1990): 1–23.

———. "Society, Morality and Religious Practice." In *Religion in Ancient Egypt: Gods, Myths and Personal Practice*, edited by Byron E. Schafer, 123–199. Ithaca, NY: Cornell University Press, 1991.

———. "Contextualising Egyptian Representations of Society and Ethnicity." In *The Study of the Ancient Near East in the Twenty-First Century: The William Foxwell Albright Centennial Conference*, edited by J.S. Cooper and G.M. Schwartz, 339–384. Winona Lake: Eisenbrauns, 1996.

———. "Temples as Symbols, Gaurantors, and Participants in Egyptian Civilization." In *The Temple in Ancient Egypt: New Discoveries and Recent Research*, edited by S. Quirke, 216–241. London: British Museum Press, 1997.
———. "Egyptian Elite Self-Presentation in the Context of Ptolemaic Rule." In *Ancient Alexandria between Egypt and Greece*, edited by W.V. Harris and G. Ruffini, 33–62. Leiden: Brill, 2004.
———. "Display of Magic in Old Kingdom Egypt." In *Through a Glass Darkly*, edited by K. Szpakowska, 1–32. Swansea: The Classical Press of Wales, 2006.
Baines, J., and C.J. Eyre. "Four Notes on Literacy." *Göttinger Miszellen* 61 (1983): 65–96.
Baines, J., and J. Malek. *Cultural Atlas of Ancient Egypt*. Revised ed. New York: Checkmark Books, 2000.
Baines, J., and R.B. Parkinson. "An Old Kingdom Record of an Oracle? Sinai Inscription 13." In *Essays on Ancient Egypt in Honour of Herman Te Velde*, edited by J. van Dijk, 9–27. Groningen: Styx Publications, 1997.
Barb, A.A. "Bois du sang, Tantale." *Syria* 29 (1952): 271–284.
Bardinet, Th. *Dents et Mâchoires dans les Représentations Religieuses et la Pratique Médicale de l'Égypte Ancienne*. Rome: Pontificio Istituto Biblico, 1990.
———. *Papyrus médicaux de l'Égypte pharaonique: Traduction intégrale et commentaire*. Paris: Fayard, 1995.
Bataille, A. "Nouveau Fragment d'un Ostracon concernant Aménothès Fils de Hapou." *Études de Papyrologie* 4 (1938): 125–131.
———. "Aménothès Fils de Hapou à Deir El Bahari." *Bulletin de la Societé française d'Égyptologie* 3 (1950): 6–14.
———. *Les Inscriptions grecques du Temple de Hatshepsout à Deir El-Bahari*. Cairo: IFAO, 1951.
———. *Memnonia: Recherches de Papyrologie et d'Epigraphie grecques sur la Nécropole de la Thebes d'Égypte aux Époques hellénistique et romaine*. Cairo: IFAO, 1952.
Battaglia, E. *'Artos': il lessico della panaficazione nei papiri greci*. Milano: *Vita e pensiero*, 1989.
Beavis, I.C. *Insects and Other Invertebrates in Classical Antiquity*. Exeter, UK: University of Exeter, 1988.
Behr, C.A. *Aelius Aristides and the Sacred Tales*. Amsterdam: A.M. Hakkert, 1968.
Benson, W.H. "Health in Pharaonic Egypt." In *Biological Anthropology and the Study of Ancient Egypt*, edited by W.V. Davies and R. Walker, 19–23. London: British Museum Press, 1993.
Bernand, A. *Le Delta égyptien d'après les Textes grecs 1: Les Confins libyques*. Cairo: IFAO, 1970.
———. *Les Inscriptions grecques et latines de Philae*. Vol. 1: Époque ptolémaique. Paris: Éditions du CNRS, 1969.
Bernand, E. *Inscriptions métriques de l'Égypte gréco-romaine*. Paris: Les Belles Lettres, 1969.
———. *Inscriptions grecques d'Égypte et du Nubie au Musée du Louvre*. Paris Éditions du CNRS, 1992.
Bertrac, P., ed. *Diodore de Sicile, Bibliothèque historique. Introduction générale. Livre I*. Paris: Les Belles Lettres, 1993.

Betz, H.D. *The Greek Magical Papyri in Translation, Including the Demotic Spells*. 2nd ed. Chicago: University of Chicago Press, 1992.

Bilson, G. "Public Health and the Medical Profession in Nineteeth-Century Canada." In *Disease, Medicine and Empire. Perspectives on Western Medicine and the Experience of European Expansion*, edited by R. Macleod and M. Lewis, 156–175. London: Routledge, 1988.

Bingen, J., A. Bülow-Jacobsen, and H. Cuvigny. *Mons Claudianus, Ostraca Graeca et Latina*. 4 vols, Documents de Fouilles de l'IFAO. Cairo: IFAO, 1992–2009.

Bisset, N.G., J.G. Bruhn, S. Curto, B. Holmstedt, U. Nyman, and M.H. Zenk. "Was Opium Known in 18th Dynasty Egypt? An Examination of Materials from the Tomb of the Chief Royal Architect Kha." *Ägypten und Levante* 6 (1996): 199–201.

Bisset, N.G., J.G. Bruhn, and M.H. Zenk. "The Presence of Opium in a 3500 Year Old Cypriote Base-Ring Juglet." *Ägypten und Levante* 6 (1996): 203–204.

Blok, H.P. "Remarques sur quelques Stéles dites "à Oreilles"." *Kemi* 1 (1928): 123–135.

Blyth, E. *Karnak: Evolution of a Temple*. London: Routledge, 2006.

Bo-Zhong, C., and K. Liljenquist. "Washing Away Your Sins: Threatened Morality and Physical Cleansing." *Science* 313, no. 5792 (2006): 1451–1452.

Bohleke, B. "An Oracular Amuletic Decree of Khonsu in the Cleveland Museum of Art." *Journal of Egyptian Archaeology* 83 (1997): 155–167.

Bonneau, D. *Le Fisc et le Nil: incidences des irrégularités de la crue du Nil sur la fiscalité foncière dans l'Égypte grecque et romaine*. Paris: Cujas, 1971.

Bonner, C. *Studies in Magical Amulets, Chiefly Graeco-Egyptian*. Ann Arbor: University of Michigan Press, 1950.

Borghouts, J.F. *The Magical Texts of Papyrus Leiden I 348*. Leiden: Brill, 1970.

———. "The Evil Eye of Apophis." *Journal of Egyptian Archaeology* 59 (1973): 114–150.

———. "Magie." In *Lexikon der Ägyptologie*, edited by W. Helck, E. Otto and W. Westendorf, 1137–1151. Wiesbaden: Harrassowitz, 1975–1992.

———. *Ancient Egyptian Magical Texts*. Leiden: Brill, 1978.

———. "Divine Intervention in Ancient Egypt and Its Manifestation (B3w)." In *Gleanings from Deir El-Medina*, edited by R.J. Demarée and J.J. Janssen, 1–70. Leiden: Nederlands Inst. voor het Nabije Oosten, 1982.

Botti, G. "Biglietti per l'oraculo di Soknebtynis in caratteri demotici." In *Studi in Memoria di Ippolito Rosellini*. Pisa, 1955.

Bouchet-Bert, L. "The Question of *Dqr* and Sterile Blades in P. Ebers 875." *Journal of Egyptian Archaeology* 84 (1998): 224–228.

Bourrieau, J. "The Second Intermediate Period." In *The Oxford History of Ancient Egypt*, edited by I. Shaw, 184–217. Oxford: Oxford University Press, 2000.

Bowen, A. *Plutarch. The Malice of Herodotus*. Warminster, UK: Aris & Phillips, 1992.

Bowman, A.K. *Egypt after the Pharaohs: 332 BC–AD 642, from Alexander to the Arab Conquest*. Oxford: Oxford University Press, 1990.

Brashear, W. "The Greek Magical Papyri: An Introduction and Survey; Annotated Bibliography." In *Aufstieg und Niedergang der römischen Welt*, edited by W. Haase, 3380–3684. Berlin and New York: Walter de Gruyter, 1995.

Braun, T. "Barley Cakes and Emmer Bread." In *Food in Antiquity*, edited by J. Wilkins, D. Harvey and M. Dobson, 25–37. Exeter, UK: University of Exeter, 1995.

Breasted, J.H. *Ancient Records of Egypt*. Vol. 3. Chicago: University of Chicago Press, 1906.

———. *The Edwin Smith Surgical Papyrus*. Vol. 1. Chicago: University of Chicago Press, 1930.

Breccia, E. *Alexandria ad Aegyptum: A Guide to the Ancient and Modern Town, and to its Graeco-Roman Museum*. Bergamo: Istituto italiano d'arti grafiche, 1922.

———. "Le Rovine e i Monumenti di Canopo." In *Monuments de l'Égypte gréco-romaine 1: Tome premier sous les Auspices de sa Majesté Fouad Ier Roi d'Égypte*, edited by Société royale d'archéologie d'Alexandrie, 35–50. Bergamo: Officine dell'istituto italiano d'arti grafiche, 1926.

Brewer, D.J., D.B. Redford, and S. Redford. *Domestic Plants and Animals: The Egyptian Origins*. Warminster, UK: Aris & Phillips, 1994.

Browne, G.M. *Documentary Papyri from the Michigan Collection*, Michigan Papyri (= *P.Mich.* X). American Studies in Papyrology. Toronto: A.M. Hakkert for the American Society of Papyrologists, 1970.

Bruyère, B. *Mert Seger à Deir el Médineh*. Cairo: IFAO, 1930.

Buikstra, J., B.J. Baker, and D.C. Cook. "What Diseases Plagued Ancient Egyptians? A Century of Controversy Considered." In *Biological Anthropology and the Study of Ancient Egypt*, edited by W.V. Davies and R. Walker, 24–53. London: British Museum Press, 1993.

Bülow-Jacobsen, A. "P. Carlsberg 24: Question to an Oracle." *Zeitschrift für Ägyptische Sprache* 57 (1984): 91–92.

Burkard, G. *Bibliotheken im alten Ägypten*. München: Saur, 1980.

Burkert, W. *The Orientalizing Revolution: Near Eastern influence on Greek culture in the early archaic age*. Cambridge, Mass.: Harvard University Press, 1992.

Burton, A. *Diodorus Siculus Book I: A Commentary*. Leiden: Brill, 1972.

Buss, D. "Sex Difference in Human Mate Preference: Evolutionary Hypotheses Tested in 37 Cultures." *Behavioral and Brain Sciences* 12 (1989): 1–49.

Calderini, A., and S. Daris. *Dizionario dei nomi geografici e topografici dell'Egitto greco-romano, e Supplementi*. Cairo, Società reale di geografia d'Egitto, 1935–1987; Milano: Cisalpina-Goliardica, 1988–2003. Pisa: F. Serra, 2006–2009.

Černy, J. *Late Ramesside Letters*. Bruxelles: Édition de la Fondation égyptologique reine Élisabeth, 1939.

———. "Ancient Egyptian Oracles." In *A Saite Oracle Papyrus from Thebes in the Brooklyn Museum* (*Papyrus Brooklyn 47.218.3*), edited by R.A. Parker, 35–48. Providence, RI: Brown University Press, 1962.

Chaniotis, A. "Illness and Cures in Greek Propitiatory Inscriptions and Dedications of Lydia and Phrygia." In *Ancient Medicine in Its Socio-Cultural Context*, edited by Ph.J. van der Eijk, H.F.J. Horstmanshoff and P.H. Schrijvers, 323–244. Amsterdam: Rhodopi, 1995.

Chapman, P.H. "Case Seven of the Smith Surgical Papyrus: The Meaning of *Tp3w*." *Journal of the American Research Center in Egypt* 19 (1992): 35–42.

Charlesworth, J. *The Lord's Prayer and Other Prayer Texts from the Greco-Roman Era*. Valley Forge, PA: Trinity Press International, 1994.

Chrisman, N.J. "Transcultural Care." In *Mosby's Comprehensive Review of Critical Care*, edited by D. Zschoche, 58–69. St. Louis: Mosby, 1986.

Chrisman, N.J., and T.M. Johnson. "Clinically Applied Anthropology." In *Medical*

Anthropology: Contemporary Theory and Method, edited by T.M. Johnson and C.F. Sargent, 93–113. New York: Praeger, 1990.

Clarysse, W. "Egyptian Scribes Writing Greek." *Chronique d'Égypte* 68, no. 186–201 (1983).

———. "Greeks and Egyptians in the Ptolemaic Army and Administration." *Aegyptus* 65 (1985): 57–66.

———. "UPZ 6a, a Reconstruction by Revillout." *Enchoria* 14 (1986): 43–49.

———. "Greeks in Ptolemaic Thebes." In *Hundred-Gated Thebes. Acts of a Colloquium on Thebes and the Theban Area in the Graeco-Roman Period*, edited by S.J. Vleeming, 1–20. Leiden: Brill, 1991.

———. "Some Greeks in Egypt." In *Life in a Multi-Cultural Society: Egypt from Cambyses to Constantine and Beyond*, edited by J.H. Johnson, 51–56. Chicago: Oriental Institute of the University of Chicago, 1992.

———. "Ethnic Diversity and Dialect among the Greeks of Egypt." In *The Two Faces of Graeco-Roman Egypt*, edited by A.M.F.W. Verhoogt and S.P. Vleeming, 1–13. Leiden: E.J. Brill, 1998.

Clarysse, W., and D.J. Thompson. *Counting the People in Hellenistic Egypt*. 2 vols. Cambridge: Cambridge University Press, 2006.

Cockburn, A., R.A. Barraco, W.H. Peck, and T.A. Reyman. "A Classic Mummy: PUM II." In *Mummies, Disease and Ancient Cultures*, edited by A. Cockburn, E. Cockburn and T.A. Reyman, 69–90. Cambridge: Cambridge University Press, 1998.

Cohn-Haft, L. *The Public Physicians of Ancient Greece*, Smith College Studies in History. Northampton, Mass.: Department of History of Smith College, 1956.

Collombert, P. "Une Statue thébaine d'Amenhotep Fils de Hapou trouvée à Esna." *Bulletin de l'Institut français d'Archéologie orientale* 102 (2002): 137–142.

Copenhaver, B.P. *The Greek Corpus Hermeticum and the Latin Asclepius in a New English Translation with Notes and Introduction*. Cambridge: Cambridge University Press, 1992.

Coulson, William D.E., I. Leventi, and J. Rehard. *Ancient Naukratis Volume II: The Survey at Naukratis and Environs. Part 1: The Survey at Naukratis*, Oxbow Monograph. Oxford: Oxbow Books, 1996.

Craik, E.M. "Hippocratic *Diaita*." In *Food in Antiquity*, edited by J. Wilkins, D. Harvey and M. Dobson, 343–350. Exeter: University of Exeter Press, 1995.

———. *Hippocrates: Places in Man*. Oxford: Clarendon Press, 1998.

Crawford, D.J. [See also Thompson, D.J.]. *Kerkeosiris; an Egyptian Village in the Ptolemaic Period*, Cambridge Classical Studies. Cambridge, U.K.: Cambridge University Press, 1971. Reprint, Pbk. 2007.

———. "Garlic-Growing and Agricultural Specialization in Graeco-Roman Egypt." *Chronique d'Égypte* 48 (1973): 350–363.

———. "The Opium Poppy: A Study in Ptolemaic Agriculture." In *Problèmes de la terre en Grèce ancienne*, edited by M.I. Finley, 223–251. Paris: Mouton & Co., 1973.

Dalby, A. *Food in the Ancient World, from A to Z*. London: Routledge 2003.

Darby, W.J, P. Ghalioungui, and L. Grivetti. *Food: The Gift of Osiris*. 2 vols. London: Academic Press, 1977.

Daressy, G. "Notes et Remarques." *Recueil de Traveux* 16 (1894): 42–60.

Daumas, F. "Le Sanatorium de Dendera." *Bulletin de l'Institut français d'Archéologie orientale* 56, no. 35–57 (1957).

Davidson, J.N. *Courtesans & Fishcakes: The Consuming Passions of Classical Athens*. London: HarperCollins, 1997.

Davis, P., B. Gribben, A. Scott, and R. Lay-Yee. "The 'Supply Hypothesis' and Medical Practice Variation in Primary Care: Testing Economic and Clinical Models of Inter-Practitioner Variation." *Social Science and Medicine* 50, no. 3 (2000): 40718.

Davoli, P. *L'archeologia urbana nel Fayyum di età ellenistica e romana*. Napoli: G. Procaccini, 1998.

———. "New Excavations at Soknopaiou Nesos: The 2003 Season." In *Tebtynis und Soknopaiou Nesos: Leben im römerzeitlichen Fajum*, edited by S. Lippert and M. Schentuleit, 29–39. Wiesbaden: Harrassowitz, 2005.

Dawson, W. "A Strange Drug." *Aegyptus* 12 (1932): 12–15.

Dean-Jones, L. "Literacy and the Charlatan in Ancient Greek Medicine." In *Written Texts and the Rise of Literate Culture in Ancient Greece*, edited by H. Yunis, 97–121. Cambridge: Cambridge University Press, 2003.

Deelder, A.M., R.L. Miller, N. de Jonge, and F.W. Krijget. "Detection of Schistosome Antigen in Mummies." *The Lancet* 335, no. 8691 (1990): 724–725.

Depauw, M. *A Companion to Demotic Studies*. Brussels: Fondation égyptologique reine Élisabeth, 1997.

Derchain, Ph. "L'authenticité de l'inspiration égyptienne dans le Corpus Hermeticum." *Revue de l'histoire des religions* 161 (1962): 175–198.

———. *Le papyrus Salt 825 (B.M. 10051): rituel pour la conservátion de la vie en Égypte. Texte, translation, introduction et commentaire*. 2 vols. Bruxelles: Palais des Académies, 1965.

———. "À propos de performativité: pensers ancients et articles récents." *Göttinger Miszellen* 110 (1989): 13–18.

Derry, D.E. "Note on Five Pelves of Women of the Eleventh Dynasty in Egypt." *Journal of Obstretrics and Gynaecology of the British Empire* 42, no. 3 (1935): 490–498.

Devauchelle, M., and M. Pezin. "Un papyrus medical démotique." *Chronique d'Égypte* 53 (1978): 57–66.

Dieleman, J. "Stars and the Egyptian Priesthood in the Graeco-Roman Period." In *Prayer, Magic and the Stars in the Ancient and Late Antique World*, edited by S.B. Noegel, J.T. Walker and B.M. Wheeler, 137–154. University Park, PA: Pennsylvania State University Press, 2003.

———. *Priests, Tongues and Rites. The London-Leiden Magical Manuscripts and Translation in Egyptian Ritual (100–300 Ce)*. Leiden: Brill, 2005.

Diels, H., ed. *Der Fragmente der Vorsokratiker*. 6th ed. rev. W. Kranz. ed. Zurich: Weidmann, 1951–1952.

Dietze, G. "Philae und die Dodekaschoinus in ptolemäische Zeit." *Ancient Society* 25 (1994): 68–72.

Dillon, M. "The Didactic Nature of the Epidaurian *Iamata*." *Zeitschrift für Papyrologie und Epigraphik* 101 (1994): 239–260.

———. *Pilgrims and Pilgrimage in Ancient Greece*. London: Routledge, 1997.

Dubuisson, M. "Remarques sur le vocabulaire grec de l'acculturation." *Revue belge de philologie et d'histoire* 60 (1982): 5–32.

Dunand, F. *Le culte d'Isis dans le Bassin oriental de la Méditerranée*. Études préliminaires aux religions orientales dans l'empire romain. Leiden: Brill, 1973.

Dzierzykay-Rogalski, T. "Paleopathology of the Ptolemaic Inhabitants of the Dakleh Oasis (Egypt)." *Journal of Human Evolution* 9, no. 1 (1980): 71–74.

Ebbell, B. *Papyrus Ebers: The Greatest Egyptian Medical Document*. Copenhagen; London: Levin & Munksgaard; Oxford University Press, 1937.

Edelstein, E.J., and L. Edelstein. *Asclepius: A Collection and Intepretation of the Testimonies*. Baltimore: The Johns Hopkins University Press, 1945. Reprint, 1998.

Edgar, C.C. *Greek Sculpture, Catalogue général des antiquités égyptiennes du musée du Caire: nos. 27425–27630*. Cairo: IFAO, 1903.

———. *Catalogue général des antiquités égyptiennes du musée du Caire, nos. 59298–59531. Zenon Papyri Vol. iii* (= *P.Cair.Zen.* III). Cairo: IFAO, 1928.

Edler, F.C. "Medical Knowledge and Professional Power: From the Luso-Brazilian Context to Imperial Brazil." In *Biomedicine as a Contested Site: Some Revelations in Imperial Contexts*, edited by P. Bala, 45–66. Lanham, MD: Lexington Books, 2009.

Edwards, I.E.S. *Hieratic Papyri in the British Museum, Fourth Series: Oracular Amuletic Decrees of the Late New Kingdom*. London: British Museum Press, 1960.

El-Farag, R., and U. Kaplony-Heckel. "Recent Archaeological Explorations at Athribis (Hw.T Rpjj.T)." *Mitteilungen des Deutschen Archäologischen Instituts, Abteilung* 41 (1985): 1–8, plates 17.

Empereur, J.-Y. *Alexandria Rediscovered*. London: British Museum Press, 1998.

Engelman, H. *The Delian Aretology of Sarapis*. Leiden: Brill, 1975.

Etkin, N.L. "Ethnopharmacology: The Conjunction of Medical Ethnography and the Biology of Therapeutic Action." In *Medical Anthropology: Contemporary Theory and Method*, edited by C.F. Sargent and T.M. Johnson, 151–165. Westport, CT: Praeger, 1996.

Evans, J.A.S. "A Social and Economic History of an Egyptian Temple in the Greco-Roman Period." *Yale Classical Studies* 17 (1961): 205–206.

Fagles, Robert. *Homer. The Odyssey*. New York: Viking Penguin, 1996.

Faraone, C.A. *Talismans and Trojan Horses: Guardian Statues in Ancient Greek Myth and Ritual*. Oxford: Oxford University Press, 1992.

Filce Leek, F. "Bite, Attrition and Associated Oral Conditions as Seen in Ancient Egyptian Skulls." *Journal of Human Evolution* 1 (1972): 289–295.

———. "Teeth and Bread in Ancient Egypt." *Journal of Egyptian Archaeology* 58 (1972): 126–132.

———. "Further Studies Concering Ancient Egyptian Bread." *Journal of Egyptian Archaeology* 59 (1973): 199–204.

———. "The Dental History of the Manchester Mummies." In *The Manchester Museum Mummy Project. Multidisciplinary Research on Ancient Egyptian Mummified Remains*, edited by A.R. David, 65–77. Manchester: Manchester University Press, 1979.

Filer, J. *Disease*. London: British Museum Press, 1995.

Flemming, R. *Medicine and the Making of Roman Women: Gender, Nature, and Authority from Celsus to Galen*. Oxford: Oxford University Press, 2000.

Fortenbaugh, W.W., and E. Schütrumpf. *Demetrius of Phalerum: Text, Translation and Discussion*. New Brunswick, N.J.: Transaction Publishers, 2000.

Fowden, G. *The Egyptian Hermes: A Historical Approach to the Late Pagan Mind*. Cambridge: Cambridge University Press, 1986.

Frankfurter, D. *Religion in Roman Egypt: Assimilation and Resistance*. Princeton, N.J.: Princeton University Press, 1998.

Fraser, P.M. "Two Studies on the Cult of Serapis." *Opuscula Atheniensia* 3, no. 3–54 (1960).

———. *Ptolemaic Alexandria*. 3 vols. Oxford: Clarendon Press, 1972.

Fraser, P.M. and E. Matthews. *A Lexicon of Greek Personal Names*. Oxford: Clarendon Press, 1987.

Gallazzi, C., G. Hadji-Minaglou, and V. Rondot. *Tebtynis 2. Le temple de Soknebtynis et son dromos*. Cairo: IFAO, 2004.

Gardiner, A.H. "The House of Life." *Journal of Egyptian Archaeology* 24 (1938): 157–179.

Gardiner, A.H., and K. Sethe. *Egyptian Letters to the Dead: Mainly from the Old and Middle Kingdoms*. London: Egypt Exploration Society, 1928.

Garnsey, P. *Famine and Food Supply in the Graeco-Roman World: Responses to Risk and Crisis*. Cambridge: Cambridge University Press, 1988.

Garofalo, I, ed. *Erasistrati Fragmenta*. Pisa: Giardini, 1988.

Gee, J.L. *The Requirements of Ritual Purity in Ancient Egypt*. PhD diss. Yale, 1998.

Geraci, G. "Ricerche sul Proskynema." *Aegyptus* 51 (1971): 3–211.

Germer, R. "Einige Bemerkungen zum angeblichen Opiumexport von Zypern nach Ägypten." *Studien zur altägyptischen Kultur* 9 (1981): 125–129.

———. *Flora des pharaonischen Ägypten*, Sonderschrift (Deutsches Archäologisches Institut. Abteilung Kairo). Mainz am Rhein: von Zabern, 1985.

———. "Ancient Egyptian Pharmaceutical Plants and the Eastern Mediterranean." In *The Healing Past: Pharmaceuticals in the Biblical and Rabbinic World*, edited by I. Jacob and W. Jacob, 69–80. Leiden: Brill, 1993.

Ghalioungui, P. *The Physicians of Pharaonic Egypt*. Cairo: Al-Ahram Center for Scientific Translations, 1983.

Ghalioungui, P., Sh. Khalil, and A.R. Ammar. "On an Ancient Egyptian Method of Diagnosing Pregnancy and Determining Foetal Sex." *Medical Historian* 7, no. 3 (1963): 241–246.2.

Girard, M.C. "L'hellébore: Panacée ou Placébo?" In *La Maladie et les Maladies dans la Collection Hippocratique: Actes du VIe Colloque International Hippocratique (Québec, du 28 Septembre au 3 Octobre 1987)*, edited by P. Potter, G. Maloney and J. Desautels, 393–405. Québec: Éditions du sphinx, 1990.

Goltz, D. *Studien zur altorientalischen und griechischen Heilkunde: Therapie, Arzneibereitung, Rezeptstruktur, Sudhoffs Archiv; Zeitschrift für Wissenschaftsgeschichte*, Beiheft 16. Wiesbaden: Steiner, 1974.

Gordon, D. "Tenacious Assumptions in Western Medicine." In *Biomedicine Examined*, edited by D. Gordon and M. Lock. Dordrecht: Kluwer Academic Publishers, 1988.

Gordon, R. "The Healing Event in Graeco-Roman Folk Medicine." In *Ancient Medicine in Its Socio-Cultural Context*, edited by Ph.J. van der Eijk, H.F.J. Horstmanshoff and P.H. Schrijvers, 363–376. Amsterdam: Rhodopi, 1995.

Goudriaan, K. *Ethnicity in Ptolemaic Egypt*, Dutch Monographs on Ancient History and Archaeology. Amsterdam: J.C. Gieben, 1988.

———. "Ethnical Strategies in Graeco-Roman Egypt." In *Ethnicity in Hellenistic Egypt*, edited by P. Bilde, T. Engberg-Pedersen, L. Hannestad and J. Zahle, 74–99. Aarhus: Aarhus University Press, 1992.

Goyon, J.-C. "Sur les formule des rituels de conjuration des dangers de l'année." *Bulletin de l'Institut français d'Archéologie orientale* 74 (1974): 75–83.

Graf, F. "Heiligtum und Ritual. Das Beispiel der griechisch-römischen Asklepieia." In *Le Sanctuaire Grec*, edited by O. Reverdin and B. Grange, 159–204. Geneva: Fondation Hardt, 1990.

Grapow, H., H. von Deines, and W. Westendorf, eds. *Grundriss der Medizin der alten Ägypter* 11 vols., (= *GdM*). Berlin: Akademie-Verlag, 1954–1973.

Grenfell, B.G., A.S. Hunt, and J.G. Smyly. *Tebtunis Papyri I* (= *P.Tebt.* I). London: Egypt Exploration Society, 1902.

Griffith, F.Ll. *Stories of the High Priest of Memphis: The Sethon of Herodotus and the Demotic Tales of Khamuas*. Oxford: Clarendon Press, 1900.

———. *Catalogue of the Demotic Graffiti of the Dodekaschoenus*. 2 vols. Vol. 1. Oxford: University Press [for] Service des Antiquités, 1935–1937.

Griffith, F.Ll., and H. Thompson. *The Demotic Magical Papyrus of London and Leiden*. London: H. Grevel, 1904.

Griffiths, A. "Democedes of Croton: A Greek Doctor at the Court of Darius." In *The Greek Sources: Proceedings of the Groningen 1984 Achaemenid History Workshop*, edited by H. Sancisi-Weerdenburg and A. Kuhrt, 37–51. Leiden: Nederlands Instituut voor het Nabije Oosten, 1987.

Griffiths, J.G. *The Conflict of Horus and Seth from Egyptian and Classical Sources*. Liverpool: Liverpool University Press, 1960.

Grmek, M.D. *Diseases in the Ancient Greek World*. Translated by M. Muellner and L. Muellner. Baltimore: Johns Hopkins University Press, 1989.

Guilmot, M. "Le Sarapeion de Memphis." *Chronique d'Égypte* 37 (1962): 359–381.

Gunn, B. "The Religion of the Poor in Ancient Egypt." *Journal of Egyptian Archaeology* 3, no. 81–94 (1916).

———. "Notes on Ammenemes I." *Journal of Egyptian Archaeology* 27, no. 2–6 (1941).

Guralnick, E. "The Egyptian-Greek Connection in the 8th to 6th Centuries BC: An Overview." In *Greeks and Barbarians: Essays on the Interactions between Greeks and Non-Greeks in Antiquity and the Consequences for Eurocentrism*, edited by J.E. Coleman and C.A. Walz, 127–154. Bethesda, MD: CDL Press, 1997.

Haeny, G. "A Short Architectural History of Philae." *Bulletin de l'Institut français d'Archéologie orientale* 85 (1985): 197–223.

Hansen, N.B. "Snakes." In *The Oxford Encyclopedia of Ancient Egypt*, edited by D.B. Redford, 296–299. Oxford: Oxford University Press, 2001.

Hanson, A.E. "The Medical Writers' Woman." In *Before Sexuality: The Construction of Erotic Experience in the Ancient Greek World*, edited by D.M. Halperin, J.J. Winkler and F.I. Zeitlin, 309–338. Princeton, N.J.: Princeton University Press, 1990.

———. "Egyptians, Greeks, Romans, Arabs and Ioudaioi in the First Century A.D. Tax Archive from Philadephia: P. Mich. Inv. 880 Recto and P. Princ. III 152, Revised." In *Life in a Multi-Cultural Society: Egypt from Cambyses to Constantine and Beyond*, edited by J.H. Johnson, 133–145. Chicago, IL.: The Oriental Institute of the University of Chicago, 1992.

———. "Talking Recipes in the Gynecological Texts of the Hippocratic Corpus." In *Parchments of Gender: Deciphering the Bodies of Antiquity*, edited by M. Wyke. Oxford: Oxford University Press, 1998.

———. "Text and Context for the Illustrated Herbal from Tebtunis." In *Atti del XXII Congresso Internazionale di Papirologia, Firenze, 23–29 agosto 1998*, edited by I. Andorlini, G. Bastianini, M. Manfredi, and G. Menci, 585–604. Firenze: Istituto Papirologico G. Vitelli, 2001.

———. "Greek Medical Papyri from the Fayum Village of Tebtunis: Patient Involvement in a Local Health-Care System?" In *Hippocrates in Context: Papers Read at the XIth International Hippocrates Colloquium; (University of Newcastle Upon Tyne, 27–31 August 2002)*, edited by Ph.J. van der Eijk, 387–402, *SAM* 31. Leiden: Brill, 2005.

———. "Doctors' Literacy and Papyri of Medical Content." In *Hippocrates and Medical Education: Selected Papers Read at the XIIth International Hippocrates Colloquium, Universiteit Leiden, 24–26 August 2005*, edited by M. Horstmanshoff, 187–204, *SAM* 31. Leiden: Brill, 2010.

Harig, G. "1975." *Deutsche Literaturzeitung* 96. Review of Goltz, D. (1974. *Studien zur altorientalischen und griechischen Heilkunde*): cols. 654–658.

Harris, W.V. "Dental Health in Ancient Egypt." In *Mummies, Disease and Ancient Cultures*, edited by A. Cockburn, E. Cockburn and T.A. Reyman, 59–68. Cambridge: Cambridge University Press, 1998.

Harrison, T. *Divinity and History*. 1st ed. Oxford: Clarendon Press, 2000.

———. "Upside Down and Back to Front: Herodotus and the Greek Encounter with Egypt." In *Ancient Perspectives on Egypt*, edited by R. Matthews and C. Roemer, 145–155. London: UCL Press, 2003.

Hartog, F. "The Greeks as Egyptologists." In *Greeks and Barbarians*, edited by T. Harrison, 211–228. Edinburgh: Edinburgh University Press, 2002.

Hawass, Z.A., and A. Senussi. *Old Kingdom Pottery from Egypt*. Cairo: Supreme Council of Antiquities, 2008.

Helck, W., E. Otto, and W. Westendorf, eds. *Lexikon der Ägyptologie*. 7 vols. Wiesbaden: Harrassowitz, 1972–1992.

Herzhoff, B. "Poppy." In *Brill's New Pauly: encyclopaedia of the ancient world*, edited by H. Cancik and H. Schneider, 615–616. Leiden: Brill, 2002–.

Heyob, S. *The Cult of Isis among Women in the Graeco-Roman World*. Leiden: Brill, 1975.

Hölbl, G. *A History of the Ptolemaic Empire. Translated by Tina Saavedra*. London: Routledge, 2001.

Holmes, B. *The Symptom and the Subject: The Emergence of the Body in Ancient Greece*. Princeton: Princeton University Press, 2010.

Hornblower, J. *Hieronymus of Cardia*. Oxford: Oxford University Press, 1981.

Humphreys, S. *Anthropology and the Greeks*. London: Routledge, 1978.

Ikram, S. "Diet." In *The Oxford Encyclopedia of Ancient Egypt*, edited by D.B. Redford, 390–395. Oxford: Oxford University Press, 2001.

Ikram, S., and A. Dodson. *The Mummy in Ancient Egypt: Equipping the Dead for Eternity*. London: Thames & Hudson, 1998.

Iversen, E. *Papyrus Carlsberg No. VIII, with Remarks on the Egyptian Origin of Some Popular Birth Prognoses*. Copenhagen: Einar Munksgaard, 1939.

Jackson, R. *Doctors and Diseases in the Roman Empire*. London: British Museum Publications, 1988.

Janssen, J.J. *Commodity Prices from the Ramesside Period: An Economic Study of the Village of Necropolis Workmen at Thebes*. Leiden: Brill, 1975.

———. "Absence from Work by the Necropolis Workmen of Thebes." *Studien zur Altägyptischen Kultur* 8 (1980): 127–152.

Jasnow, R. "Insinger Papyrus." In *The Oxford Encyclopedia of Ancient Egypt*, edited by D.B. Redford, 167–169. Oxford: Oxford University Press, 2001.

———. "Recent Trends and Advances in the Study of Late Period Egyptian Literature." *Journal of the American Research Center in Egypt* 39 (2002): 207–216.

Jeffreys, D.G., H.S. Smith, M. Price, and L.L. Giddy. *The Anubieion at Saqqâra*. 2 vols. Vol. 1, Excavation Memoirs. London: Egypt Exploration Society, 1988.

Johnson, J.H. "The Demotic Chronicle as a Historical Source." *Enchoria* 4 (1974): 1–18.

———. "Is the Demotic Chronicle an Anti-Greek Tract?" In *Grammata demotika: Festschrift für E. Lüddeckens zum 15. Juni 1983*, edited by H.-J. Thissen and K.-T. Zauzich, 107–124. Würzburg: G. Zauzich Verlag, 1983.

Johnson, J.H., and R.K. Ritner. "Multiple Meaning and Ambiguity in the 'Demotic Chronicle'." In *Studies in Egyptology Presented to Miriam Lichtheim*, edited by S. Israelit-Groll, 494–506. Jerusalem: Magnes Press, Hebrew University, 1990.

Johnston, S.I. *Restless Dead: Encounters between the Living and the Dead in Ancient Greece*. Berkeley: University of California Press, 1999.

Jonckheere, F. "Prescriptions médicales sur Ostraca hiératiques." *Chronique d'Égypte* 29 (1954): 46–61.

———. *Les medecins de l'Égypte pharaonique: essai de prosopographie*. Brussels: Fondation égyptologique reine Elisabeth, 1958.

Jones, W.H.S. *The Medical Writings of Anonymus Londinensis*. Cambridge: Cambridge University Press, 1947.

Jouanna, J. *Hippocrates*. Baltimore: Johns Hopkins University Press, 1999.

———. *Hippocrate. Maladie sacrée*. Paris: Les Belles Lettres, 2003.

———. "L'archéologie de l'école de Cnide et le nouveau témoignage du P. Köln 356 (Inv. 6067)." In *Testi medici su papiro: atti del seminario di studio*, edited by I. Andorlini, 221–236. Firenze: Istituto Papirologico G. Vitelli, 2004.

———. "Médecine égyptienne et médecine grecque." In *La médecine grecque antique: Actes du 14e colloque de la Villa Kérylos*, edited by J. Jouanna and J. Léclant. Paris: Académie des inscriptions et belles-lettres, 2004.

Jutikkala, E., and M. Kauppinen. "The Structure of Mortality During Catastrophic Years in a Pre-Industrial Society." *Population Studies* 25, no. 2 (1971): 283–285.

Kákosy, L. "New Studies in Magical Healing Statues." *Annales Universitatis Scientiarum Budapestinensis, Sectio Classica* 9 (1982–1985): 57–62.

———. "Some Problems of the Magical Healing Statues." In *La magia in Egitto ai tempi dei faraoni*, edited by A. Roccati and A. Siliotti, 171–186. Milan: Rassegna internazionale di cinematografia archeologica, 1987.

Kanawati, N., and A. Hassan. *The Teti Cemetery at Saqqara 2. The Tomb of Ankhmahor*. 9 vols. Vol. 2, *The Teti Cemetery at Saqqara. Reports, Australian Centre for Egyptology*. North Ryde, N.S.W.: Australian Centre for Egyptology; Warminster, UK: Aris and Phillips, 1997.

Kater-Sibbes, G.J.F., and M.J. Vermaseren. *Apis*. Leiden: Brill, 1975.

Kayser, F. "Oreilles et couronnes à propos des cultes de Canope." *Bulletin de l'Institut français d'Archéologie orientale* 91 (1991): 207–230.

Kellert, S. "A Sociocultural Concept of Health and Disease." *The Journal of Medicine and Philosophy* 1, no. 3 (1976): 222–228.

Kemp, B.J. *Ancient Egypt: Anatomy of a Civilization*. 2nd ed. London: Routledge, 2006.

Kessler, D. *Die heilige Tiere und der König. Teil 1, Beiträge zu Organisation, Kult und Theologie der spätzeitlichen Tierfriedhöfe*. Wiesbaden: Harrassowitz, 1989.

———. "Das hellenistische Serapeum in Alexandria und Ägypten in ägyptologischer Sicht." In *Ägypten und der östliche Mittelmeerraum im 1. Jahrtausend v. Chr.*, edited by M. Görg and G. Hölbl, 163–230. Wiesbaden: Harrassowitz, 2000.

King, H. *Hippocrates' Woman: Reading the Female Body in Ancient Greece*. London: Routledge, 1998.

Kleinman, A. *Patients and Healers in the Context of Culture: An Exploration of the Borderland between Anthropology, Medicine and Psychiatry*. Berkeley: University of California Press, 1980.

Kleinman, A., L. Eisenberg, and B. Good. "Culture, Illness and Care: Clinical Lessons from Anthropologic and Cross-Cultural Research." *Annals of Internal Medicine* 88, no. 2 (1978): 251–258.

Koschel, K. "Opium Alkaloids in a Cypriote Base-Ring I Vessel (Bilbil) of the Middle Bronze Age from Egypt." *Ägypten und Levante* 6 (1996): 159–166.

La'da, C.A. *Foreign Ethnics in Hellenistic Egypt, Prosopographia Ptolemaica; Studia Hellenistica*. Leuven, Belgium: Peeters, 2002.

———. "Encounters with Egypt: The Hellenistic Greek Experience." In *Ancient Perspectives on Egypt*, edited by R. Matthews and C. Roemer, 157–169. London: UCL, 2003.

Lacua, P. "Les statues 'guérisseuses' dans l'anciente Égypte." *Académie des inscriptions et belles-lettres. Commission de la fondation Piot. Monuments et mémoires* 25 (1921–1922): 189–209.

Lajtar, A. *Deir El-Bahari in the Hellenistic and Roman Periods: A Study of an Egyptian Temple Based on Greek Sources*. Warsaw: Warsaw University, Institute of Archaeology, Department of Papyrology/The Raphael Taubenschlag Foundation, 2006.

Lambert, M. "Ancient Greek and Traditional Zulu Medicine: A Question of Balance." *Acta Classica* 38 (1995): 71–87.

Laskaris, J. *The Art Is Long: On the Sacred Disease and the Scientific Tradition*, *SAM* 25. Leiden: Brill, 2002.

———. "Error, Loss and Change in the Generation of Therapies." In *Hippocrates in Context.: Papers Read at the XIth International Hippocrates Colloquium, University of Newcastle Upon Tyne 27–31 August 2002*, edited by Ph.J. van der Eijk, 173–189, *SAM* 31. Leiden: Brill, 2005.

Laskowska-Kusztal, E. *Le sanctuaire ptolémaïque de Deir El-Bahari*. Warsaw: PWN, 1984.

———. "Une stele du sanctuarie ptolémaïque de Deir El-Bahari." In *Les civilisations du Bassin Méditerranéen: hommages à Joachim Sliwa*, edited by K.M. Cialowitz. Cracovie: Inst. d'Archéologie, 2000.

Lauer, J.-Ph., and Ch. Picard. *Les statues ptolemaiques du Sarapieion de Memphis*. Paris: Presses universitaires de France, 1955.

Lefkowitz, M.K. "Some Ancient Advocates of Greek Cultural Dependency." In *Greeks and Barbarians: Essays on the Interactions between Greeks and Non-Greeks in Antiquity and the Consequences for Eurocentrism*, edited by J.E. Coleman and C.A. Walz, 237–253. Bethesda, MD: CDL Press, 1997.

Leitz, C. *Magical and Medical Papyri of the New Kingdom*. London: British Museum Press, 1999.

Lewis, N. *Life in Egypt under Roman Rule*. Oxford: Clarendon Press, 1983.

Lichtheim, M. *Ancient Egyptian Literature*. 3 vols. Berkeley: University of California Press, 1973–1978.

———. *Late Egyptian Wisdom Literature in the International Context: A Study of Demotic Instructions*. Göttingen: Vandenhoeck & Ruprechtw, 1983.

LiDonnici, L.R. *The Epidaurian Miracle Inscriptions: Text, Translation and Commentary*. Atlanta, GA: Scholars Press, 1995.

Littré, É. *Oeuvres complètes d'Hippocrate*. Paris: J.B. Bailliére, 1839–1861.

Lloyd, A.B. *Herodotus Book II*. 3 vols. Vol. 2: Commentary 1–98, *Études préliminaires aux religions orientales dans l'Empire romain*. Leiden: E.J. Brill, 1976.

———. "Nationalist Propaganda in Ptolemaic Egypt." *Historia* 31 (1982): 33–55.

———. "The Late Period." In *The Oxford History of Ancient Egypt*, edited by I. Shaw, 369–394. Oxford: Oxford University Press, 2000.

———. "The Ptolemaic Period (332–30 BC)." In *The Oxford History of Ancient Egypt*, edited by I. Shaw, 395–421. Oxford: Oxford University Press, 2000.

———. "*Heka*, Dreams and Prophecy in Ancient Egyptian Stories." In *Through a Glass Darkly*, edited by K. Szpakowska, 71–94. Swansea: The Classical Press of Wales, 2006.

Lloyd, G.E.R. *Magic, Reason and Experience: Studies in the Origin and Development of Greek Science*. Cambridge: Cambridge University Press, 1979.

———. *Science, Folklore and Ideology: Studies in the Life Sciences in Ancient Greece*. Cambridge: Cambridge University Press, 1983.

———. *The Revolutions of Wisdom: Studies in the Claims and Practice of Ancient Greek Science*, Sather Classical Lectures. Berkeley: University of California Press, 1987.

———. *Methods and Problems in Greek Science*. Cambridge: Cambridge University Press, 1991.

———. *Ancient Worlds, Modern Reflections: Philosophical Perspectives on Greek and Chinese Science and Culture*. Oxford: Oxford University Press, 2004.

Long, A.A., and D.N. Sedley. *The Hellenistic Philosophers*. 2 vols. Cambridge: Cambridge University Press, 1987.

Long, A.R. "Cardiovascular Renal Disease." *Archives of Pathology* 12 (1931): 92–96.

Longrigg, J. *Greek Rational Medicine. Philosophy and Medicine from Alcmaeon to the Alexandrians*. London: Routledge, 1993.

Lonie, I.M. "Literacy and the Development of Hippocratic Medicine." In *Formes de pensée dans la collection hippocratique: Actes du IVe Colloque international hippocratique (Lausanne, 21–26 septembre 1981)*, edited by F. Lassere and Ph. Mudry, 145–161. Genève: Librairie Droz, 1983.

Loprieno, A. "Defining Egyptian Literature: Ancient Texts and Modern Theories." In *Ancient Egyptian Literature: History and Forms*, edited by A. Loprieno, 39–58. Leiden: Brill, 1996.

Macke, A., and C. Macke-Ribet. "Les Recherches Anthropologiques. Vallée des Reines, Vallée des Rois, Vallée des Nobles." *Les Dossiers d'Archéologie* 149–150 (1990): 34–39.

Makler, P.T. "New Information on Nutrition in Ancient Greece." *Klio* 62 (1980): 317–319.

Malinine, M. *Choix de textes juridiques en hiératique anormal et en démotique*. 2 vols. Vol. 1 (XXVe–XXVII dynasties). Cairo: IFAO, 1953.

———. "Une lettre démotique à Amenothès, fils de Hapou." *Revue d'Ègyptologie* 14 (1962): 37–43.

Malkin, I. *Ancient Perceptions of Greek Ethnicity, Center for Hellenic Studies Colloquia* 5. Washington D.C.: Center for Hellenic Studies, 2001.

Manetti, D. "'Aristotle' and the Role of Doxography in the Anonymus Londiniensis (PBrLib inv. 137)." In *Ancient Histories of Medicine: Essays in Medical Doxography and Historiography in Classical Antiquity*, edited by Ph.J. van der Eijk, 95–141, *SAM* 20. Leiden: Brill, 1999.

Manniche, L. *An Ancient Egyptian Herbal*. London: British Museum Press, 1989.

Manning, J.G. *Land and Power in Ptolemaic Egypt: The Structure of Land Tenure*. Cambridge: Cambridge University Press, 2003.

Mansfeld, J. "Theoretical and Empirical Attitudes in Early Greek Scientific Medicine." In *Hippocratica: Actes du Colloque hippocratique de Paris (4–9 septembre 1978)* edited by M.D. Grmek, 371–390. Paris: Éditions de CNRS, 1980.

Marciniak, M. *Deir el-Bahari I: Les inscriptions hiératiques du temple de Thoutmosis III*. Warsaw: Editions Scientifiques de Pologne, 1974.

———. "Un Text Inédit de Deir El-Bahari." *BIFAO* 81, no. supplément (1981): 283–291.

Marganne, M.-H. *Inventaire analytique des papyrus grecs de médecine*. Genève: Droz, 1981.

———. "Les instruments chirurgicaux de l'Égypte gréco-romaine." In *Archéologie et Médecine*. Juan-les-Pins: Association pour la promotion et la diffusion des connaissances archéologiques, 1987.

———. "Links between Egyptian and Greek Medicine." *Forum: trends in experimental and clinical medicine* 3, no. 5 (1993): 35–43.

———. *L'ophtalmologie dans l'Égypte gréco-romaine d'après les papyrus littéraires grecs*, *SAM* 8. Leiden: Brill, 1994.

———. *La chirurgie dans l'Égypte gréco-romaine d'aprés les papyrus littéraires grecs*, *SAM* 17. Leiden: Brill, 1998.

Mariette, A. *Le Sérapeum de Memphis*. Paris: Vieweg, 1888.

Marr, J.L., and P.J. Rhodes, eds. *The 'Old Oligarch': The Constitution of the Athenians: Attributed to Xenophon*. Oxford: Aris & Phillips, 2008.

Martin, G.T. *The Sacred Animal Necropolis at North Saqqara: The Southern Dependencies of the Main Temple Complex*. London: Egypt Exploration Society, 1981.

Martin, V. "L'onomastique comme indice des rapports entre indigènes et occupants dans l'Égypte gréco-romaine." In *Akten Des VIII. Internationalen Kongresses für Papyrologie*, edited by H. Gerstinger, 85–90. Wien: Rohrer, 1956.

Masali, M., and B. Chiarelli. "Demographic Data on the Remains of Ancient Egyptians." *Journal of Human Evolution* 1 (1972): 161–169.

Mattern, S.P. *Galen and the Rhetoric of Healing*. Baltimore: Johns Hopkins University Press, 2008.

McDowell, A.G. *Village Life in Ancient Egypt: Laundry Lists and Love Songs*. 1st ed. Oxford: Oxford University Press, 1999. Reprint, 2001.

McKenzie, J.S., S. Gibson, and A.T. Reyes. "Reconstructing the Serapeum in Alexandria from the Archaeological Evidence." *Journal of Roman Studies* 94 (2004): 73–121.

McKenzie, J.S. *The Architecture of Alexandria and Egypt 300 B.C.–A.D. 700*. New Haven, CT: Yale University Press, 2007.

Meiggs, R., and D. Lewis. *A Selection of Greek Historical Inscriptions*. Oxford: Oxford University Press, 1988.

Merlin, M.D. *On the Trail of the Ancient Opium Poppy*. Rutherford; London: Fairleigh Dickinson University Press; Associated University Presses, 1984.

Merrillees, R.S. "Opium Trade in the Bronze Age Levant." *Antiquity* 36 (1962): 287–292.

Miller, R.L. "*Dqr*, Spinning and the Treatment of Guinea Worm in P. Ebers 875." *Journal of Egyptian Archaeology* 75 (1989): 249–254.

———. "Counting Calories in Egyptian Ration Texts." *Journal of the Economic and Social History of the Orient* 34 (1991): 257–269.

Miller, R.L., S. Ikram, G.J. Armelagos, R. Walker, W.B. Harer, C.J. Shiff, D. Baggett, N. Carrigan, and S.M. Maret. "Diagnosis of Plasmodium Falciparum. Infections in Mummies Using the Rapid Manual *Para*sight™-F Test." *Transactions of the Royal Society of Tropical Medicine and Hygiene* 88, no. 1 (1994): 31–32.

Millet, N.B., G.D. Hart, T.A. Reyman, M.R. Zimmerman, and P.K. Lewin. "*ROM* I: Mummification for the Common People." In *Mummies, Disease and Ancient Cultures*, edited by A. Cockburn, E. Cockburn and T.A. Reyman, 91–105. Cambridge: Cambridge University Press, 1998.

Milne, J.S. "The Sanatorium of Deir El-Bahri." *Journal of Egyptian Archaeology* 1 (1914): 96–98.

Möller, A. *Naukratis: Trade in Archaic Greece*, Oxford Monographs on Classical Archaeology. Oxford: Oxford University Press, 2000.

Monnais, L. "Rejected or Elected? Processes of Therapeutic Selection and Colonial Medicine in French Vietnam, 1905–1939." In *Biomedicine as a Contested Site: Some Revelations in Imperial Contexts*, edited by P. Bala, 115–133. Lanham, MD: Lexington Books, 2009.

Morgan, G. ""Nourishing Foods": Herodotus 2.77." *Mnemosyne* 44, no. 3/4 (1991): 415–417.

Morini, A. *Bibliografia del Fayyum*. Bologna: La mandragora, 2004.

Morkot, R. "Archaism and Innovation in Art from the New Kingdom to the Twenty-Sixth Dynasty." In *"Never Had the Like Occurred": Egypt's View of Its Past*, edited by J. Tait, 79–100. London: UCL Press, 2003.

Mueller, K. *Settlements of the Ptolemies: City Foundations and New Settlement in the Hellenistic World, Studia Hellenistica*. Leuven, NL, and Dudley, MA: Peeters, 2006.

Murray, O. "Herodotus and Hellenistic Culture." *Classical Quarterly* 22 (1972): 200–213.

———. "Review of A. Burton, *Diodorus Siculus Book I: A Commentary*." *Journal of Hellenic Studies* 95 (1975): 214–215.

Naville, E. *Ägyptische Todtenbuch der XVIII. bis XX. Dynastie aus verscheidenen Urkunden*. Berlin: A. Asher, 1886.

Nerlich, A.G., A. Zink, U. Szeimies, and H.G. Hagedorn. "Ancient Egyptian Prosthesis of the Big Toe." *The Lancet* 356, no. 9248 (2000): 2176–2179.

Nielsen, E.R. "Honey in Medicine." In *Sesto congresso internazionale di egittologia: Atti*, edited by S. Curto, S. Donadoni, A.M. Donadoni Roveri and B. Alberton, 415–419. Torino, 1993.

Nijhuis, K. "Greek Doctors and Roman Patients: A Medical Anthropological Approach." In *Ancient Medicine in Its Socio-Cultural Context*, edited by Ph.J. van der Eijk, H.F.J. Horstmanshoff and P.H. Schrijvers, 49–68. Amsterdam: Rhodopi, 1995.

Nock, A.D., and A.J. Festugière. *Corpus Hermeticum*. 4 vols. Paris: Les Belles Lettres, 1946–1954.

Nunn, J. *Ancient Egyptian Medicine*. London: British Museum Press, 1996.

Nutton, V. "The Seeds of Disease." *Medical History* 27 (1983): 1–34.

———. "Medicine in Late Antiquity and the Early Middle Ages." In *The Western Medical Tradition: 800 B.C.–1800 A.D.*, edited by L.I. Conrad and The Wellcome Institute for the History of Medicine, 71–87. Cambridge: Cambridge University Press, 1995.

———. *Ancient Medicine*. London: Routledge, 2004.

O'Connor, D. "Egypt's View of 'Others'." In *"Never Had the Like Occurred": Egypt's View of Its Past*, edited by J. Tait, 155–186. London: UCL Press, 2003.

Oppenheim, A.L. "The Interpretation of Dreams in the Ancient Near East." In *Transactions of the American Philological Society*, 179–373. Philadelphia: American Philological Society, 1956.

Pahl, W.M. *Altägyptische Schädelchirurgie*. Stuttgart: G. Fischer, 1993.

Pahl, W.M., and F. Parsche. "Rätselhafte Befunde an anthropoligischen Untersuchungsmaterial aus Ägypten. Addenda zu Herodots 'Historien', Lib. II, 86–88 und zum ägyptischen Sparagmos?" *Anthropologische Anzeiger* 49 (1991): 39–48.

Panofsky, E. "'Canopus Deus': The Iconography of a Non-Existent God." *Gazette des Beaux-Arts* 57 (1961): 193–216.

Parke, H.W. *The Oracles of Zeus: Dodona, Olympia, Ammon*. Oxford: Blackwell, 1967.

Parker, R. *Miasma: Pollution and Purification in Early Greek Religion*. Oxford: Clarendon, 1983.

Parkinson, R.B. *Voices from Ancient Egypt: An Anthology of Middle Kingdom Writings*. London: British Museum Press, 1991.

———. *The Tale of the Eloquent Peasant*. Oxford: Griffith Institute and Ashmolean Museum, 1991.

———. *Poetry and Culture in Middle Kingdom Egypt: A Dark Side to Perfection*. London: Continuum, 2002.

Parsons, P.J. "Ulpius Serenianus." *Chronique d'Égypte* 49 (1974): 135–157.

Perdrizet, P., and G. Lefebvre. *Les graffites grecs du Memnion d'Abydos. Inscriptiones Graecae Aegypti* 3. Nancy; Paris: Berger-Levrault, 1919.

Peremans, W. "Egyptiens et étrangers dans l'administration civile et financière de l'Égypte ptolémaïque." *Ancient Society* 2 (1971): 33–45.

———. "Un groupe d'officiers dans l'armée des Lagides." *Ancient Society* 8 (1977): 175–185.

———. "Les Égyptiens dans l'armée de terre des Lagides." In *Althistorische Studien Hermann Bengtson: zum 70. Geburtstag dargebracht von Kollegen und Schulern*, edited by H. Heinen, K. Stroheker and G. Walser, 92–101. Wiesbaden: F. Steiner, 1983.

Peremans, W., and E. Van't Dack. *Prosopographia Ptolemaica, Studia Hellenistica*. Louvain: Université catholique de Louvain, 1950–1981.

Pestman, P.W. "Who Were the Owners, in the "Community of Workmen", of the Chester Beatty Papyri?" In *Gleanings from Deir El-Medina*, edited by R.J. Demarée and J.J. Janssen, 155–172. Leiden: Brill, 1982.

———. "The Offical Archive of the Village Scribes of Kerkeosiris: Notes on the So-Called Archive of Menches." In *Festschrift zum 100-jährigen Bestehen der Papyrussammlung der Österreichischen Nationalbibliothek: Papyrus Erzherzog Rainer*, 127–134. Wien: In Kommission bei Verlag Brüder Hollinek, 1983.

———. "Haronnophris and Chaonnophris: Two Indigenous Pharaohs in Ptolemaic Egypt (205–186 B.C.)." In *Hundred-Gated Thebes: Acts of a Colloquium on Thebes and the Theban Area in the Graeco-Roman Period*, edited by S.P. Vleeming, 101–137. Leiden: Brill, 1995.

Pilchen, H. "The Science of Voodoo: When Mind Attacks Body." *New Scientist* 2708 (2009): 30–33.

Pillet, M. "Les scènes de naissance et de circoncision dans le temple nord-est de Mout, à Karnak." *Annales du Service des Antiquités de l'Égypte* 52 (1952): 93–104.

Pinault, J.R. *Hippocratic Lives and Legends, SAM* 4. Leiden: Brill, 1992.

Pinch, G. *Magic in Ancient Egypt*. London: British Museum Press, 1994.

Plaumann, G. *Ptolemais in Oberägypten: Ein Beitrag zur Geschichte des Hellenismus in Ägypten*. Leipzig: Quelle & Meyer, 1910.

Posener, G. "Un papyrus d'El Hibeh." *Journal of Egyptian Archaeology* 68 (1982): 134–138.

Potter, P. "Epidemien I/III: Form und Absicht der zweiundvierzig Fallbeschreibungen." In *Die Hippokratischen Epidemien: Theorie, Praxis, Tradition*, edited by G. Baader and R. Winau, 9–19. Stuttgart: Franz Steiner Verlag, 1989.

Preaus, A. "Greek Philosophy in Egypt." In *Greeks and Barbarians: Essays on the Interactions between Greeks and Non-Greeks in Antiquity and the Consequences for Eurocentristism*, edited by J.E. Coleman and C.A. Walz, 155–174. Bethesda, MD: CDL Press, 1997.

Préaux, Cl. "Esquisse d'une histoire des révolutions égyptiennes sous les Lagides." *Chronique d'Égypte* 11 (1936): 522–552.

———. "Les prescriptions médicales des ostraca grecs de la bibliothèque Bodléenne." *Chronique d'Égypte* 31 (1956): 135–148.

———. *Le monde hellénistique: la Grèce et l'Orient de la mort d'Alexandre à la conquête romaine de la Grèce (323–146 av. J.-C.), Nouvelle Clio*. Paris: Presses universitaires de France, 1978.

Quack, J. "A Black Cat from Your Right, and a Scarab on Your Head." In *Through a Glass Darkly*, edited by K. Szpakowska, 175–187. Swansea: University of Wales Press, 2003.

Quaegebeur, J. "Tëephibis, dieu oraculaire?" *Enchoria* 5 (1975): 19–24.

Quibell, J.E. *The Ramesseum*. London: Egypt Exploration Society, 1896.

Quirke, S. *Ancient Egyptian Religion*. London: British Museum Press, 1992.

———. "Review of S. Sauneron, Un Traité Égyptien d'Ophiologie." *Journal of Egyptian Archaeology* 83 (1997): 243–245.

Rathbone, D.W. "Villages, Land and Population in Graeco-Roman Egypt." *Proceedings of the Cambridge Philological Society* n.s. 36 (1990): 103–142.

Raven, M.J. "A Rare Type of Osiris Canopus." *Oudheidkundige Mededelingen uit het Rijksmuseum van Oudheden te Leiden, Supplement* 66 (1986): 21–27.

Ray, J.D. "Papyrus Calsberg 67: A Healing-Prayer from the Fayum." *Journal of Egyptian Archaeology* 61 (1975): 181–188.

———. *The Archive of Hor.* London: Egypt Exploration Society, 1976.

———. "Observations on the Archive of Hor." *Journal of Egyptian Archaeology* 64 (1978): 113–120.

———. "Ancient Egypt." In *Divination and Oracles*, edited by M. Loewe and C. Blacker, 174–190. London: George Allen and Unwin, 1981.

———. "Phrases Used in Dream-Texts." In *Aspects of Demotic Lexicography: Acts of the Second International Conference for Demotic Studies, Leiden, 19–21 September, 1984*, edited by S.P. Vleeming, 85–93. Leiden: Brill, 1987.

———. "Jews and Other Immigrants in Late Period Egypt." In *Life in a Multi-Cultural Society: Egypt from Cambyses to Constantine and Beyond*, edited by J.H. Johnson, 273. Chicago: The Oriental Institute of the University of Chicago, 1992.

———. "Literacy and Language in Egypt in the Late and Persian Periods." In *Literacy and Power in the Ancient World*, edited by A.K. Bowman and G. Woolf, 51–66. Cambridge: Cambridge University Press, 1994.

———. "Dreams before a Wise Man: A Demotic Ostracon in the Nicholson Museum, University of Sydney Inv. T. 98." In *Studies on Ancient Egypt in Honour of H.S. Smith*, edited by A. Leary and J. Tait, 241–247. London: Egypt Exploration Society, 1994.

———. "The Dreams of the Twins in St. Petersburg." In *Through a Glass Darkly*, edited by K. Szpakowska, 189–203. Swansea: The Classical Press of Wales, 2006.

Redford, D.B. *Pharaonic King-Lists, Annals and Day-Books.* Mississauga, Canada: Benben Publications, 1986.

Rémondon, R. "Problèmes de bilingualisme dans l'Égypte lagide (*UPZ* I 148)." *Chronique d'Égypte* 39 (1964): 126–146.

Renberg, G.H. "Was Incubation Practised in the Latin West?" *Archiv für Religionsgeschichte* 8 (2003): 105–147.

Renehan, R. "The Staunching of Odysseus' Blood." *American Journal of Philology* 113, no. 1 (1992): 1–4.

Reymond, E.A.E. *A Medical Book from Crocodilopolis: P. Vindob. D. 6257, From the Contents of the Libraries of the Suchos Temples in the Fayyum.* Wien: in Kommission bei Verlag Brüder Hollinek, 1976.

Riad, H. "Egyptian Influence on Daily Life in Ancient Alexandria." In *Alexandria and Alexandrianism*, 29–39. Malibu, CA: The J. Paul Getty Museum, 1996.

Riddle, J.M. *Dioscorides on Pharmacy and Medicine.* Austin, TX: University of Texas Press, 1985.

Ritner, R.K. "A Uterine Amulet in the Oriental Institute Collection." *Journal of Near Eastern Studies* 43, no. 3 (1984): 209–221.

———. "Review of D. Wildung, Imhotep und Amenhotep." *Journal of Near Eastern Studies* 44, no. 4 (1984): 353–355.

———. "Horus on the Crocodiles: A Junction of Religion and Magic in Late Dynastic Egypt." In *Religion and Philosophy in Ancient Egypt*, edited by W.K. Simpson, 103–116. New Haven: Yale University Press, 1989.

———. "O. Gardiner 363: A Spell against Night Terrors." *Journal of the American Research Center in Egypt* 27 (1990): 25–41.

———. "Implicit Models of Cross-Cultural Interaction: A Question of Noses, Soap, and Prejudice." In *Life in a Multi-Cultural Society: Egypt from Cambyses to Constantine and Beyond*, edited by J.H. Johnson, 283–290. Chicago: The Oriental Institute of the University of Chicago, 1992.

———. *The Mechanics of Ancient Egyptian Magical Practice*. Chicago: The Oriental Institute of the University of Chicago, 1993.

———. "The Religious, Social and Legal Parameters of Traditional Egyptian Magic." In *Ancient Magic and Ritual Power*, edited by M. Meyer and Paul Mirecki, 43–60. Leiden: Brill, 1995.

———. "Innovations and Adaptations in Ancient Egyptian Medicine." *Journal of Near Eastern Studies* 59 (2000): 107–117.

———. "Medicine." In *The Oxford Encyclopedia of Ancient Egypt*, edited by D.B. Redford, 353–356. Oxford: Oxford University Press, 2001.

———. "'And Each Staff Transformed into a Snake': The Serpent Wand in Ancient Egypt." In *Through a Glass Darkly*, edited by K. Szpakowska, 205–255. Swansea: The Classical Press of Wales, 2006.

———. "The Cardiovascular System in Ancient Egyptian Thought." *Journal of Near Eastern Studies* 65, no. 2 (2006): 99–109.

Roberts, C., C. Bourbou, A. Lagia, S. Triantaphyllou, and A. Tsaliki. "Health and Disease in Greece." In *Health in Antiquity*, edited by H. King, 32–58. London: Routledge, 2005.

Roberts, C.H. *Catalogue of the Greek and Latin Papyri in the John Rylands Library, Manchester. Volume 3: Theological and Literary Texts* (*Nos. 457–551* = *P.Ryl.* III). Manchester, UK: The University of Manchester Press, 1938.

Rocca, J. "The Brain Beyond Kühn." *Bulletin of the Institute of Classical Studies* (2002): 87–100.

Roebuck, C. *The Asklepieion and Lerna, Based on the Explorations and Preliminary Studies of F.J. de Waele*. Princeton: The American School of Classical Studies at Athens, 1951.

Roeder, G. *Kulte, Orakel und Naturverehrung im alten Ägypten*. Zurick; Stuttgart: Artermis-Verlag, 1960.

Rose, J.C., G.J. Armelagos, and L.S. Perry. "Dental Anthropology of the Nile Valley." In *Biological Anthropology and the Study of Ancient Egypt*, edited by W.V. Davies and R. Walker, 61–67. London: British Museum Press, 1993.

Rossi, C. *Architecture and Mathematics in Ancient Egypt*. Cambridge: Cambridge University Press, 2004.

Roth, A.M. "Erasing a Reign." In *Hatshepsut: From Queen to Pharaoh*, edited by C.H. Roehrig, R. Dreyfus and C.A. Keller, 227–281. New York/New Haven: Metropolitan Museum of Art / Yale University Press, 2006.

Rottrof, S.I. "The Greeks and the Other." In *Greeks and Barbarians: Essays on the Interactions between Greeks and Non-Greeks in Antiquity and the Consequences for Eurocentrism*, edited by J.E. Coleman and C.A. Walz. Bethesda, MD: CDL Press, 1997.

Roussel, P. *Les cultes égyptiens à Delos du IIIe au Ier siècle av. J.-C.* Paris, Nancy: Berger-Levrault, 1916.

Rowe, A. *Discovery of the Famous Temple and Enclosure of Serapis at Alexandria. Supplément aux Annales du Service des Antiquités de l'Égypte, Cahier No. 2*. Cairo: IFAO, 1946.

Rowe, A., and B.R. Rees. "A Contribution to the Archaeology of the Western Desert 4: The Great Serapeum of Alexandria." *Bulletin of the John Rylands Library Manchester* 39, no. 2 (1957): 485–520.

Rowlandson, J., ed. *Women and Society in Greek and Roman Egypt: A Sourcebook*. Cambridge: Cambridge University Press, 1998.

Rowling, J.T. "Respiratory Disease in Egypt." In *Diseases in Antiquity: A Survey of the Diseases, Injuries and Surgery of Early Populations*, edited by D.R. Brothwell, A.T. Sandison and with a foreword by W.R. Dawson, 489–493. Springfield, Ill.: Thomas, 1967.

———. "The Rise and Decline of Surgery in Dynastic Egypt." *Antiquity* 63, no. 239 (1989): 312–319.

Rübsam, W.J.R. *Götter und Kulte in Faijum während der griechisch-römisch-byzantinischen Zeit*. Bonn: Habelt, 1974.

Ruffer, M.A. "Note on the Presence of 'Bilharzia Haematobia' in Egyptian Mummies of the Twentieth Dynasty (1250–1000 B.C.)." *British Medical Journal* 1 (2557) (1910): 16.

———. "Remarks on the Histology and Pathological Anatomy of Egyptian Mummies." *Cairo Scientific Journal* 3 (1910): 1–5.

Rutherford, I. "Kalasiris and Setne Khamwas: A Greek Novel and Some Egyptian Models." *Zeitschrift für Papyrologie und Epigraphik* 117, no. 203–209 (1997).

———. "Island of the Extremity: Space, Language and Power in the Pilgrimage Tradition of Philae." In *Pilgrimage and Holy Space in Late Antique Egypt*, edited by D. Frankfurter, 229–256. Leiden: Brill, 1998.

———. "Pilgrimage in Greco-Roman Egypt: New Perspectives on Graffiti from the Memnonion at Abydos." In *Ancient Perspectives on Egypt*, edited by R. Matthews and C. Roemer, 171–189. London: UCL Press, 2003.

Ryholt, K. "A Parallel to the Inaros Story of P. Krall (P. Carlsberg 456 + P.CtYBR 4513)." *Journal of Egyptian Archaeology* 84 (1998): 151–169.

———. "A Demotic Version of Nectanebo's Dream (P. Carlsberg 562)." *Zeitschrift für Papyrologie und Epigraphik* 122 (1998): 197–200.

———. "Nectanebo's Dream or the Prophecy of Petesis." In *Apokalyptik und Ägypten: eine kritische Analyse der relevanten Texte aus dem griechisch-römischen Ägypten*, edited by A. Blasius and B.U. Schipper, 221–241. Leuven: Peeters, 2002.

———. "On the Contents and Nature of the Tebtunis Temple Library: A Status Report." In *Tebtynis und Soknopaiu Nesos: Leben im römerzeitlichen Fajum*, edited by S. Lippert and M. Schentuleit, 141–170. Wiesbaden: Harrassowitz, 2005.

Sadek, A.I. "An Attempt to Translate the Corpus of the Deir El-Bahari Hieratic Inscriptions." *Göttinger Miszellen* 71–72, no. 68–91; 65–84. (1984).

———. *Popular Religion in Egypt During the New Kingdom, Hildesheimer ägyptologische Beiträge* 27. Hildesheim: Gerstenberg, 1987.

Salazar, C.F. *The Treatment of War Wounds in Graeco-Roman Antiquity, SAM* 21. Leiden: Brill, 2000.

Sallares, R.P. *The Ecology of the Ancient Greek World.* London: Duckworth, 1991.

———. *Malaria and Rome: A History of Malaria in Ancient Italy.* Oxford and New York: Oxford University Press, 2002.

Samuel, A.E. *The Shifting Sands of History: Interpretations of Ptolemaic Egypt*, Publications of the Association of Ancient Historians. Lanham, MD: University Press of America, 1989.

Sandison, A.T. "Evidence of Infective Disease." *Journal of Human Evolution* 1, no. 2 (1972): 213–224.

Sandison, A.T., and E. Tapp. "Disease in Ancient Egypt." In *Mummies, Disease and Ancient Cultures*, edited by A. Cockburn, E. Cockburn and T.A. Reyman, 38–58. Cambridge: Cambridge University Press, 1998.

Sandy, D.B. *The Production and Use of Vegetable Oils in Ptolemaic Egypt, BASP Supplement* 6. Atlanta, GA: Scholars Press, 1989.

Sauneron, S. "Les songes et leur interprétation dans l'Égypte ancienne." In *Sources orientales*, 17–61. Paris: Éditions du Seuil, 1959.

———. *Le papyrus magique illustré de Brooklyn: Brooklyn Museum 47.218.156, Wilbour monographs* 3. New York: Brooklyn Museum, 1970.

———. *Un traité égyptien d'ophiologie: papyrus du Brooklyn Museum No. 47.218.48 et .85.* Cairo: IFAO, 1989.

Scarborough, J. "Theoretical Assumptions in Hippocratic Pharmacology." In *Formes de pensée dans la collection hippocratique: actes du IVe colloque international hippocratique (Lausanne, 21–26 Septembre 1981)*, edited by F. Lassere and Ph. Mudry, 307–325. Genève: Librairie Droz, 1983.

———. "The Pharmacology of Sacred Plants, Herbs, and Roots." In *Magika Hiera: Ancient Greek Magic and Religion*, edited by C.A. Faraone and D. Obbink, 138–174. Oxford: Oxford University Press, 1991.

———. "The Opium Poppy in Hellenistic and Roman Medicine." In *Drugs and Narcotics in History*, edited by R. Porter and M. Teich, 4–23. Cambridge: Cambridge University Press, 1995. Reprint, 1997; 2001.

Scheidel, W. *Death on the Nile: Disease and the Demography of Roman Egypt, Mnemosyne Supplementum* 228. Leiden: Brill, 2001.

———. "Creating a Metropolis: A Comparative Demographic Perspective." In *Ancient Alexandria between Egypt and Greece*, edited by W.V. Harris and G. Ruffini, 1–31. Leiden, Boston and Cologne: Brill, 2004.

Schöne, H.I. "Hippokrates Περὶ Φαρμάκων." *Rheinisches Museum* 73 (1924): 434–448.

Schubart, W. "Orakelfragen." *Zeitschrift der ägyptische Sprache* 67 (1931): 110–115.

Seele, K.C. "Horus on the Crocodiles." *Journal of Near Eastern Studies* 6 (1947): 43–52.

Serpico, M., and R. White. "Oil, Fat and Wax." In *Ancient Egyptian Materials and Technology*, edited by P.T. Nicholson and I. Shaw, 390–429. Cambridge: Cambridge University Press, 2000.

Sherwin-White, S. *Ancient Cos: An Historical Study from the Dorian Settlement to the Imperial Period.* Göttingen: Vandenhoeck und Ruprecht, 1978.

Smith, G.E., and R. Dawson. *Egyptian Mummies.* London: George Allen and Unwin, 1924. Reprint, London: Kegan Paul International, 1991.

Smith, G.E., and F.W. Jones. *Archaeological Survey of Nubia—Report 1907–1908*, Volume II: *Human Remains.* Cairo: National Printing Dept., 1910.

Smith, G.E, and M.A. Ruffer. *Potts'che Krankheit an einer ägyptischen Mumie aus der Zeit der 21. Dynastie (um 1000 v. Chr.)*. Giessen: A. Töpelmann, 1910.
Smith, H.S. *A Visit to Memphis: Life at Memphis and Saqqara, C. 500–30 B. C.* Warminster, UK: Aris & Phillips, 1974.
Smith, H.S., and S. Davies. "Sacred Animal Temples at Saqqara." In *The Temple in Ancient Egypt*, edited by S. Quirke, 112–131. London: British Museum Press, 1997.
Smith, H.S., and A. Smith. "A Reconsideration of the Kamose Texts." *Zeitschrift der ägyptische Sprache* 103 (1976): 48–76.
Smith, W.D. *The Hippocratic Tradition*. Ithaca: Cornell University Press, 1976.
Spiegelberg, W. "Ägyptologische Randglossen zu Herodot." *Zeitschrift der ägyptische Sprache* 43 (1906): 84–96.
———. "Zwei Kalksteinplatten mit demotischen Texten." *Zeitschrift der ägyptische Sprache* 50–51 (1912–1913): 32–36; 137–138.
———. "Briefe der 21. Dynastie aus El-Hibe (mit 16 Abbildungen und Tafel I–VIII)." *Zeitschrift der ägyptische Sprache* 53 (1917): 13–14.
———. *Die demotischen Denkmäler*. Vol. 3, Catalogue général des antiquités égyptiennes du musée du Caire, Nos. 30601–31270, 50001–50022, 50023–50165. Leipzig: W. Druguin, 1932.
Stambaugh, J. *Sarapis under the Early Ptolemies*. Leiden: Brill, 1972.
Steckerl, F. *The Fragments of Praxagoras of Cos and His School, Philosophia Antiqua* 8. Leiden: Brill, 1958.
Steuer, R.O. *Aetiological Principle of Pyaemia in Ancient Egyptian Medicine*. Baltimore: Johns Hopkins Press, 1948.
Steuer, R.O., and J.B. de C.M. Saunders. *Ancient Egyptian and Cnidian Medicine: The Relationship of Their Aetiological Concepts of Disease*. University of California Press: Berkeley, 1959.
Sullivan, R. "The Identity and Work of the Ancient Egyptian Surgeon." *Journal of the Royal Society of Medicine* 89 (1996): 467–473.
Sweeney, D. "Illness and Healer in Combat in Middle Kingdom and Early New Kingdom Medical Texts." In *Feinde und Aufrührer: Konzepte von Gegnerschaft in ägyptischen Texten besonders des Mittleren Reiches* edited by H. Felber, 139–155. Leipzig: Verlag der Sächsischen Akademie der Wissenschaften zu Leipzig, 2006.
Szpakowska, K. *Behind Closed Eyes: Dreams and Nightmares in Ancient Egypt*. Swansea: The Classical Press of Wales, 2003.
———. "Playing with Fire: Some Initial Observations on the Use of Clay Cobras from Amarna." *Journal of the American Research Center in Egypt* 40 (2003): 113–122.
———. *Daily Life in Ancient Egypt: Recreating Lahun*. Oxford: Blackwell, 2008.
———. "Demons in the Dark: Nightmares and Other Nocturnal Enemies of Ancient Egypt." In *Ancient Egyptian Demonology: Studies on the Boundary Between the Demonic and the Divine in Egyptian Magic*, edited by P. Kousoulis, 63–76. Leuven: Peeters, 2011.
Tait, J. *Papyri from Tebtunis in Egyptian and Greek* (*P. Tebt. Tait*). London: Egypt Exploration Society, 1977.
———. "Demotic Literature and Egyptian Society." In *Life in a Multi-Cultural Society: Egypt from Cambyses to Constantine and Beyond*, edited by J.H. Johnson, 303–310. Chicago: The Oriental Institute of the University of Chicago, 1992.

———. "The "Book of the Fayum": Mystery in a Known Landscape." In *Mysterious Lands*, edited by D. O'Connor and S. Quirke, 183–202. London: UCL Press, 1993.

———. "The Wisdom of Egypt: Classical Views." In *The Wisdom of Egypt: Changing Visions through the Ages*, edited by P. Ucko and T. Champion, 23–37. London: UCL Press, 2003.

———. "P. Carlsberg 230: Eleven Fragments from a Demotic Herbal." In *The Carlsberg Papyri I. Demotic Texts from the Collection*, edited by P.J. Frandsen. Copenhagen: Museum Tusculanum Press, 1991.

Tapp, E. "Disease in the Manchester Mummies: Multidisciplinary Research on Ancient Egyptian Mummified Remains." In *The Manchester Museum Mummy Project*, edited by A.R. David, 95–102. Manchester, UK: Manchester University Press, 1979.

———. "The Unwrapping of a Mummy." In *The Manchester Museum Mummy Project*, edited by A.R. David, 83–93. Manchester, UK: Manchester University Press, 1979.

———. "Disease and the Manchester Mummies—the Pathologist's Role." In *Evidence Embalmed: Modern Medicine and the Mummies of Ancient Egypt*, edited by A.R. David and E. Tapp, 78–95. Manchester, UK: Manchester University Press, 1984.

———. "Histology and Histopathology of the Manchester Mummies." In *Science in Egyptology*, edited by A.R. David, 247–350. Manchester, UK: Manchester University Press, 1986.

Tapp, E., A. Curry, and C. Anfield. "Sand Pneumoconiosis in an Egyptian Mummy." *British Medical Journal* 2 (1975): 276.

Tapp, E., and K. Wildsmith. "The Autopsy and Endoscopy of the Leeds Mummy." In *The Mummy's Tale: The Scientific and Medical Investigation of Natsef-Amun, Priest in the Temple at Karnak*, edited by A.R. David and E. Tapp, 132–153. London: Michael O'Mara Books, 1992.

Taylor, J. "The Third Intermediate Period." In *The Oxford History of Ancient Egypt*, edited by I. Shaw, 339–341. Oxford: Oxford University Press, 2000.

Te Velde, H. *Seth, God of Confusion: A Study of His Role in Egyptian Mythology and Religion*. Leiden: Brill, 1967.

Teeter, E. "Amenhotep Son of Hapu at Medinet Habu." *Journal of Egyptian Archaeology* 81 (1995): 232–236.

Thissen, H.-J. *Studien zum Raphiadekret*. Meinsenheim am Glan: A. Hain, 1966.

Thomas, R. *Herodotus in Context: Ethnography, Science and the Art of Persuasion*. Cambridge: Cambridge University Press, 2000.

Thompson, D.J. [See also Crawford, D.J.]. "Agriculture." In *Cambridge Ancient History*, edited by F.W. Walbank, 363–370. Cambridge: Cambridge University Press, 1984.

———. *Memphis under the Ptolemies*. Princeton: Princeton University Press, 1988.

———. "Language and Literacy in Early Hellenistic Egypt." In *Ethnicity in Hellenistic Egypt*, edited by P. Bilde, T. Engberg-Pedersen, L. Hannestad and J. Zahle, 39–52. Aarhus: Aarhus University Press, 1992.

———. "Literacy and Power in Hellenistic Egypt." In *Literacy and Power in the Ancient World*, edited by A.K. Bowman and G. Woolf, 67–83. Cambridge: Cambridge University Press, 1994.

———. "Food for Ptolemaic Temple Workers." In *Food in Antiquity*, edited by J. Wilkins, D. Harvey and M. Dobson, 316–325. Exeter, UK: University of Exeter, 1995.

———. "The Infrastructure of Splendour: Census and Taxes in Ptolemaic Egypt." In *Hellenistic Constructs: Essays in Culture, History, and Historiography*, edited by P. Cartledge, P. Garnsey and E.S. Gruen, 242–257. Berkeley: University of California Press, 1997.

———. "New and Old in the Ptolemaic Fayum." In *Agriculture in Egypt: From Pharaonic to Modern Times*, edited by A.K. Bowman and E. Rogan, 107–122. Oxford: Oxford University Press for the British Academy, 1999.

———. "Alexandria: The City by the Sea." In *Alexandrian Studies in Honour of Mostafa El-Abbadi. Bulletin of the Société d'Archéologie d'Alexandrie*, 73–79, 2001.

———. "*Ethnê*, Taxes and Administrative Geography in Early Ptolemaic Egypt." In *Atti des XXII Congresso Internazionale di Papirologia, Firenze, 23–29 Agosto 1998*, edited by I. Andorlini, G. Bastianini, M. Manfredi and G. Menci, 1255–1263. Firenze: Istituto Papirologico G. Vitelli, 2001.

———. "Hellenistic Hellenes: The Case of Ptolemaic Egypt." In *Ancient Perceptions of Greek Ethnicity*, edited by I. Malkin, 301–322. Washington D.C.: Center for Hellenic Studies, 2001.

Thompson, H. "A Demotic Ostracon." *Proceedings of the Royal Society of Biblical Archaeology* 35 (1931): 95–96.

———. "Two Demotic Self-Dedications." *Journal of Egyptian Archaeology* 26, no. 68–78 (1940).

Thornton, F. "Oral Pathological Comparison of Discrete Ancient Nile Valley and Concurrent Populations." University of Bradford, 1990.

Tieleman, T. *Galen and Chrysippus on the Soul: Argument and Refutation in the De Placitis, Books II–III*. Leiden: Brill, 1996.

Tod, M. "The Scorpion in Graeco-Roman Egypt." *Journal of Egyptian Archaeology* 3 (1939): 55–61.

Totelin, L.M.V. *Hippocratic Recipes: Oral and Written Transmission of Pharmacological Knowledge in Fifth- and Fourth-Century Greece, SAM* 34. Leiden: Brill, 2009.

Tran Tam Tinh, V. *Le culte des divinités orientales à Canope*. Leiden: Brill, 1971.

———. *Sérapis debout: corpus des monuments de Sérapis debout et étude iconographique*. Leiden Brill, 1983.

Traunecker, C. "Une chapelle de magie guérisseuse sur le parvis du temple de Mout à Karnak." *Journal of the American Research Center in Egypt* 20 (1983): 65–92.

Turner, E.G. "The Greek Papyri from Saqqara." In *Proceedings of the XIV International Congress of Papyrologists, Oxford 24–31 July 1974*, 250–251. London: Egypt Exploration Society, 1975.

Valbelle, D., and G. Husson. "Les questions oraculaires d'Égypte: histoire de la recherche, nouveautés et perspectives." In *Studies in Egyptian Religion: The Last Thousand Years*, edited by W. Clarysse, A. Schoors and H. Willems, 1055–1071. Leuven: Peeters, 1998.

Vallance, J.T. *The Lost Theory of Asclepiades of Bithynia*. Oxford: Clarendon Press, 1990.

van der Eijk, Ph.J. "Towards a Rhetoric of Ancient Scientific Discourse: Some Formal Characteristics of Greek Medical and Philosophical Texts (Hippocratic Corpus,

Aristotle)." In *Grammar as Interpretation: Greek Literature in Its Linguistic Contexts*, edited by E.J. Bakker, 77–129. Leiden: Brill, 1997.

———. *Diocles of Carystus: A Collection of the Fragments with Translation and Commentary*. *SAM* vols. 22 and 23. Leiden: Brill, 2000–2001.

———. *Medicine and Philosophy in Classical Antiquity*. Cambridge: Cambridge University Press, 2005.

van Dijk, J. "The Birth of Horus According to the Ebers Papyrus." *Jaarbericht van het Vooraziatisch-Egyptisch Genootschan: Annuaire de la Société Orientale "Ex Oriente Lux"* 26 (1979–1980): 10–25.

———. "The Amarna Period and the Later New Kingdom." In *The Oxford History of Ancient Egypt*, edited by I. Shaw, 272–313. Oxford: Oxford University Press, 2000.

van Minnen, P. "Boorish or Bookish? Literature in Egyptian Villages in the Fayum in the Graeco-Roman Period." *Journal of Juristic Papyrology* 28 (1998): 99–184.

———. "Dietary Hellenization or Ecological Transformation." In *Atti del XXII Congresso Internazionale di Papirologia, Firenze, 23–29 agosto 1998*, edited by I. Andorlini, G. Bastianini, M. Manfredi, and G. Menci, 1265–1280. Firenze: Istituto Papirologico G. Vitelli, 2001.

van Straten, F.T. "Gifts for the Gods." In *Faith, Hope and Worship: Aspects of Religious Mentality in the Ancient World*, edited by H.S. Versnel, 62–151. Leiden: Brill, 1981.

———. "Votives and Votaries in Greek Sanctuaries." In *Le Sanctuaire Grec*, edited by O. Reverdin and B. Grange, 247–290. Geneva: Vandoeuvres, 1990.

Vanderlip, V.F. *The Four Greek Hymns of Isidorus and the Cult of Isis*, *ASP* 12. Toronto: A.M. Hakkert, 1972.

Varille, A. *Inscriptions concernant l'architecte Amenhotep, fils de Hapou*. Cairo: IFAO, 1968.

Varille, A., and C. Robichon. *Le Temple du scribe royale Amenhotep, fils de Hapou*. Cairo: IFAO, 1936.

Vassilika, E. *Ptolemaic Philae*. Leuven: Peeters, 1989.

Vasunia, P. *The Gift of the Nile: Hellenizing Egypt from Aeschylus to Alexander*. Berkeley: University of California Press, 2001.

Vegetti, M. "L'épistémologie d'Érasistrate et la technologie hellénistique." In *Ancient Medicine in Its Socio-Cultural Context: Papers Read at the Congress Held at Leiden University, 13–15 April 1992*, edited by Ph.J. van der Eijk, H.F.J. Horstmanshoff and P.H. Schrijvers, 461–472. Amsterdam: Rodopi, 1995.

———. "Between Knowledge and Practice: Hellenistic Medicine." In *Western Medical Thought from Antiquity to the Middle Ages*, edited by M.D. Grmek, 72–103. Cambridge, MA: Harvard University Press, 1998.

Verhoogt, A.M.F.W. *Menches, Komogrammateus of Kerkeosiris: The Doings and Dealings of a Village Scribe in the Late Ptolemaic Period (120–110 B.C.)*, *Pap.Lugd.-Bat.* 29. Leiden: Brill, 1998.

Verity, A., translator, *Idylls: Theocritus*, with an introduction and notes by R. Hunter, editor. Oxford: Oxford University Press, 2003 (pbk.).

Volokhine, Y. "Le Dieu Thot au Qasr El-Agoüz, *Dd-Hr-Pj-Hb, Dhwty-Stmd*." *Bulletin de l'Institut français d'Archéologie orientale* 102 (2002): 405–423.

Volten, A. *Das Demotische Weisheitsbuch*. Copenhagen: Einar Munksgaard, 1941.

———. *Das Demotische Traumdeutung* (*Pap. Carlsberg XIII und XIV Verso*). Copenhagen: Einar Munksgaard, 1942.

von Känel, F. *Les prêtres-ouâb de Sekhmet et les conjurateurs de Serket, Bibliothèque de l'école des hautes études, section des sciences religieuses* 87. Paris: Presses Universitaires de France, 1984.

von Staden, H. "Hairesis and Heresy: The Case of the 'Haireseis Iatrikai'." In *Jewish and Christian Self-Definition 3: Self-Definition in the Greek and Roman World*, edited by B.F. Meyer and E.P. Sanders, 76–100. London: SCM Press, 1982.

———. *Herophilus: The Art of Medicine in Early Alexandria*. Cambridge: Cambridge University Press, 1989.

———. "Incurability and Hopelessness: The *Hippocratic Corpus*." In *La maladie et les maladies dans la Collection hippocratique: actes du VIe Colloque international hippocratique* (*Québec, du 28 septembre au 3 octobre 1987*), edited by P. Potter, G. Maloney and J. Desautels, 75–112. Québec: Éditions du sphinx, 1990.

———. "Women and Dirt." *Helios* n.s. 19 (1992): 7–30.

———. "Body and Machine: Interactions between Medicine, Mechanics and Philosophy in Early Alexandria." In *Alexandria and Alexandrianism. Papers Delivered at a Symposium Organized by the J. Paul Getty Museum and the Getty Center for the History of Art and the Humanitites and Held at the Museum April 22–25, 1993*, 85–106. Malibu, CA: The J. Paul Getty Museum, 1996.

Walker, J.H. *Studies in Ancient Egyptian Anatomical Terminology*. Warminster, UK: Aris & Phillips 1996.

Weeks, K.R. "Art, Word and the Egyptian World View." In *Egyptology and the Social Sciences: Five Studies*, edited by K.R. Weeks, 59–81. Cairo: American University in Cairo Press, 1979.

Wente, E. *Late Ramesside Letters*. Chicago: University of Chicago Press, 1967.

———. *Letters from Ancient Egypt*. Atlanta, GA: Scholars Press, 1990.

West, S. "The Greek Version of the Legend of Tefnut." *Journal of Egyptian Archaeology* 55 (1969): 161–183.

Westendorf, W. *Papyrus Edwin Smith: Ein medizinisches Lehrbuch aus dem alten Ägypten*. Bern: H. Huber, 1966.

———. "Beiträge aus und zu den medizinischen Texten." *Zeitschrift der ägyptische Sprache* 92, 96 (1966; 1970): 128–154; 45–51.

———. *Handbuch der altagyptischen Medizin*. 2 vols. Leiden: Brill, 1999, c. 1998.

Wickkiser, B.L. *Asklepios, Medicine and the Politics of Healing in Fifth-Century Greece*. Baltimore: Johns Hopkins University Press, 2008.

Wilcken, U. *Urkunden der Ptolemäerzeit* (*ältere Funde*), *I, Papyri aus Unterägypten*. Berlin: De Gruyter, 1927.

Wild, R.A. *Water in the Cultic Worship of Isis and Sarapis*. Leiden: Brill, 1981.

Wilde, S. "Submitting to Surgery in the 1890s: Four Vignettes." In *Biomedicine as a Contested Site: Some Revelations in Imperial Contexts*, edited by P. Bala, 171–189. Lanham, MD: Lexington Books, 2009.

Wildung, D. *Imhotep und Amenhotep: Gottwerdung im alten Ägypten, Münchner ägyptologische Studien* 36. München: Deutscher Kunstverlag, 1977.

———. *Egyptian Saints: Deification in Pharaonic Egypt*. New York: New York University Press, 1977.

Wilkinson, A. *The Garden in Ancient Egypt*. London: The Rubicon Press, 1998.

Wilson, H. *Egyptian Food and Drink*. Aylesbury, UK: Shire Publications Ltd., 1988.

Wilson, J. "A Note on the Edwin Smith Surgical Papyrus." *Journal of Near Eastern Studies* 11 (1952): 76–80.

Wilson, P. *Sacred Signs*. Oxford: Oxford University Press, 2003.

Winkler, E.-M., and H. Wilfing. *Tell El-Dab'a VI: anthropologische Untersuchungen an den Skelettresten der Kampagnen 1966–1969, 1975–1980, 1985*. Wien: Verlag der Österreichischen Akademie der Wisschenschaften, 1991.

Winnicki, J. "Amenhotep Son of Hapy and Imhotep at Deir El-Bahari—Some Reconsiderations." *Mitteilungen des Deutschen Archäologischen Instituts, Abteilung* 39 (1983): 93–105.

Winter, E. *Der Apiskult im alten Ägypten*. Mainz: Novo Industrie, 1983.

Wittern, R. "Die Unterlassung ärztlicher Hilfeleistung in der griechischen Medizin der klassischen Zeit." *Münchener medizinische Wochenschrift* 121, no. 21 (1979): 731–734.

Yoyotte, J. "Les pélerinages dans l'Égypte ancienne." In *Les Pélerinages: Égypte ancienne, Isräel, Islam ....* 17–74. Paris: Seuil, 1960.

———. "Une théorie étiologique des médecins égyptiens" *Kemi* 18 (1968): 79–84.

Zakbar, L.V. "Six Hymns to Isis in the Sanctuary of Her Temple at Philae and Their Theological Significance: Part 1." *Journal of Egyptian Archaeology* 69 (1983): 115–137.

———. *Hymns to Isis in Her Temple at Philae*. Hanover: Brandeis University Press, 1988.

Zecchi, M. *Geografia Religiosa del Fayyum: dalle origini al IV seculo a.C.* Bologna: La mandragora, 2001.

Zivie, C.M. *Giza au deuxième millénaire, Bibliothèque d'étude* 70. Cairo: IFAO, 1976.

SUBJECT INDEX

INDEX OF PROPER NAMES

INDEX OF PLACES

INDEX OF CITATIONS

Papyri (Greek; Demotic Egyptian, Hieratic, and Hieroglyphic)

Inscriptions (*Greek and Egyptian*)

Ostraka (*Greek and Demotic Egyptian*)

www.ingramcontent.com/pod-product-compliance
Lightning Source LLC
LaVergne TN
LVHW010656300926
849161LV00005B/1140